I0125724

Half Doctor

Understanding Medical Science: Patient's Perspective

Dr Sandeep Kumar

Ajay Kumar Agrawal

STARDOM BOOKS

www.StardomBooks.com

STARDOM BOOKS

112 Bordeaux Ct.

Coppell, TX 75019, USA

Copyright © 2025 by Dr Sandeep Kumar &
Ajay Kumar Agrawal

All rights reserved. No part of this book may be reproduced or used in any manner
without written permission of the copyright owner except for the use of quotations
in a book review.

FIRST EDITION MAY 2025

STARDOM BOOKS, LLC.
112 Bordeaux Ct. Coppell, TX 75019, USA

www.stardombooks.com

Stardom Books, United States
Stardom Alliance, India

The author and publishers have made all reasonable efforts to contact copyright holders for permission and apologize for any omissions or errors in the form of credits given. Corrections may be made to future editions.

HALF DOCTOR

Understanding Medical Science: Patient's Perspective

Dr Sandeep Kumar & Ajay Kumar Agrawal

p. 543

cm. 16.24 X 22.86

Category: HEA039000 - Health & Fitness: Diseases – General
HEA028000 - Health & Fitness: Health Care Issues

ISBN: 978 - 1 - 957456 - 73 - 7

Contents

If I am not for myself, who will be for me?
If I am only for myself, what am I?

And, if not now…. when?

Hillel the Elder

Foreword

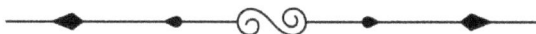

In the vast and ever - evolving landscape of medicine, where information is abundant yet often confusing, there emerges a rare book that bridges the gap between professional medical knowledge and everyday health awareness. Half Doctor by Dr Sandeep is precisely such a book - a remarkable endeavor to empower individuals with the wisdom and insight necessary to navigate their health with confidence and clarity.

Dr Sandeep, a distinguished doctor and surgeon with over four decades of experience, has not only mastered the art of healing but also the art of explaining complex medical concepts in a way that is both engaging and accessible. His journey, inspired by the deep - rooted wisdom of his grandmother - who, despite her limited formal education, exhibited an intuitive understanding of health - demonstrates the power of knowledge when shared with purpose and passion. Her influence as the family's "half doctor" was a testament to the profound impact that awareness and proactive healthcare can have on a community.

This book is more than just a guide to understanding medical conditions; it is an exploration of the intricate relationship between modern scientific medicine and traditional healing systems, patient rights and medical ethics, public health policies, and the transformative role of technology in healthcare. With meticulous attention to detail, Dr Sandeep has structured the book in a way that takes the reader on an enlightening journey - starting from the fundamentals of healthcare systems in India to the nuances of diagnosis, treatment, and preventive care.

One of the standout qualities of Half Doctor is its ability to address the diverse needs of readers. Whether you are a patient seeking to make informed medical decisions, a caregiver supporting a loved one, or even a young medical student stepping into the world of healthcare, this book offers invaluable insights. It demystifies medical terminologies, sheds light on the significance of evidence - based medicine, and offers practical guidance on selecting the right doctor, understanding medical tests, and recognizing early symptoms of diseases.

The book does not shy away from challenging subjects, including quackery, the role of artificial intelligence in healthcare, and the growing concerns around antibiotic resistance. In a time when misinformation spreads rapidly, Dr Sandeep presents a balanced and scientifically grounded perspective, advocating for a more informed and health - conscious society.

Beyond the science, Half Doctor is also a book of wisdom - one that reminds us that good health is not merely the absence of disease but the presence of holistic well - being. From mental health to nutrition, from preventive medicine to dealing with chronic illnesses, it serves as a trusted companion for anyone who values health as their greatest wealth.

As we step into an era where technology and healthcare are increasingly intertwined, Half Doctor stands as a beacon of knowledge, encouraging individuals to take charge of their health with informed choices and a proactive mindset. I wholeheartedly believe that this book will serve as a timeless resource, enriching lives and reshaping the way we approach healthcare in India and beyond.

Dr Sandeep has given us a gift - a comprehensive, compassionate, and compelling guide that will empower generations to come. It is an honor to present Half Doctor to you, and I am confident that it will not only educate but also inspire you to take a more active role in your own well - being and that of your loved ones.

Raam Anand
Founder, Stardom Circle

Preface

"Half Doctor"

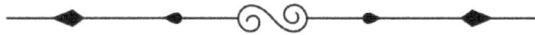

My grandmother, born in 1914, got married at the age of 16. She studied only up to class 5 but raised a family of highly qualified doctors and engineers - both among her children and grandchildren. She was able to detect her own cancer at an early stage and had it treated with radium therapy. She ensured that all the domestic workers and their families were cared for by her two doctors - sons and daughters - in - law. She absorbed a lot from the conversations in the house and the advice given to relatives and visitors. In those early days, she insisted on antenatal check - ups for young women working in the house and made sure they received iron, folic acid, and calcium supplements. She taught us all about hygiene, healthy eating habits, and the importance of exercise. We all affectionately called her "**half - doctor.**"

The idea of writing a book that explains common medical knowledge had been in my mind for many years. As a busy doctor and surgeon, I often heard my patients request, "**Doctor Sahib, please give me the best treatment.**" The Indian ethos is that patients put themselves completely in their doctors' hands. Of course, every doctor wants the best for their patients. We strive to provide the most suitable treatment tailored to the patient's circumstances. However, medical science also has its limits. Therefore, patients would benefit greatly from knowing more about the science of medicine.

Listening to patients' concerns and beliefs, I strongly felt there was a need for such a book for the Indian public. To this end, I first started writing in Hindi and published the book *"Achche Ilaj ke 51 Nuskhe"* along with my co - author, Mr Ajay Agrawal, a versatile reader and litterateur who provided the layperson's perspective to the book. Although, in my opinion, the Hindi version has several shortcomings, I am surprised by how much interest it has generated in India and abroad. We have received letters from various states requesting translations into different Indian languages. This encouraged us to work on an improved English version, which we hope will also address some of the shortcomings.

Medicine - and indeed, biology - is a fascinating science! On one hand, nature shows an almost mind - boggling precision where one considers how cells, tissues, and organ systems function, or the structure of DNA and its effects on individuals. On the other hand, there is endless - perhaps even infinite - variation within species, meaning no two individuals are exactly alike. This variation affects how diseases manifest, how treatments work, and what outcomes we see, which are often expressed through statistics.

Another important concept for readers to understand is that vast and largely unexplored areas (like the functioning of the human mind) remain in human biology and medicine. Modern medicine acknowledges these deficiencies and makes no unfounded claims about them.

This book represents the essence, summary, and gist of the medical and surgical knowledge I have acquired over 40 years. It is primarily written for the Indian public, with the goal of empowering them with knowledge about the human body and illness. The choice and sequence of chapters follow a logical flow. The book is **based entirely on science** and adopts an empirical approach - starting with the structure of healthcare in India and the types of medical care available. It combines public health and personal health practices, explaining how doctors operate, how medical histories are taken, how clinical examinations are performed, how a diagnosis is made, and how treatments are planned. These steps define the doctor - patient encounter.

The book also covers 'challenging' issues like medical ethics, patients' rights, quackery, spurious and generic drugs, and triage. It traces the evolution of scientific medicine through the ages and introduces readers to the latest technology in medicine - including the internet, telemedicine, Google, WhatsApp, and artificial intelligence. There is no area of medical science that has been left untouched by the ceaselessly advancing modern technology. The book also attempts to explain the concept of **Randomized Controlled Trials** (RCTs), which are used to validate new drugs before they are introduced to the market.

Both the Indian population and government have a strong belief in Indigenous Knowledge (IK) and Traditional Medicine (TM). International health agencies are moving toward developing Traditional Complementary and Integrative Medicine (TCIM) as a holistic system for wellbeing. This book emphasizes that our ancient systems should be brought into the mainstream, after undergoing the 'litmus test' of RCTs.

Additionally, we have included some relatively new topics in medicine, such as the gut microbiome, DALYs, QALYs, metabolic syndrome, health - seeking and illness - breeding behaviors, the triple burden of disease and epidemiologic transitions. Subjects like diabetes, high blood pressure, balanced diet, and obesity are particularly important in the Indian context.

The second half of the book covers the major organ systems one by one. After briefly describing the structure and function of each system, the book explains the major maladies affecting them. Finally, the last section discusses preparation for old age and death.

In a world brimming with medical information - often containing unfounded advice - the journey toward maintaining health and well - being can feel overwhelming. **"Half Doctor"** invites readers to embark on a transformative journey toward empowerment and enlightenment in the realm of personal health. This book serves as a compass to guide common citizens through wellness procedures, fostering resilience and adaptation to a balanced lifestyle. It equips readers with knowledge to help them seek and secure quality medical treatment for themselves and their loved ones.

Of course, social and environmental determinants of health, as well as patients' own knowledge and concerns, also play a significant role in medical outcomes. We believe this book will be useful reading not only for the general public but also for paramedics and even medical students in the early stages of their careers.

Lastly, I am deeply grateful to my co - author for his hard work and insightful contributions, which provided the consumer's perspective to this interdisciplinary knowledge. My wife, **Rashmi**, offered valuable ideas for content and additional chapters, as well as editing and proofreading the book. She added more 'science' to each chapter. **Varsha** provided logistical support at every step and assisted with proofreading, and **Indu Sharma** offered secretarial help. I am also thankful to **Raam Anand** of **Stardom Books** for his publishing guidance.

SANDEEP KUMAR

profsandeepsurgeon@gmail.com Lucknow, February 2025

Whispering Vibrations

It was a cool night. My eyes witnessing different thoughts…, perturbed with feelings enamoring for past few years…sting on brain. Feelings intermixed with optimistic vision and somewhat frustrating events…feeling to achieve something great in future…feeling to be doomed in nothingness. Today in this cool night I was taking sound sleep when a nightmare appeared, "I am talking to a doctor – I am too feeble to win over. Different organs are vanquishing over me – mind, heart, kidneys…leaving my company. Deprived of vibrations, sensing and feeling, I am losing consciousness. Better to leave this world!" My eyes opened …nothing is permanent, all existences are momentary and ethereal.

Sometimes, disorder in the mind or the body is **sensed** but testing shows no traces. Sometimes, a disorder is **felt**, but no disease is diagnosed– the doctor may prescribe vitamins, minerals, follow diet schedules and perform a few exercises etc. When disease strikes, it is **experienced** more intensely. Disease may result from any of the reasons like eating unhygienic or harmful food, infection, accident, climatic transmutation or genetic pre - disposition. **Sensing** a disorder, **feeling** a disease and **experiencing** a disease are different phenomena – here sensing shows no clinical signs, feeling comes with certain mute or soft symptoms but experiencing comes out with severe symptoms. Sensing a disorder is the result of vibration in the mind, vicious or unhealthy thinking bears unhygienic atmosphere, foul and vile lifestyle ultimately result in diseases.

This book from beginning to end instructs the reader to develop a lifestyle harmonized with chaste thinking, balanced speech and virtuous deeds to avoid diseases in everyday life. I hope that readers will go through the book with the pragmatic - empirical approach. Incredulous thinking and skeptic approach now and then leads to the condition of hallucination or delusion and sometimes towards obsessive compulsive disorder. Sometimes, these disorders result in somatoform disorder, impulse control disorder and many other diseases of body and mind. **Illness anxiety disorder** in its acute form alters into hypochondriasis and such conditions may prevail throughout the routine or life like various undiagnosed medical conditions. Carry the book throughout all your activities and consult it like a dictionary of health.

The book **Half Doctor** teaches the reader not to be over swayed by every type of adverse situation, rather the book instructs the reader to watch oneself against infections and unfavorable circumstances so that health may be maintained aptly, and unnecessary expenditure may be saved. The book pleads the principle of self - healing and naturopathy, yet it champions the cause of only evidence - based medicines on the ground that patients should not be harmed at any cost. The book invites the conscience of the reader to judge the working of the doctor, that is how and in what manner he follows the principles of medical ethics and patient - right. The book elucidates that a conscientious medical practitioner condescends the patient and their caregiver to develop a cognitive approach towards fast developing technological medical services. The book evokes the reader in many different ways from chapter to chapter that treatment should be procured for accomplishing sumptuous health wherein the treating physician establishes uniformity with the feelings and values of the patient and their family. This book comes up before the reader as a protagonist in fostering wellness which is essential in capacity building the people growing old – strong generation assembles strong society and fabricates strong nation.

Pleading for wellness from chapter-to-chapter **Half Doctor** communicates firmly that societies where people live long conserve posterity and the cultural composition of the nation – early death leads to dearth of treasure in the nation. At the outset, I express my utmost gratitude towards **Dr Sandeep Kumar,** who, despite knowing my less familiarity with biology, offered me the opportunity to co - author the book along with him because of my precision and aptitude. I am grateful to my late father, Sri Gopal Krishna Agrawal, and my late mother, **Smt. Laxmi Devi Agrawal** for enabling this succinct to blossom out with creativity. **Varsha Dwivedi,** a witty, deliberative, and discreet companion, made an edge by spotting illustrations in the book. Last but not least, **Indu Sharma** stands a preferential place in extracting invaluable material from the internet and devised word processing throughout the book. My wife **Shikha** has played a commendable role, otherwise, I would have deviated from the creative purposes. I congratulate **Raam Anand** of Stardom for bringing out a publication suiting our aspirations.

Ajay Kumar Agrawal MA Political Science Retd. Joint Director Department of Culture, Government of UP.

Chapter 1

Health Care Structure in India & Types of Medical Facilities

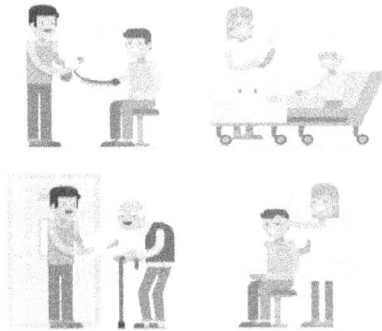

Learning Objectives:

- Primary, Secondary, and Tertiary level medical care

- Different types of medical facilities viz; outreach service, dispensary, hospital, hospice, ambulatory care, nursing home, clinic, etc.

- Where to contact for appropriate medical care and treatment

- Specialized therapy clinics viz; rehabilitation and palliative care

- National Medical Commission

Health care can be divided into three levels: **Primary, Secondary,** and **Tertiary**. In India, health care is provided through two parallel systems: the state - run or government system and the private sector. The government system caters to rural areas through **Sub - Centers, Primary Health Centers** and **Community Health Centers.**

Recently the government is taking special measures in improving public health and opening **Wellness Centers** at rural and district levels.

District Hospitals deliver secondary care, while medical colleges offer tertiary care. The private sector is structured with individual practitioners for primary care, polyclinics and nursing homes for secondary care, and expansive corporate hospitals for tertiary care.

The Central Government, Indian Army, and Employees State Insurance Corporation provide special clinics and hospitals in major cities for their beneficiaries.

Primary Health Care – One of the government's significant responsibilities is providing primary health care. This includes preventive, promotive services, vaccinations, nutritional support, managing minor health issues, epidemic control, health education, maternal care, child health and survival, emergency management, referrals, and patient transport. Additionally, the implementation of programs to combat public health concerns like malaria and filaria, diarrhea, and encephalitis falls in the realm of primary care. The **Alma - Ata Declaration** of 1978 reinvigorated the focus on primary care globally, paving the way toward the objective of **"health for all**."

Secondary Care - This level includes in its fold disease diagnosis and treatment of severe infections and chronic conditions like diabetes, hypertension, arthritis, and depression. Surgical procedures, both minor and significant, such as Caesarean sections, hernia repairs, gall bladder surgeries, uterus removal (hysterectomy), and bone fracture treatments, are usually conducted in district hospitals, urban nursing homes, and specialized institutions. Modern government community health centers in rural areas are now equipped with pathology labs and X - ray facilities. Secondary care also offers physiotherapy, rehabilitation, labor, and delivery services. Rapid advancements and expansions in secondary care services like ultrasound and CT scan facilities are taking place.

Tertiary Care – This type of medical care is given to patients who are suffering from both acute and chronic diseases, communicable and non - communicable. This type of medical care may be given by big, comprehensive hospitals with specialized departments.

Tertiary care hospitals often have intensive care units (ICU) and Critical Care Units. Conditions such as kidney failure, dialysis, and cardiac and liver diseases are treated. Major surgeries on vital organs are conducted at this level. Esteemed medical institutions, including various medical colleges, state - run postgraduate medical institutes, and several All India Institutes of Medical Sciences - AIIMSs are equipped with state - of - the – art infrastructure.

These include services like Trauma and Medical Emergency (TEM), burn treatment centers, neonatology care units, organ transplant units, radiation oncology units, physical medicine, and rehabilitation centers, all types of major surgeries, and sophisticated bone marrow, liver, kidney, and lung transplantation, etc.

Types of Medical Services

1. **Outreach Medical Care -** This refers to the delivery of diverse medical services to remote or distant communities and those hesitant or incapable of visiting a hospital or primary health care center. Outreach care is particularly effective for door - to - door vaccination, prenatal care, deworming, treatment for malaria and filaria, and caring for the elderly. Care of pregnant women, dispensing of calcium, iron, and folic acid pills, and care of sick elderly are a special focus of outreach medical care. Home - based newborn care is also a notable outreach service. Both government and private entities sometimes offer specialty treatments on the go using medically equipped vehicles or by setting up temporary clinics in suitable locations.

2. **Ambulance -** Over the past five years, state governments have successfully introduced pivotal ambulance services, notably numbers 108 and 112. In developed nations, ambulances usually have a crew comprising one or two paramedics trained in first aid and basic life support. Immediate on - site assessment allows for quick interventions such as clearing airways, managing bleeding, and supporting broken limbs.

   The principle is often *'scoop and run'* - rapid transport to a medical facility after initiating basic care. Comprehensive training programs are underway to prepare paramedics who can perform critical first - response actions, from ensuring open airways, stopping external bleeding, splinting and supporting fractured bones, and safe transport of patients to appropriate hospitals.

3. **Primary Health Center/Dispensary/Doctor's Clinic** – These facilities, commonly found in rural areas and smaller towns, play a crucial role in delivering Primary Health Care. Certain state governments are establishing out - patient, diagnostic and treatment facilities called *Mohalla* Clinics.

4. **Hospitals** – These are essential establishments where patients receive care from a team of professionals, including specialist doctors, resident doctors, nurses and other healthcare staff. Hospitals can be categorized as:

   a. Rural - based Primary Health Care (PHC) and Community Health Care (CHC) centers operate around the clock.

   b. State - run District hospitals, as well as smaller private hospitals and Nursing Homes, are common in urban areas.

   c. Large - scale government institutions like AIIMS, Post Graduate Medical Institutes (PGI), and Medical Colleges, along with expansive corporate hospitals, offer general, specialty, and super - specialty services. A sizable hospital typically features distinct Emergency, Outpatient, Inpatient, Operation theatres and Intensive Care departments, complemented by diagnostic services such as pathology, microbiology, and radiology. Some might also host day - care wards, and a blood bank is a vital component. It is noteworthy that in many regions, the term "Nursing Homes" refers to long - term care facilities, often catering to the elderly or those with disabilities.

5. **Trauma and Emergency Management** – Patients experiencing medical emergencies, such as acute abdominal pain, chest discomfort, shortness of breath, loss of consciousness, paralysis, unexpected bleeding, high fever, severe diarrhea, vomiting, poisoning or envenomation, drowning, etc. are promptly attended to in Emergency & Trauma Departments.

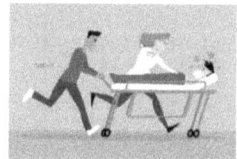

Emergencies requiring surgical intervention – like burns, road accidents, head injuries, intestinal ruptures, complications during childbirth, critical stages of cancer, mental health crises, and suicide attempts – result in immediate hospital admissions. Here, a coordinated team of doctors offers swift, life - saving interventions.

The government of India has recently emphasized training doctors in emergency medical care, leading to the establishment of Emergency Medicine Departments in all Indian medical colleges. However, it is not just doctors who are at the forefront; nurses, ambulance drivers, police officers, and even the general public benefit from understanding basic life - saving techniques.

Life support training has become mandatory in hospitals and has advanced into standardized protocols like **Advanced Trauma Life Support (ATLS).**

The ATLS protocol, along with others, is strictly observed in Trauma & Emergency Medicine (TEM) departments. For critical cardiac patients, **Advanced Cardiovascular Life Support (ACLS)** is employed. Numerous protocols cater to a variety of illnesses and conditions. Once a patient's condition stabilizes, they may be directed to a specialty department for continued care.

6. **CCU/ICU Critical Intensive Care Unit** – Hospitals designated for tertiary - level care are obligated to maintain ICU facilities. Patients who are critically ill, especially those with heart conditions, are swiftly moved to the CCU/ICU after receiving immediate and necessary care in trauma and emergency centers. Such patients may need a range of support, from ventilators for artificial respiration and heart monitoring systems to kidney dialysis and intravenous nutrition. Once their critical condition stabilizes, they are transitioned from the ICU to a 'Step Down' ward or **High Dependency Unit** and eventually to the Inpatient Department (IPD). This could be either a general ward or a specialized one, depending on the patient's needs. ICUs are manned by a dedicated team, including critical care specialists, anesthetists, specialized nurses, and trained attendants. They are equipped with advanced amenities such as motorized beds, cardiac monitors, ventilators, infusion pumps, and more beside each bed.

Notably, the expenses associated with ICU care tend to be considerably high in private hospitals.

7. **Outpatient Department** – The OPD, or Outpatient Department, is a vital component of any general hospital across the country. While some doctors exclusively offer outpatient or ambulatory care, others operate within larger institutions. Major hospitals in India witness approximately 5000 to 10,000 patients daily, coming as follow - up and new patients. Care provided in the OPD is termed **"ambulatory,"** meaning patients can walk in, consult, or receive treatment and then walk out without an overnight stay.

In addition to the General OPD, there are specialized OPDs catering to specific ailments. Specialists typically schedule their consultations on designated days. Patients with serious conditions that warrant comprehensive examination, repeated observation, detailed investigations, or surgery are recommended for inpatient care.

The OPD roster comprises a variety of physicians and specialists proficient in treating a diverse range of conditions: from eye, ear, nose, and throat ailments to metabolic and thyroid disorders, from gastrointestinal issues to conditions of the kidney, heart, and respiratory system. They also cater to dental care, obstetrics and gynecology, pediatrics, cancer, and long - term infections such as HIV and leprosy.

A primary objective is to diagnose and treat these ailments. Modern OPDs now feature on - site laboratory equipment for immediate on the spot testing, often referred to as **"point of care tests."**
This practice of instant testing in OPD itself provides efficient and quality medical treatment, less sorties for the patient and high patient satisfaction.

8. **Day Care** – Large general hospitals offer 'day - care' services for the monitoring and diagnostic evaluation of patients, including cancer chemotherapy and the administration of intravenous medications. Daycare services encompass procedures that don't require an extended hospital stay. Patients are discharged on the same day.

Additionally, outpatient departments in these hospitals boast efficient operating theaters. They handle a range of surgical procedures, from cataract surgeries and endoscopies to minor general surgeries like treating abscesses, wounds, in - growing toenails, anorectal issues, and cysts.

These procedures are often performed under local anesthesia and, in some cases, brief general anesthesia. Notably, patients typically return home the same day after these treatments. Family planning operations of vasectomy in men and tubectomy in women can generally be performed on a daycare basis. Several procedures like surgery of gall bladder due to technological development can now be done in daycare.

9. **In Patient Department or Indoor Patient** – Patients can be admitted to a general ward, a partially paying ward, or a fully paying ward. During their daily rounds, attending or specialist doctors oversee the patients and assess the ward's management. As they make their rounds, senior doctors attend to the patients, engage with their families and provide guidance to the attending staff and nurses. This guidance is then executed by resident doctors and nurses.

    Primary and community health centers, located at village and block levels, typically have two or three medical officers and an obstetrician on staff. Often, patients from distant villages travel to urban general hospitals or larger cities to diagnose their ailments and receive appropriate medical or surgical treatment.

    A key measure of a country's development in healthcare is the doctor - population ratio i.e. number of qualified doctors per thousand population. The number of available indoor beds in community hospitals for the concerned population is a normative parameter of any country's development.

10. **Specialty Hospital** – Specialty hospitals are established to cater to specific population groups, such as children or the elderly. Alternatively, they can focus on the treatment of specific diseases or organ systems, such as cancer, leprosy, TB, psychiatric disorders, or eye conditions. Specialty hospitals for the treatment of specific diseases or organ systems are stand - alone hospitals.

11. **Hospice** – Hospices provide care for patients facing incurable, terminal diseases. Their existence in various nations reflects the unique cultural and social values of each society. Rooted in principles of social justice and advocacy, hospices offer a sanctuary for those burdened with profound suffering and sorrow.

In contemporary times, hospices have evolved to care for patients in advanced stages of cancer, Alzheimer's, and incurable conditions of the heart, lungs, liver, kidney, or brain, especially when most medical interventions have been exhausted.

When a patient's life nears its end, physicians often advise families to consider hospice care, which emphasizes tender loving care, pain relief, and palliative treatments. Hospices also offer end - of - life care and bereavement services. Ideally, resources should be optimized to support those with terminal illnesses, rejuvenating their desire for life and allowing them to cherish past memories. Such hospices are called nursing homes in Australia and Veterans hospitals in the USA.

12. **Telemedicine** – With the advent of the internet, fiber optics, satellite technology, and 4G, 5G, and 6G networks, coupled with the rise of artificial intelligence, telemedicine and diagnostics have soared to new heights. Telemedicine has not only transformed the landscape of ambulatory care but has also diversified its applications. Today, specialists from urban areas can provide comprehensive care to patients in remote regions. In emergency situations, these specialists can extend their expertise beyond traditional settings, offering consultations and treatments to patients in rural clinics, factories, and community centers through video conferencing, ensuring timely interventions. Telemedicine adeptly handles tasks like drug dosage adjustments, prescription clarifications, addressing concerns of anxious parents, consultations related to sexual health, inquiries about vaccinations, dietary advice, and more. Telemedicine is serving remotely living patients with their ailments, providing both primary care and follow - up consultation.

13. **Therapy Clinic** – Adults and children grappling with various physical and mental challenges can find tailored solutions at specialized therapy centers.

Here are a few examples of therapies provided for these conditions:

a.   **Physical Medicine and Rehabilitation (PMR)** – Also called the physiotherapy department. It is imperative for all medical colleges to have this department operational.

As individuals transition into adulthood or advance in age, ailments like pain in the neck, shoulder, back, knee joints, or other musculoskeletal discomforts become prevalent. Physiotherapy offers effective treatments for such conditions, as well as for post - fracture care, post - operative joint care, or after joint replacements.

Another significant role of PMR is the provision and fitting of prosthetic limbs to enhance mobility in individuals with disabilities. Currently, the domain of physiotherapy is expanding exponentially. Patients benefit from holistic treatments that include multi - faceted exercises and therapies utilizing ultrasound, diathermy, and other innovative tools.

b.   **Psychosomatic Therapy** – When an individual experiences a decline in mental or physical flexibility or a reduction in endurance due to events such as a major accident, paralytic stroke, brain injury, Alzheimer's disease, depression, psychosis, or neurosis, they can be rehabilitated through psychosomatic therapy.

c.   **Occupational Therapy** – The objective of this therapy is to train and rehabilitate individuals, equipping them with the skills to carry out daily activities such as sitting, walking, managing finances, engaging in social interactions, achieving self - reliance, and reintegrating into suitable employment.

d.   **Speech Therapy** – Individuals facing challenges such as stuttering, pronunciation difficulties, issues with sentence formation and lacking confidence in speaking can benefit from speech therapy. Speech therapy sessions are typically conducted in day care settings, lasting around 2 - 4 hours daily.

14. **Disaster Management and Medicine** – Disasters, whether natural or man - made, demand specialized responses. Events like earthquakes, landslides, cloud bursts, building collapses, fires, tsunamis, toxic gas leakages and tornadoes can result in mass casualties, with many injured, immobilized, or killed instantly. These situations necessitate intervention by specialist doctors and adept paramedic teams.

Immediate medical attention is provided on - site for those in need, while those requiring extensive care are administered basic life support and transported to suitable medical facilities. Effective disaster response teams often consist of doctors, ambulance services, firefighters, and debris removal specialists who converge at the disaster site for rapid action. Medical teams utilize disaster triage to prioritize treatment.

Additionally, helicopter and drone services can play a pivotal role in rescue operations and delivering medical aid. Historical events, such as the Bhopal gas tragedy, the cloud burst in Kedarnath, and various fire accidents and landslides, highlight the importance and effectiveness of organized disaster response systems. The National Disaster Management Authority (NDMA) is the apex body for disaster management in India, headed by the Prime Minister. It is responsible for framing policies, laying down guidelines, and coordinating with State Disaster Management Authorities (SDMAs) to ensure effective disaster response and management.

15. **Wilderness Medicine** – Adventurous endeavors, whether trekking the towering Himalayan peaks like Everest or traversing wild deserts, can pose significant risks. Similarly, engineers and laborers dispatched on expeditions to extract vital resources from oceans, deserts, or icy landscapes face environmental hazards. These areas are characterized by extreme weather conditions, encounters with wild animals, and other life - threatening challenges, making conventional medical aid inaccessible.

This specialized care termed **Wilderness Medicine** (Hindi term - *Aranya Chikitsa*), prioritizes immediate response in challenging terrains. The Indian Army, stationed at some of the world's highest battlefronts, faces extreme cold and isolation, which can lead to physical and mental challenges. Their well - being in such inhospitable terrains is an embodiment of the principles of wilderness medicine.

Individuals dispatched to such remote sites are often equipped with GPS tracking systems connected to satellites. In emergencies, medical teams can pinpoint their location and provide on - site treatment or evacuate them to a more equipped facility. Notably, Australia has made significant advancements in this medical domain.

16. **Warfare Medicine** – The Army Medical Corps, an integral component of national armies worldwide, is staffed with physicians, surgeons, nursing professionals, and paramedics. Through continual research and study, the Corps refines and establishes updated medical protocols tailored for warfare. This ongoing development ensures that the treatments and battlefield medical facilities adhere to the latest standards and best practices. Battlefield medical protocols are rigorously tested to ensure they can be swiftly and effectively applied during combat situations.

For instance, immediate actions to control bleeding, such as tight bandaging, are vital. Protocols also cover the "**scoop - and - run**" system, where the primary objective is to quickly evacuate an injured soldier from the frontline.

The transportation of injured personnel is systematic: they are initially taken to a nearby camp hospital. Depending on the severity of injuries, they may then be transferred to a base hospital and subsequently to specialized Command hospitals for comprehensive care.

The National Medical Commission (NMC) earlier the Medical Council of India is a national regulatory body for medical education and practice. The roles of the NMC are to

(i)   ensure adequacy of high - quality medical professionals in all parts of the country

(ii)   improve access to quality medical education,

(iii) promote equitable and universal healthcare

(iv)   encourage medical professionals to adopt the latest medical research in their work

(v)   to maintain high standard of medical institutions

(vi)   maintain a medical register for medical professionals in India

(vii)   enforce high ethical standards in all aspects of medical services;

(viii) have an effective grievance redressal mechanism.

In conclusion, many people in our country may not be aware about the health care structure and types of medical care available to them. A citizen aware of the facilities available for health care can make best use of these.

Chapter 2

Patient Rights, Medical Ethics and Moral Dilemmas

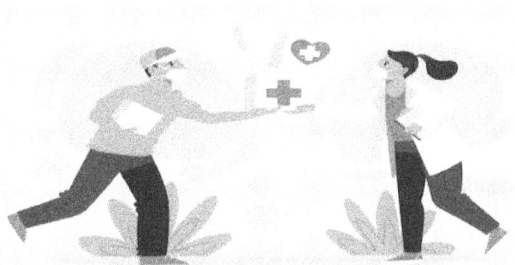

Learning Objectives:

- Development of the Principles of Medical ethics and Patient Rights

- Awareness about the rights of patients and responsibilities of patients

- Examples of moral dilemmas in medical practice

This chapter delves into the commitment to uphold and protect the rights of patients receiving care in the medical facilities available in India. Historically, fundamental rights include the basic needs: *Roti* (food), *Kapda* (clothing), and *Makaan* (shelter). However, by the mid - 20th century, equal access to education and healthcare joined the roster of fundamental rights available to every man from his birth.

Development of Patients' Rights – With the development of civilization, nations of the world moved along to guarantee all the citizens certain basic needs like food, clothing, and shelter as fundamental rights that are undeniable to them from birth.

Medical scientists, jurists, and various scholars and luminaries started pleading for the cause of humanity, and these basic needs or fundamental rights were safeguarded. The violence and hostilities in World War II resulted in the holocaust with systematic extermination of Jews. The acts of brutality and savagery cast a dark shadow on humanity. In the aftermath of this large - scale violence at the global level, the United Nations Organization (UNO) was formed in the year 1948. Central to its mission was to safeguard humanity from the future scourge of war. Thus, the **Universal Declaration of Human Rights 1948** came into being to fulfill the aspirations of humankind. The dark chapter placed greater importance on human dignity in all spheres. Efforts paved the way to eliminate the scars left by discrimination based on religion, race, caste, and gender and the destruction brought to humanity and environmental heritage. Numerous attempts were made to restore the intrinsic dignity of all humans who were devastated by the war, giving humankind a new wave of freedom. All these efforts culminated in a new age of human development.

In this new world, the belief that patients belonging to any caste, creed, or sex are entitled to equal protection and dignity during their treatment and well - being has surfaced. Organizations like the UNO and others around the world believed that no patient should be denied healthcare based on any discriminatory factors, ensuring that the rights of patients are protected globally.

Rights of Patients in India – Article 21 of the Indian Constitution guarantees every citizen the right to seek treatment from any hospital or doctor as they deem appropriate for their well - being. Any discrimination made by the doctor or the hospital on the basis of gender, caste, color, creed, or religion is a violation of this right. If any harm is inflicted upon the patient due to discrimination or negligence mentioned above, the doctor or hospital shall be held legally accountable. Stringent provisions may be invoked against those not adhering to Article 21 or the regulations therein.

The primary goal of any medical treatment is to uphold the rights and dignity of the patient while striving to achieve the best possible health outcomes.

Consequently, a doctor's moral responsibility entails offering a spectrum of care - from basic to emergency services - and ensuring that the patient and their caregivers are well informed about potential recovery pathways and strategies to enhance the quality of life. Guided by international standards set by organizations like the UNO and WHO, various nations have formulated their own Patients' Rights Charters. In India, many of these provisions pertaining to Patients' Rights are found dispersed across several legislative documents.

These include the Drugs and Cosmetics Act 1940, the Constitution of India (Article 21), the Consumer Protection Act 1986, the Indian Medical Council (Professional Conduct, Etiquette, and Ethics) Regulations 2002, the Right to Information Act 2005, the Clinical Establishments Act 2010, and the National Health Policy 2017. Furthermore, the judgments of the Hon'ble Supreme Court of India and decisions from the National Consumer Disputes Redressal Commission (NCDRC) play a pivotal role in shaping and reinforcing these rights. The latest comprehensive Patients' Rights Charter of India has been proposed by the National Human Rights Commission and vetted by the Ministry of Health and Family Welfare.

Patients' Rights Charter of India (NHRC 2019): The full document is available at https://nhrc.nic.in/document/charter - patient - rights and http://clinicalestablishments.gov.in/WriteReadData/9901.pdf

An abridged version with salient features is given below:

1. **Right to Information** - The patient and their attendants have the right to know, in simple regional or English language, regarding their cause of illness, proposed investigations, diagnosis, test reports, expected results, identity and professional status of doctors of the hospital, and the expected cost of the treatment.

2. **Information on rates and charges -** Each type of service, rate, and available facilities should be displayed conspicuously in regional and English languages.

3. **Right to Receive Records and Reports -** Outpatient and admitted patients shall be able to access and obtain copies of their records, test reports, and treatment bills.

4. **Right of Consent -** Informed consent prior to specific tests/treatments (surgery, chemotherapy, biopsy, etc.) is mandatory.

5. **Right to seek a second opinion -** The patient or their attendants shall have the right to obtain a second opinion or get treatment from a second or other specialist doctor, who shall be provided with full information and all the records created by the previous treating team.

6. **Right to Confidentiality, human dignity, and privacy -** Every doctor is obliged to maintain confidentiality regarding the disease and treatment provided to the patient. Upholding the dignity of the patient and the privacy thereof is the core of care providers.

7. **Privacy of female patients -** Male doctors should ensure the presence and assistance of female personnel during the examination of a female patient.

8. **Right to Non – Discrimination -** Every patient is entitled to procure the treatment if suffering from HIV and AIDS - without being discriminated against.

9. **Right to treatment according to one of the available alternatives as selected by the patient -** Patients have the right to choose one of the alternatives offered to them for treatment options.

10. **Right to receive a dead body -** The patient and his attendants shall have the right to receive the dead body without any maneuvering, and this right shall not be denied.

11. **Right to settle the agreed - upon payment -** It was recommended that patients seeking transfer to another hospital/discharge from a hospital will have the responsibility to "settle the agreed - upon payment."

12. **Right to no discrimination in treatment -** Treatment should be based solely on illness or conditions, including HIV status or other health conditions, and not on ethnicity, gender (including transgender), age, sexual orientation, linguistic, or geographical/social origins.

13. **Digitization of medical records -** Informed consent of the patient shall be included mandatorily in the digitization of medical records.

14. **Right to care according to prescribed rates -** Care shall be provided

according to the rates as displayed on the display board or fixed by the National Pharmaceutical Pricing Authority (NPPA).

15. **Right to choose the source for obtaining medicines or tests -** Hospitals, especially corporate hospitals and other clinical establishments, should not force patients to purchase medicines from their in - house pharmacies. If patients procure medicines from outside at a lower price/cost, they shall not be subjected to rejection. Similarly, the patients requiring their tests to be done from outside shall be facilitated by the concerned hospitals or clinical establishments.

16. **Right to protection and compensation for patients -** Patients involved in clinical trials are protected under the Drugs and Cosmetics Act, ICMR, and other Government Guidelines.

17. **Right to protection and compensation for participants -** Participants involved in biomedical and health research are protected as per the National Medical Commission, ICMR, and other Government guidelines.

18. **Right to Patient Education -** All patients shall have the right to be provided with the relevant information regarding their disease and its treatment procedures.

19. **Right to be heard and seek redressal -** Every hospital shall be equipped with a time - bound **Grievance Redressal mechanism** to address the grievances of the patients. A Grievance Redressal Officer shall be designated, and their name and contact details should be displayed in a conspicuous place in the local language and in English. The records of grievances received and resolved shall be maintained in their original form.

20. **Right to proper referral and transfer free of perverse commercial influences**

a. In case of referral by the hospital, the referring hospital shall provide a proper referral transport facility in the most appropriate vehicle/ambulance for the transfer of the patient to an appropriate hospital where facilities for management of the patient are available.

b.   Such transfer of a patient shall not be refused if the same is not referred to by the previously treating hospital and even if the patient is leaving against medical advice (LAMA). The applicable reasonable charges may be levied by the clinical establishment for such transfers. However, in case of an emergency situation, such referral transport shall be provided free of cost as far as possible and shall not be refused for want of any payment.

c.   State/UT Government may consider defining various charges for different types of ambulances for compliance by the hospitals and other clinical establishments. The clinical establishments will be required to display the rates/charges of ambulance(s).

         The referring hospital shall provide the assistance of a qualified and trained person to monitor and manage the condition of the patient enroute till the patient is received by the referee hospital.

The information about the above additional rights shall be **widely disseminated** by the Ministry and State Governments among hospitals, doctors, patients, and the public to make them aware of the above existing rights.

All of the above patient rights are an integral part of the policies declared by the Indian Council of Medical Research (ICMR) and the Medical Council of India (now the National Medical Commission). Adopting all of the above patient rights as the operational standards of hospital functioning ought to be observed in India.

However, above all considerations, the goodwill and dedication of the treating physician remain paramount.

Responsibilities of Patients - NHRC 2019

1. All required health - related issues should be informed to the doctor by the patient to achieve quick and quality treatment.

2. Patients should follow the doctor's advice and cooperate with the doctor during examinations, diagnostic tests, and treatment.

3. Hospital instructions like appointment time, cooperation with hospital

staff, fellow patients, maintaining discipline and cleanliness, and not causing disturbances enhance the dignity of the patient and his caregivers.

4. Settling the dues of the hospital well within time.

5. Patients should respect the dignity of the doctor and other hospital staff as human beings and as professionals. Patients are expected to be aware of their responsibility regarding treatment alternatives agreed upon or refused by them.

6. **Never resort to violence**. Whatever the grievance may be, patients/caregivers should not resort to violence in any form and should not damage or destroy any property of the hospital or service provider. Patients and their caregivers should be aware of the legal consequences of resorting to violence or destruction of hospital property in lieu of their grievances.

Medical Ethics

The primary goal of all medical treatments is to restore optimal physical and mental health to the patient. No harm should be inflicted on the patient as this is the essence of medical ethics. Physicians should consistently uphold human values while executing treatment for their patients.

Providing treatment to all patients equally, regardless of their race, religion, caste, gender, or socio - economic status, is the prime, basic obligation of the doctor. All types of medical research activities must proceed according to the norms of medical ethics.

Safeguarding human dignity and values in the medical examination of human cadavers is also dictated by medical ethics. The concept of medical ethics can be traced to the following sources:

1. **Hippocratic Oath** – The foundational methodology for consulting and treating patients is credited to the Greek physician Hippocrates (460 - 370 BC). Modern medical science remains deeply indebted to the high standards and ideals that Hippocrates established, practiced, and promoted.

To this day, young doctors in some medical colleges worldwide take the Hippocratic Oath upon graduation, reflecting his enduring influence and the pivotal role he played in shaping the ethics of modern medicine.

2. **Nuremberg Code – 1947** – During the Second World War, Nazi physicians conducted medical experiments and research on Jewish prisoners and cadavers of Jewish soldiers. Actions by the Nazi physicians were later deemed deeply unethical and in gross violation of human dignity. In the subsequent Nuremberg Trials, these Nazi doctors were prosecuted and held accountable for their heinous crimes.

   Out of these trials, the Nuremberg Code was established, setting clear guidelines on the ethical conduct of medical research and experimentation. This pivotal moment in history paved the way for the Helsinki Declaration in 1964, further elaborating on these ethical principles for medical research.

3. **Universal Declaration of Human Rights – December 10, 1948** – A charter of human rights rolled out after the pages of history against atrocities and felonies committed worldwide by the Nazis against Jews. The Declaration of Human Rights was adopted by the United Nations Organization in 1948. This served as a milestone in safeguarding human rights, including the right to a life with dignity and mental health. It also provided a framework for ethical medical practice.

Principles of Medical Ethics

Respect for Autonomy – The patient has the freedom and right to choose or refuse his treatment. This principle also includes consent of the patient as to why, how, and when his treatment should be carried out or what is the most appropriate course of his treatment according to his preference.

Principle of Beneficence – The doctor should treat the patient to bring him to the best possible state of physical and mental health while trying to meet the expectations of the patient and family. During the process of treatment, the patient should be respected as 'end' and not to be taken as a 'means' of the medical examination. Treating the patient as a means is against the value of humanity.

Principle of Non - Maleficence – Primum Non - Nocere – This means that first, do not inflict harm to the patient, even if he cannot be benefited as such.

Principle of Justice – The doctor should ensure justice in the treatment of any patient so that treatment should be fair, equitable, and appropriate.

When, due to any emergency situation or disaster, many patients reach the hospital all of a sudden, the necessary treatment of the hospital extends to take care of severely ill emergency patients while not delaying the less seriously ill patients in queues of waiting. Thus, taking care of patients as a priority while treating the disease and distributing medicines and services to them without losing time is the principle of justice that the doctor and healthcare staff are obliged to fulfill at that time. Prioritizing patients for treatment according to the seriousness of their illness is called "Triage."

Consumer Protection Act (CPA), 1986 (replaced by CPA, 2019) is an act passed by the Parliament of India to protect the interests of consumers in India. The liability of the medical professional arises when an injury results due to conduct that is below the standards of 'reasonable' care.

It includes private and government hospitals, as well as independent and employed medical practitioners, but does not apply to hospitals and practitioners that provide free services to all patients. The patient can report the incident within 2 years from the date of occurrence by filing a complaint with the National Medical Commission, local police station, or consumer court.

Moral Dilemmas – Ethical and moral dilemmas can arise in the minds of doctors during the treatment of their patients. Examples of such dilemmas are…

Case (1) – Sunita, a teenage girl in a village near Chandigarh, was suffering from liver failure. Sunita's father took her to a big teaching hospital's emergency in Chandigarh. The resident doctor realized the girl was serious. Only a liver transplant could possibly save her, but this treatment was extremely expensive. Her father did not have a single penny in his pocket. Admission to a liver transplant unit was deferred. No intensive care could be carried out. The doctor explained the facts to the father.

Consideration – Poverty overruled the right of treatment. Human life was relegated to nothingness before money. Should the doctor or father bear this burden on his mind?

Case (2) – Bhavana's father Jagatnarayan, a 62 - year - old Chief Executive Officer, gradually developed jaundice… eyes turning yellow, appetite diminishing day by day with no other apparent sign of disease or pain.

An oncologist, Dr. Bhumi, diagnosed advanced stage pancreatic cancer and advised stenting to overcome bile duct obstruction and undergo chemotherapy. She had informed me that this treatment was likely to achieve some life prolongation of 1 or 2 years only. Hoping for a good outcome, Bhavana gave consent for treatment. However, the bile started to get infected.

Despite some temporary relief from chemotherapy, the overall condition of the patient deteriorated. Bhavana was later convinced that the quality of life was not good - days mostly spent in and out of the hospital, he was admitted 17 times with recurrent attacks of cholangitis and pancreatitis before dying.

Consideration – Bhavana was neither pragmatic nor analytical regarding her father's situation… imposing the burden of guilt on Dr. Bhumi, who could have been more assertive. Several other members of the family should have been involved in decision - making. Even with the best efforts and money, life - prolonging measures without improvement in quality of life may not be worthwhile. Dr. Bhumi was disheartened too.

Case (3) – Dr. Chandrashekhar, Chief Medical Officer (CMO), was battling with the consequences of Japanese encephalitis in the district headquarters for the last few years. Several successive officers of the district called him to do his utmost and to lead the staff in eradicating the disease.

There was pressure on him to report less number of cases reports. But the CMO's professional integrity would not allow him to tamper with the truth, which antagonized him with dire consequences of either transfer or resignation.

Case (4) – A 39 - year - old woman, Dharmishtha, a resident of Andhra Pradesh, was suffering from acute cholecystitis. She was brought to the nearby corporate hospital by her three children on a trolley - she had low blood pressure, anemia, and imminent septic shock.

Her husband was working in Mumbai. Meanwhile, she was infused with bottles of fluids and given antibiotics. Surgery was essential - no surgeon was available in a nearby government hospital. Dr. Deepak, the surgeon on duty, requested the hospital authorities to allow him to operate on this patient at the cost of the hospital, which was denied. The doctor still performed the operation, and the cost was deducted from his salary.

Consideration – Human suffering could not surpass the rules of the hospital. Thus, Dr. Deepak was baffled with the rules on one side and morality on the other side.

Case (5) – Dr. Anshul, a retired professor of pathology and molecular biology, was visiting the charges of a private hospital in Gujrat - Covid - 19 was treated here. Senior government officers who visited the hospital praised Dr. Anshul for his prompt and skilled work. Later, the Chief Executive Officer requested the laboratory to under - report Covid - 19 positivity to stop the panic. Ignoring this advisory, Dr. Anshul lost his job.

Consideration – The direction of the Chief Executive Officer was contrary to human values and medical ethics.

Note: The above case scenarios are true incidents (names changed). Many such ethical - moral dilemmas occur in doctors' lives - the readers should be aware.

Ultimately, medical ethics and the rights of the patients are two sides of the same coin. On the one hand, if the patients seek their treatment on the basis of their rights, they must also fully cooperate and trust the doctors. Quality treatment and medical ethics appear to be different issues, but both are interconnected. If doctors and patients complete their duties well, mutual trust will develop. Responsible patients should cooperate fully with their treating physicians and have confidence in their treatment.

Chapter 3

Public Health, Preventive, Curative, Social, Family & Community Medicine

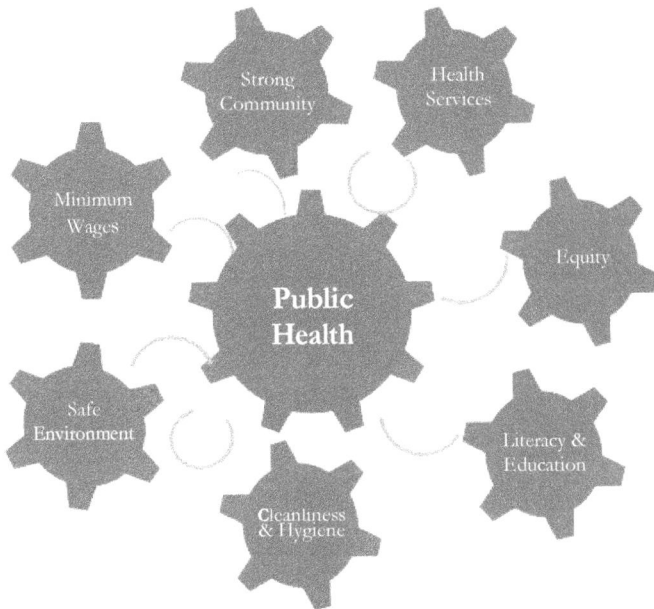

Learning Objectives:

- Recognition and significance of Health for All

- Significance of Public Health and State Medicine

- Significance of Preventive, Curative, Community, Social and Family Medicine

---

Health is Wealth is an old adage. The health of individuals may be protected from diseases only when healthy habits and practices are followed. Societies indifferent to standards of hygiene and health are overwhelmed by diseases.

Here the role of the Government becomes significant. It is incumbent upon the government to implement measures to prevent and combat diseases pervading the efficiency of society. This may be achieved by creating and maintaining appropriate infrastructure of Public Health. Public health is delivered through outreach programs to reach the 'last person in the queue.'

It includes diverse activities such as dissemination of health education, imparting hands - on training on public health programs, restricting pollution, provision of sanitation and safe drinking water, appropriate disposal of garbage, and medical waste of hospitals, provision of nutrition, etc. Vaccination and provision of medicines during epidemics by Government programs are important activities to combat diseases spreading in the society.

History of Public Health – The concept of public health started about 150 years ago, when industrial revolutions and rapid urbanization were at their peak. People in Europe, lacking hygiene, were dying prematurely in large numbers.

Many infectious diseases like TB, typhoid, cholera (these diseases were not known in those days) overpowered Europe.

Life expectancy in Britain was only 20–40 years. The great cholera epidemic in England of 1832 prompted the British lawyer **Edwin Chadwick** to write his report on the unsanitary conditions of the working class. Chadwick led the "sanitary movement," through which the Public Health Act was passed in Britain in the year 1848. Surveys were conducted to search for the cause of these epidemics, as a result of which it was detected that many diseases are caused due to overcrowding, polluted drinking water, and small dwellings with scanty sunlight and ventilation, and infections spread by mosquito bites, etc. In 1860, the French bacteriologist

Louis Pasteur confirmed the presence of bacteria in the air. He propounded the **Germ Theory of disease.** In 1877, **Robert Koch** demonstrated that a bacterium caused anthrax, further confirming this theory. Following this, more and more disease - causing microorganisms) were discovered in quick succession. Gonococcus, Typhoid bacillus, and Pneumococcus were proven to be the cause of gonorrhea, typhoid, and pneumonia, respectively, by the year 1880.

Similarly, bacteria causing TB was detected in sputum smears, and pneumonia in 1882, and bacteria like Cholera vibrio and Diphtheria bacillus were detected, respectively, in 1883 and 1884.

The last decade of the 19th century brought a flood of discoveries and inventions in the field of medical science when surgeon Major Ronald Ross verified that the Tsetse Fly was the cause of sleeping sickness in Africa.

Ross confirmed that malaria was spread by Anopheles mosquitoes, and Walter Reed detected that Aedes aegypti mosquitoes spread yellow fever.

With knowledge of transmission, measures to reduce the spread and treat these diseases became possible. Control activities like quarantine, water purification, milk pasteurization, vaccination, sanitary engineering, vector control, disposal of sewage, and monitoring of sewer lines, etc. were developed. These preventive measures reduce disease outbreaks in society. People started becoming aware of infections as well as their prevention.

The chemicals acting as agents of disinfection and pollution control were used to prevent the spread of infections. Diseases spread by insects are called **vector - borne diseases**. Examples are malaria, yellow fever, dengue, filaria, and encephalitis. Therefore, the control of vectors like mosquitoes, flies, etc. are recognized as a measure in preventive medicine.

In the past, these diseases were prevented by chemicals like DDT, malathion, etc. By the end of the 19th century, many other effective preventive measures against disease - like good nutrition, vaccines, handwashing and disinfectants were discovered. This was the threshold of Preventive Medicine.

Preventive Medicine – Identifying the germs, viruses, and bacteria causing infection and studying the methods for their prevention gained importance.

It was recognized that infectious diseases like Smallpox, Polio, Rabies (hydrophobia), Diphtheria, Typhoid, etc., may be prevented by immunization or vaccination. By the end of the 19th century, the concept of preventive medicine was mostly restricted to control infections, which later expanded to the prevention of non - communicable diseases like heart disease, stroke, etc., by measures like keeping blood pressure and diabetes under control and restricting the use of tobacco to prevent many diseases.

These could not be explained on the basis of germ theory. Surgery was performed as a practice for treating disease for many years, but the wounds were prone to catch infection after surgery. Dr. Joseph Lister of Great Britain – an experimental surgeon was called "father of modern surgery." Surgery got a great boost after the invention of antiseptics and disinfectants.

After 1900, medicine moved toward rational, scientific approaches to disease diagnosis. The next thinking that evolved was that of **multifactorial causation of disease** i.e., multiple factors - genetic, social, economic, ecological, and psychological - in causing disease. Public Health Acts were passed in various countries with the objective to prevent infectious diseases, control pollution, establish primary health care services, community health programs, provide medication for life - style diseases like chronic diseases (high blood pressure, diabetes, etc.), provide treatment in cancer and mental illnesses, etc. Efforts were made aware of harmful effects of drug addiction, tobacco, alcohol, and other illness breeding behaviors. Medicine branched off into **Preventive, Curative, and Palliative**.

In this era, emphasis on precise testing, diagnostics, and therapies took center stage, and patient - specific treatment plans, personalized medicine, and the promotion of preventive healthcare were more widely embraced.

Social Medicine, State Medicine, Community Medicine, Family Medicine, and Public Health – These are some names given to modern preventive and curative medicine, and they more or less focus on similar issues and objectives. The aim of preventive medicine is to focus mainly on how to prevent the disease itself.

In the same manner, the thrust area of curative medicine is to provide relief and cure when the disease has already occurred. However, Public Health is a broader term and focuses more on the social and economic structure of communities and educational factors, to improve all the levels of health.

Public health is defined as "the science and art of preventing disease, prolonging life and promoting health through organized efforts and informed choices of society, organizations, public and private, communities and individuals."

Social Medicine and State Medicine – Social medicine is an area in which financial resources and values of people are given priority only up to a considerable level. The objective of social medicine is making the people aware of morbid rituals, customs, living standards, etc., which create impediments in hygienic living.

The scope of social medicine encompasses the whole society along with physicians doing private practice according to the norms and rules fixed by the State.

Community Medicine – Community medicine is a branch of medicine which aims to protect and promote the health and well - being of communities and populations. This branch of medicine includes all the components of public health, community health, social medicine, etc.

Community health gives priority to the prevention of diseases. WHO recognizes the significance of national cultures, traditions, geography, and economic resources and validates the role of community medicine in the overall development of a disease - free society. Recently, the Government of India is establishing **Wellness Centers** throughout the country.

Family Medicine – Family medicine is a specialty in itself. The practitioners of family medicine are skilled and accomplished in providing preventive, promotional, and curative medicine. Practitioners of family medicine are also recognized as Family Physicians. They are proficient in dealing with Maternal - Child welfare, minor surgery, common infectious diseases, and lifestyle and chronic diseases like hypertension, diabetes, rheumatism, etc.

Thus, the family physician acts as the bridge between the patient and specialist doctors. Family doctors provide vaccinations for children and the elderly. He sometimes carries out complementary and supplementary treatment of his patients as prescribed by the specialist doctor.

Scope of Public Health – As of now, prevention in modern medicine is not limited only to vaccination and quarantine. Public health includes all activities at community level aimed at screening for diseases (so that they can be diagnosed early), study of epidemiology of diseases - communicable, nutritional, and noncommunicable, investigation and containment of epidemics, planning and implementing programs for disease control or eradication, demography, environment, occupational health, disaster management, health planning, and international health.

Four stages of preventive medicine

1. **Primordial Prevention** – Primordial prevention is a concept that precedes primary prevention and focuses on **risk factor prevention**. Complete restriction on tobacco agriculture and production and declaration of tobacco as illegal substance would be the primordial prevention of oral and lung cancer. Another example of primordial prevention is that of genetic diseases by identifying and not marrying carriers of defective genes.

2. **Primary Prevention** – Prevention of disease in a healthy population is e.g., disseminating information on vaccination against Japanese encephalitis and taking measures to vaccinate the people. Restricting tobacco addiction, promoting a law regulating the use of tobacco in public places, and awakening the people to stop smoking is primary prevention of lung cancer. To stop chewing tobacco or gutkha is primary prevention of oral cancer.

3. **Secondary Prevention** – Identifying disease at an early stage and giving the appropriate treatment early, thereby minimizing its effects or curing it, e.g., screening of the female population for breast cancer by a mammogram is an example of secondary prevention.

4. **Tertiary Prevention** – Providing all the procedural treatment completely to the patient and giving him comfort is tertiary prevention This means taking such measures during the treatment so that the patient may not get disabled, and no further impairment or harm is inflicted on him. Ensuring that no delays occur in biopsies if suspicious of cancer, expedited pathological tests, and early treatment institutions are procedures adapted to tertiary prevention.

World Health Organization (WHO) – This international body came into being with the end of World War II. Witnessing the insufficient collaboration between countries of the world in controlling the spread of dangerous diseases, the World Health Organization (WHO) was formed.

WHO provides **advisory and recommendatory role** in health research and development activities and accordingly keeps member countries informed about the outcome of research activities. This body also issues important **guidelines** for the countries of the world on how to safeguard public health. The **International Classification of Diseases** (ICD) was introduced in 1948, in which inactivated and live attenuated polio vaccines, a list of essential medicines, **international health regulations**, etc., were included. In 1978, the **International Conference on Primary Health Care** was held in **Alma - Ata, Kazakhstan**. **Health was defined as a "state of complete physical, mental and social well - being and not merely the absence of disease or infirmity."** The aspirational goal, **"Health for All," by the year 2000,** was set, calling for universal health coverage through Primary Health Care. Smallpox was given a death blow and eliminated from the world by 1979. The call for polio eradication was made in 1988, and since then, polio is eradicated from most countries of the world - India was declared polio - free in 2014. In 1995, the **Integrated Management for Childhood Illnesses (IMCI)** was launched.

In 1999, the **Global Alliance for Vaccines & Immunization (GAVI)** was instituted, and the **Global Action Plan on the Prevention and Control of Noncommunicable Diseases** (NCDs) was launched and accelerated.

In the year 2000, the **Millennium Development Goals (MDGs)** were set to be reached by 2015.

Of the 8 MDGs, 3 were health - related goals - namely, to

(i)   Reduce child mortality,

(ii)   Improve maternal health, and

(iii)   Combat HIV/AIDS, malaria, and other diseases.

The MDGs have been followed up by **Sustainable Development Goals (SDGs)** to be met by 2030 for the prosperity of the modern world and future generations.

Seventeen goals enshrined in MDG and SDG goals are included in the Health Act and Policies of Governments in almost all the countries of the world.

Alleviation of poverty and hunger, growth of per capita income, growth of GDP, equality in education and sex, supply of pure water, removal of ecological imbalance, nutrition, and discrimination in religion and caste are the few objectives that are given significance in the distribution of community medicine and health services. It was recommended and determined by these memoranda that the objective of multinational organizations is to promote and strengthen the resources of community medicine in each country. The following are self - explanatory United Nation's Sustainable Development goals aimed at achieving all round progress and well - being in the world.

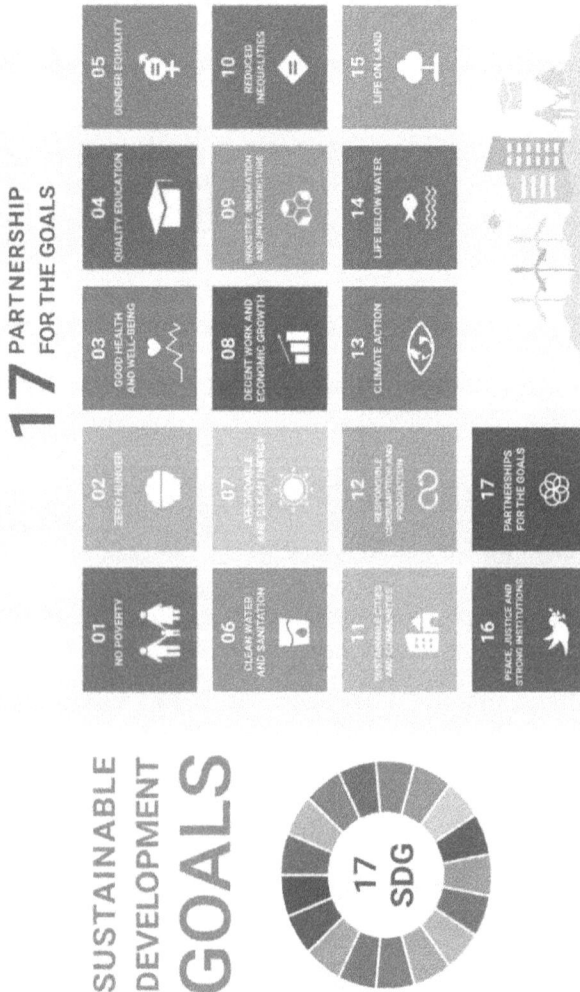

Chapter 4

National Health Care Policy and Programs

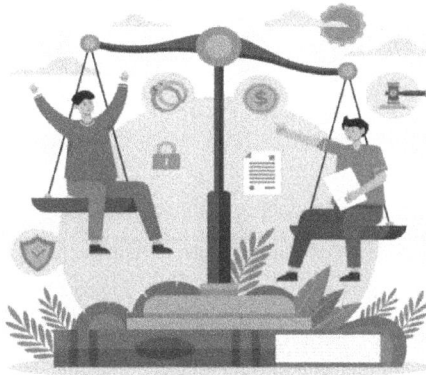

Learning Objectives:

- **Human Development Index** is central to a country's development

- Evolution of Indian Health Policy

- Health care programs for improving social and public health in India

---

Alongside the **UNO Charter of 1948** on Human Rights, the constitutions of many countries have drafted their respective health policies health programs for their citizens. The Indian Constitution entrusts the responsibility of formulating the nation's healthcare policy to the Central Government. In India, the sector of health is the subject of state lists.

Union Government formulates, revises, and amends health care policy, but implementation of these health policies locally at the state level is carried out by different state governments according to local requirements.

Of late, necessity was felt to bridge the health sector to the concurrent list in which both the union and the state governments participate. Despite this, India's expenditure on health and nutrition remains at a mere 1% to 2% of the Gross Domestic Product (GDP), which is considerably low in comparison to other countries.

The Indian Government formulated the **first National Health Policy in 1983,** which was later **amended in 2002 and then in 2017**. This policy aims to ensure the best possible health and well - being for all citizens, regardless of age. The motto of India's National Health Policy has been to strengthen the health of all citizens of India. It emphasizes a preventive and promotive health care approach, allowing for universal accessibility to quality health care services without causing financial hardship.

This ambition accords with reducing the cost, improving the quality, and expanding the accessibility of healthcare delivery. Moreover, the policy acknowledges the significance of the Sustainable Development Goals (SDGs) set for 2030, to which India is committed.

The **Human Development Index (HDI)** was created in 1990 to underline the importance of people of the country and their capabilities rather than just economic growth alone as the ultimate measure of development. **HDI is a summary measure incorporating life expectancy at birth, expected years of schooling, and per capita income.** As per the Human Development Index Report from the United Nations Development Program (UNDP) in 2018, India ranks 130th out of 189 countries. With a view to augmenting the efficiency of Indian citizens, the revised National Health Policy of 2017 was launched by the Government of India.

Basic objectives of National Health Care Policy 2017:

1. Increase health expenditure from the current GDP 1.15% to 2.5% by 2025.

2. Increase the life expectancy at birth from 67.5 years to 70 years by the year 2025.

3. Bring down the total fertility rate (TFR) per woman in India to 2.1 by 2025.

4. Reduce the mortality rate among children under five years to achieve the goal of 25 deaths per 1000 children by the year 2025.

5. Reduce the maternal mortality rate (MMR) to 100 women per every 1 lakh deliveries.

6. Reduce stunting among children under 5 years by up to 40% by the year 2025.

7. Bring down the infant mortality rate to 23/1000 live births by 2025.

8. Reduce neonatal mortality rate (NMR) from 25/1000 to 18/1000 in India by 2025.

9. Reduce blindness up to 0.25 per thousand by the year 2025 and bring down the number of blind patients to one - third.

10. Eliminate Kala - azar (Leishmaniasis) and Lymphatic Filariasis by 2017, and Leprosy by the year 2018.

11. Reduce the death rate due to diseases such as heart diseases, chronic respiratory diseases, and cancer by 25% by the year 2025.

12. Ensure the eradication of tuberculosis by 2025.

13. Extend the utilization of government hospitals by 50% by the year 2025.

14. Vaccination of 90% infants below 1 year by the year 2025.

15. Increase the number of trained nurses for delivery to 90% babies by 2025.

16. Reduce the consumption of tobacco by 15% and 30% respectively by the years 2020 and 2025.

17. Reduce the number of people falling into occupation of tobacco manufacturing and trade by 50% by the year 2025.

18. To ensure the expenditure of 8% on health services in all the state budgets of India by the year 2020.

19. Reduce the health expenditure of various families of India by 25% by 2025.

To achieve the objectives of the National Health Policy, the Government of India has implemented several programs. Remarkably, two major infectious diseases, smallpox and polio, have been eliminated from India. Some key programs include:

1. **Mid - Day Meal Program (1956)** – Originally launched to enhance child nutrition by providing balanced cooked meals, this program also aims to boost school enrollment.

2. **Integrated Child Development Scheme (ICDS, 1975)** – Recognized as the world's largest community - based program, ICDS is directed at children up to the age of six, pregnant and lactating mothers, and women aged 16–44. Its goal is to improve the health, nutrition, and education of these target groups.

3. **Expanded Program of Immunization (EPI, 1978)** – Initially rolled out against six diseases: tuberculosis, polio, diphtheria, tetanus, pertussis, and measles – the EPI has since expanded to cover several other infectious diseases.

4. **National Health Mission (NHM, 2005)** – This mission was initiated by the Central Government to bolster health systems in both rural and urban settings of various states of India.

5. Its primary areas of focus include Reproductive, Maternal - Neonatal - Child and Adolescent Health (RMNCH+A) and addressing both Communicable and Non - Communicable Diseases.

Various initiatives taken under NHM are:

a. **ASHA (Accredited Social Health Activists)** – Drawn from local communities, ASHAs serve as frontline providers, facilitators, and community health mobilizers, with a specific focus on the wellbeing of women and children.

b. **Grants to Sub - Centers (SC)** – As part of the national health mission, untied grants are given through which sub - centers are being revamped and equipped with advanced medical appliances to provide better services.

c. **Village Health Sanitation and Nutrition Committee (VHSNC)** – This committee plays a pivotal role in community empowerment and participation. It addresses issues related to environmental and social determinants of health at the grassroots level.

d. **Healthcare Service Delivery** – To bridge the gap in human resources, NHM has incorporated approximately 1.88 lakh additional health workers into the healthcare system.

e. **Reproductive, Maternal, Neonatal, Child and Adolescent Health (RMNCH+A, 2013)** – The primary goal is to curtail the mortality rates of women and children by enhancing their overall health. This is achieved by monitoring pregnant women's health, making scorecards in government hospitals, distributing iron and folic acid supplements to address maternal and child anemia under the National Iron Initiative Program, raising awareness about congenital conditions like cleft lips and cleft palate, malformation of heart valves, club foot, spina bifida (disorders of spinal cord), etc.

    This program is also focused on implementing screening for curing vitamin and mineral deficiencies. Various programs under RMNCH+A are discussed in Chapter 22.

f. **Janani Suraksha Yojana (JSY)** – This initiative aims to decrease maternal mortality by giving monetary incentives to pregnant women to opt for deliveries in healthcare institutions.

g. **Janani Shishu Suraksha Karyakram (JSSK, 2011)** – Inaugurated on 1st June 2011, JSSK entitles pregnant women choosing public health institutions for delivery to absolutely free and no expense delivery, including both normal and Caesarean deliveries. A similar facility is extended to infants up to 12 months of age.

h. **National AIDS Control Organization (NACO - 1992)** – NACO takes measures for diagnosis and treatment of HIV - AIDS according to global standards. This program has been instrumental in keeping HIV - AIDS in check in the country.

i. **Revised National Tuberculosis Control Program – RNTCP/** Recently changed to National Tuberculosis Elimination Program – NTEP

The following measures were undertaken for TB elimination, viz:

(i)   Detection,

(ii)   treatment,

(iii)   prevention,

(iv)   building labs,

(v)   Directly Observed Treatment,

(vi)   Short - course (DOTS), etc.

All of these measures yielded envisaged results. Issuing TB patient notification was made mandatory for all health institutions in India.

Incentives amounting from ₹250.00 to ₹750.00 per case were fixed for TB care, treatment, drug sensitivity, and drug resistance testing to private sector hospitals and institutions being monitored by RNTCP under the "Nikshay" (TB elimination) program. The Government of India is distributing services and medicines for treating TB free of cost to build a "TB free India."

j. **National Leprosy Eradication 1983** – Along with the campaign of leprosy eradication measures, effective treatment of the patient suffering from this disease is undertaken by all the government hospitals. At present, by preventing leprosy infection, patients are being kept safe by all the procedural treatments so that they may not be disfigured. The government is taking all the effective measures to keep the patient working efficiently in society. Multi - drug therapy is provided free of cost at all government hospitals.

The Leprosy program is an essential part of the National Health Mission. Leprosy treatment is an integral part of government hospital services.

k. **National Vector Borne Disease Control Program (NVBDCP-2002)** – This program integrates the National malaria control program with other Vector Borne Diseases such as Kala - Azar, Dengue, Lymphatic Filariasis, Japanese Encephalitis, and Chikungunya.

l. **Mission Indradhanush** – In this scheme, 12 vaccines are given to all the children of the country (earlier only 7 vaccines were given).

These include – TB, Diphtheria, Whooping cough, Tetanus, Polio, Measles, Hepatitis - B, Meningitis (due to H. Influenza type - b - Hib), Pneumonia, Rubella, and Japanese Encephalitis (in selected districts) and rotavirus.

m. **National Mental Health Program (NMHP)** – The World Bank report (1993) revealed that the Disability - Adjusted Life Year (DALY) loss due to neuro - psychiatric disorders is much higher than diarrhea, malaria, worm infestations, and tuberculosis if taken individually. According to the estimates, the DALY loss due to mental disorders is expected to represent 15% of the global burden of diseases by 2020. **NMHP has three components:**

1. Treatment of Mentally ill

2. Rehabilitation

3. Prevention and promotion of positive mental health.

n. **Pulse Polio Immunization Program** – This was a very high - level program that started in 1995 and went on until polio was finally eliminated in 2011. Polio vaccination is being given under routine immunization now. Branding of this immunization was undertaken by the government with a view to awakening the people towards this disabling disease.

o. **Pradhan Mantri Swasthya Suraksha Yojana, 2006** – The objective of this scheme is to remove social inequality, provide affordable health care to the general public in under - served areas of the country, and to give a fillip to the expansion of medical education. Under this scheme, many new AIIMS have been started, and government medical institutions have been upgraded.

p. **Rashtriya Arogya Nidhi** – This fund was set up in the year 1997 by the Ministry of Health and Family Welfare.

The purpose of this fund is to provide financial assistance to patients below the poverty line for the treatment of serious diseases from super specialty hospitals for which the required amount is remitted to the Hospital.

q. **National Tobacco Control Program 2003** – This scheme intends to make the populace aware of the serious and chronic diseases caused by tobacco consumption. The Tobacco Use Control Act was passed in the year 2004.

r. **Ayushman Bharat Scheme 2018** – Ayushman Bharat is a paramount initiative by the Government of India, designed to realize the ambition of Universal Health Coverage (UHC) for the population of India. Moving away from a segmented and sectoral method of health service delivery, this scheme embraces a comprehensive, need - based healthcare service paradigm.

It aims to introduce groundbreaking changes that holistically address every facet of the healthcare system - spanning prevention, promotion, and ambulatory care - across primary, secondary, and tertiary levels.

Curative tertiary level care up to Rs 5 lacs per annum per family is provided as health insurance to half the population of the country from private hospitals and clinics.

Catering to the vast population, the scheme envelopes 10 crore families, translating to approximately 50 crore individuals. Ayushman Bharat reposes on a continuum of care philosophy, which is manifested and elucidated in two interwoven components:

Health and Wellness Centers (HWCs) – 1.5 lacs Ayushman Bharat Health and Wellness centers to be established throughout the country that can be accessed by all to seek positive and quality health.

Pradhan Mantri Jan Arogya Yojana (PM - JAY) – It is a national public health insurance scheme that aims to provide free access to health insurance coverage for low - income earners eventually to cover 50% of the country's population. Up to Rs five lac treatment per family per annum can be obtained from empaneled private hospitals and nursing homes.

Poshan Abhiyaan (2018) – This program was launched with the aim to reduce malnutrition, through a life - cycle approach. The objective is to bring down stunting in children 0 - 6 years of age. Reduce anemia among women and adolescent girls in the age group of 15 - 49 years and reduce low
birth weight.

In conclusion, the journey of Bharatvarsh from slavery to independence, from poverty towards economic growth, from backwardness towards multidimensional technological development, from a plethora of diseases towards strong health and immunity, from dogmatism towards scientific temper are the features that have made it complete and fulfilled.

Thus, India may improve a lot if the people living in this country are taught and shown as to how to attain the benefits of the health programs being run by our government. The Central and the State Governments' commitment and honest implementation of the healthcare policy and healthcare programs will go a long way in developing strong nation clinics.

Chapter 5

Recognize the Disorders in Your Body

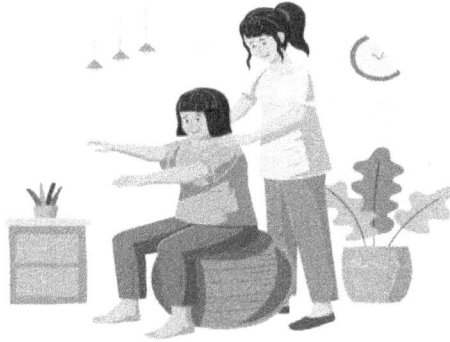

Learning Objectives:

- Understanding the overall structure and functions of the body

- Understanding terms – symptoms, signs, disorders, disease, disability, acute, and chronic

- Recognizing and distinguishing the disorders and diseases appearing in the body

---

Often, we either overlook minor ailments in our bodies or become overly concerned about a trivial disorder. Sometimes, we might become confused by information sourced from the internet. On certain occasions, we might exacerbate a small problem through unscientific self - treatment or by resorting to quackery.

In reality, quackery can lead us into a dangerous situation where a little knowledge becomes harmful, and a disease that could have been treated in its initial stage escalates into something more serious.

A **symptom** is a manifestation of a disease that the patient experiences, such as pain or a cough. In contrast, a **sign** is a discernible manifestation of the disease that a physician detects upon **examination,** such as an enlarged liver, a lump in the abdomen, raised blood pressure, or a hemorrhage in the retina. A **disease** represents a distinct abnormal process - a departure from a healthy state in the body with a specific cause and characteristic symptoms. On the other hand, a **disorder** signifies an irregularity or minor disruption of normal functions, typically temporary, and which generally resolves on its own.

While diseases may present with certain disorders, not every disorder is a disease. For instance, constipation may simply be a disorder commonly caused by changes in lifestyle, travel, or diet. However, constipation can also be a symptom of a more serious disease, such as growth or cancer in the large intestine. Despite these distinctions, the terms "disease" and "disorder" are often used interchangeably.

Disability can be mental or physical. Complete impairment or any significant restriction in mental or physical capability is defined as a disability.

Syndrome: This term refers to a group of symptoms and signs that occur together, potentially due to various underlying causes. For example, nephrotic syndrome, characterized by body swelling, protein in the urine, low levels of albumin in the blood, and increased cholesterol, occurs due to many kidney disorders.

Symptoms or diseases are classified as **acute** when they develop rapidly over a short period or **chronic** when they persist over an extended time. If one or more symptoms persist for more than 4 - 5 days, seeking proper medical treatment is advisable.

Atmospheric pollution, changing lifestyles, imbalanced diets, food prepared in unsanitary conditions, excessive consumption of white sugar, salt, refined flour (*maida*), and junk food such as pizzas, noodles, patties, *samosas*, sodas, chocolates, etc., combined with a sedentary lifestyle lacking regular exercise and increasing dependency on others, contribute to the onset of various diseases and health complications.

Dietary guidelines are preached in nearly every culture, with physicians often providing diet charts tailored to individual needs. Some general dietary guidelines endorsed by *Ayurveda* - the ancient system of medicine originating in India - can be adopted by people across different societies.

These guidelines include:

1. **Eat Seasonal Food**: Each season brings its own agricultural produce to the market, offering a variety of fresh vegetables, fruits, grains, and more. Consuming these seasonal foods is preferable, as they are fresh and align with the body's natural needs during that time of year.

2. **Eat Less**: Eating up to 80% of your hunger helps maintain proper digestion - "Eat less, escape worries" (*Kam khayein, gam khayein*). People in Okinawa, Japan, and other Blue Zones follow this principle and are known for their longevity.

3. **Eat Nutritious Food – *Hita - Bhukh***: Consuming nutritious food has long been a fundamental principle for maintaining good health. Avoiding foods that can trigger common disorders like gastric irritation, acidity, and belching can help keep such ailments at bay. The age - old adage "one man's meat is another man's poison" (*kisi ko baigan bawale, kisi ko baigan pathya* - किसी को बैगन बावले, किसी को बैगन पथ्य*) means avoiding foods that do not agree with your system.

Our bodies are composed of millions of cells, which are microscopic and invisible to the naked eye. **Cells** with similar structures and functions come together to form **tissues** (e.g., epithelium or lining). These tissues combine to form **organs**, each comprising different tissues and serving a distinct purpose (e.g., kidneys, lungs, heart). These organs collectively form **organ systems**. Notable organ systems include the gastrointestinal system, responsible for digestion and assimilation of food; the cardiovascular system, which comprises the heart and blood vessels responsible for blood circulation, delivering nutrients and oxygen to every cell while removing harmful waste; the nervous system, including the brain, spinal cord, and nerves, which governs thinking, behavior, actions, and balance, and also controls other systems; the renal system, responsible for waste excretion; and the endocrine system, which includes various glands like the thyroid and adrenal glands.

The hematologic system (blood) and the integumentary system (skin) are also classified as organ systems. The lymph nodes, liver, and spleen collectively form the reticuloendothelial system.

Our body is always in a state of motion and momentum. Activity and dynamism are the essential pillars around which life revolves. The body undertakes three types of actions:

1. **Voluntary Actions** are those performed willingly by the mind, such as routine physical work, walking, running, physical exercise, reading, practicing music, etc.

2. **Involuntary Actions** are performed spontaneously by the body, such as breathing, blinking, or heartbeats. Our intestines work continuously, 24 hours a day, in the processes of digestion, assimilation, and excretion.

3. **Reflex Actions** are instinctive reactions to stimuli, such as suddenly applying brakes to avoid a collision or closing the eyes in response to an approaching object.

Any noticeable change in these voluntary, unwilling, involuntary, or reflex actions should be observed carefully, as they may indicate a disorder or disease.

Changes in our body, such as nausea, vomiting, loose motions, fever or a feverish sensation, headaches, coughs, stomach cramps, blood in stool, or any other pain, weight loss, etc., should not be ignored for extended periods.

While spontaneous recovery from such symptoms is possible, they might also serve as early warning signs of a more serious ailment. Ignoring these signs is akin to "illness - breeding behavior." Diseases can invade our bodies stealthily, like burglars, and neglecting them may have long - term consequences. English proverbs such as "a stitch in time saves nine" and "nipping it in the bud" hold true when considering early disease symptoms.

Pay attention to your body's signals and seek medical advice to prevent potential complications. Medical science supports the idea that proactive "health - seeking behavior" maintains our vitality and well - being.

For instance, a lump in a woman's breast that feels new, mainly if it is growing, irregular in shape, and firm, should always be checked by a qualified doctor. Similarly, an ulcer that doesn't heal within two weeks or bleeding from any natural orifice - such as the mouth, nose, anus, or ears - should also be examined by a physician.

Common Symptoms of Diseases Affecting Different Systems of the Body:

1. **Pain**: Pain is the most common symptom prompting a person to seek medical advice. It denotes uncomfortable sensations conveyed by nerves to the brain and can manifest as a sharp stab, dull ache, throbbing, burning, stinging, pinching, or soreness. Pain can be sudden, acute, chronic, intermittent, localized, or generalized, and each person's tolerance to pain varies. It often indicates some disorder in the body. Pain is not typically a symptom of cancer, especially in its early stages.

2. **Fever**: Fever is a prevalent symptom, often resulting from **inflammation** in a part of the body.

3. **General Symptoms**: Lethargy, loss of appetite, weight loss, and generalized body aches can indicate infections or chronic diseases. Changes in the skin, such as scaling and abnormalities in nails, should be noticed. Swelling, especially around the eyes and feet, may indicate an underlying disease.

4. **Gastrointestinal Symptoms**: These include vomiting, nausea, jaundic, abdominal pain, diarrhea, belching, and bloating.

5. **Respiratory Symptoms**: These encompass cough (with or without sputum), sore throat, nasal discharge or blockage, breathlessness, and chest pain.

6. **Cardiovascular Symptoms**: Chest pain and breathlessness are the primary symptoms, while signs may include high or low blood pressure, swelling of the ankles and feet, and irregular pulse. Additional tests may indicate cardiovascular disease.

7. **Nervous System Symptoms**: These range from headaches, convulsions (fits), altered consciousness, muscle weakness, muscle

tightness, paralysis, pain or tingling sensations, or loss of sensation or balance Recent memory loss, incoherent speech, delayed development in children, and poor scholastic performance are also indicative of nervous system disorders.

8. **Hematologic Symptoms/Signs**: Signs of blood - related diseases might include anemia, uncontrolled bleeding, spontaneous appearance of tiny hemorrhages under the skin, and enlargement of the spleen and liver.

In conclusion, it is crucial to consult a doctor rather than succumbing to undue worry or panic. Both inaction and excessive alarm can be harmful.

Moderation in all things is key - a principle captured by the Hindi proverb: *"Ati Sarvatra Varjayet (अति सर्वत्र वर्जयेत्)"* meaning "Avoid excess in everything."

Avoid harmful habits such as tobacco, bidi, cigarettes, pan masala, drugs, and alcohol, which are known to be detrimental to health and harbingers of untoward symptoms. Nurture your body with the habits of a regulated life: eat wisely as described above, engage in plenty of physical activity and exercise, and cultivate a positive, fun - loving attitude, avoiding excessive worry about worldly gains. At the same time, be mindful of what is happening to your body and its systems.

Chapter 6

How to Treat Day - to - Day Health Problems

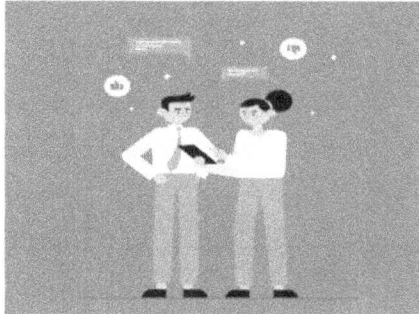

Learning objectives:

- Treatment of cough, cold, fever, diarrhea, dysentery, acidity, belching, hiccups, frequent sneezing

- Treatment of aches and pains in the head, back, neck, or shoulders

- Prevention and treatment of cracks in feet, ankles, hair loss or acne, etc.

- Treating disorders occurring due to deficiency of vitamins, minerals, etc.

Nature has endowed humans and animals with an innate ability to fend off diseases and heal themselves. Common ailments like coughs, colds, mild fevers, diarrhea, indigestion, acidity, nervousness, weakness, headaches, sore throats, and constipation frequently occur `but often resolve on their own.

Rest and fasting may be all that's needed. Many of these issues arise due to 'microbes' - tiny organisms invisible to the naked eye.

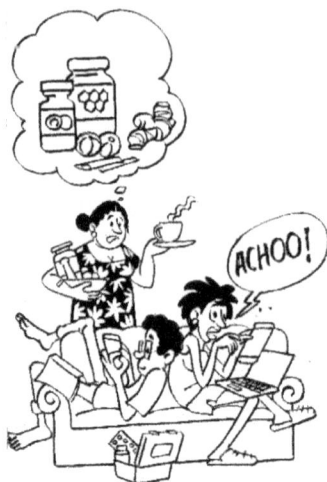

For example, the common cold is caused by a viral upper respiratory tract infection and is typically self - limiting. It's rare to find someone who has never caught a cold, hence the term "common cold." In most cases, the body's immune system effectively combats these infections without needing medical intervention. As the saying goes, "A cold lasts for a week if treated and seven days if not," meaning active treatment might not significantly speed up recovery. Bacterial infections affecting the skin, respiratory system, and gastrointestinal tract are also common.

Symptoms and health concerns often vary across different age groups, influenced by changes in time, climate, environment, and diet.

Age - specific health issues are common. Below are a few examples across different age groups:

Babies:

Newborns may occasionally struggle with breastfeeding or may regurgitate after feeding. These challenges are generally not indicative of severe illness. Techniques like kangaroo care, proper holding, and ensuring the baby burps post - feeding can be beneficial. If the baby is gaining weight appropriately, these concerns are usually not serious. Avoid inserting fingers into a baby's mouth, as regurgitated milk could lead to ear or respiratory infections. Given a baby's delicate skin, only gentle, non - irritating products should be used for skin care and massage.

Growing Children:

Playful and active children are prone to falls and injuries. In cases of minor abrasions, rinsing the wound with clean, running water is advisable. Having a first - aid kit at home, equipped with essentials like paracetamol, is good practice. For children experiencing leg or foot pain (called growing pains) after prolonged physical activity, pain relief medication, and warm compresses can be beneficial.

Some children might exhibit the habit of consuming substances like clay or chalk, a condition known as '**Pica.**' This may be due to deficiencies in iron, calcium, or certain psychological factors.

Dry skin might indicate a deficiency in vitamin A, while anemia may suggest an iron deficiency.

If symptoms persist, consulting a physician is recommended. Parents and teachers should also be vigilant in recognizing eye refractory errors, such as myopia (nearsightedness) or hypermetropia (farsightedness).

Adolescence (10 - 19 years):

This phase brings significant physiological changes, including the onset of menstruation in girls and nocturnal emissions (night falls) in boys.

Adolescents often grapple with academic pressures, competitive dynamics, fears of failure, self - image concerns, and peer influence, all of which can lead to mental and emotional distress. It is crucial for parents, teachers, and caregivers to offer guidance, support, and counseling during these formative years.

Unfortunately, this age group also has a concerning rate of suicides, emphasizing the need for robust emotional and psychological support systems. Family, peers, and educational institutions significantly influenced the values and judgments formed during this period.

Day - to - Day Problems

Headache – Headaches can vary in intensity and origin, manifesting differently in each individual. Regular occurrences of severe headaches may indicate conditions such as **migraine**. Other common causes of headaches include muscle tension, dehydration, hunger, and sleep deprivation.

It is essential to consult a physician if the headache is persistent, associated with vision disturbances or vomiting, or if it interferes with daily activities. In some cases, the underlying cause of a headache might be psychological, requiring intervention and consultations with mental health professionals.

Lower Back Ache, Neck, and Shoulder Pain – Pain in the neck, shoulder, and lower back are common across all age groups. These pains are often triggered by daily stressors, muscle spasms, poor posture (both during sitting and sleeping), high pillows,

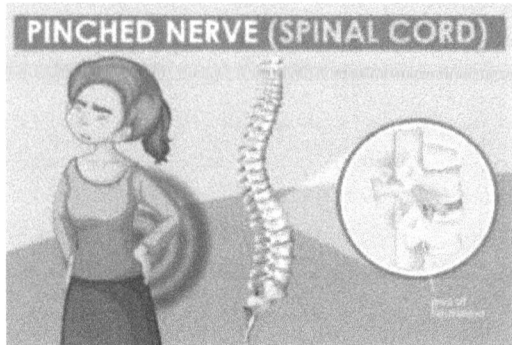

and deficiencies in nutrients like vitamins and calcium.

Understanding and applying ergonomics in daily activities can help prevent these issues. This includes maintaining proper posture, adjusting seating, and ensuring adequate distance between the eyes and reading material.

Solutions such as adequate rest, pain - relieving topical applications, regular exercise, physiotherapy, and practices like *Yoga* and *Pranayama* can be beneficial. In some cases, medications like painkillers and muscle relaxants may be prescribed to manage the pain.

Cracks and Fissures in Feet – Working barefoot, especially in moist environments, can lead to painful cracks and fissures in the heels and toes. These cracks may sometimes become infected with fungi like Tinea pedis.

While short durations of barefoot walking are recommended for health, proper foot care is crucial. This includes washing the feet with clean running water or using warm water in colder seasons before bedtime, which is both relaxing and preventive. Regular foot soaks in lukewarm water, exfoliation using a pumice stone, and application of moisturizers can promote healing. If fungal infections are suspected, using antifungal medications or creams is recommended.

Snoring – Light snoring is common, but persistent and loud snoring, especially in individuals who are overweight, short - necked, or have a thick tongue, may lead to a severe health issues. The narrowing of the airway during sleep due to a repositioned tongue, and lax soft palate tissues can result in heavy snoring. Congenital bony deformities can also contribute to a narrowed air passage.

Around 20% of individuals who snore heavily experience reduced oxygen levels in their blood during sleep, known as **hypoxemia**.

This condition can escalate to high blood pressure (hypertension) and even cause heart attacks during sleep. Another consequence is **sleep apnea** or interrupted breathing during sleep. Maintaining good sleep hygiene is vital for overall health. Disturbances in sleep patterns can lead to morning headaches, irritability, and excessive daytime sleepiness, also known as somnolence. This condition is particularly hazardous when performing activities like driving, as it increases the risk of accidents.

To diagnose and treat heavy snoring, individuals might need to visit a sleep laboratory where interventions like sleep respiratory pumps can be prescribed.

Acidity, Belching, Intestinal Gas, Hiccups, and Frequent Sneezing – Many individuals experience excessive belching, hiccups, and persistent sneezing. These issues can arise from various factors, including stress, spicy food, overconsumption of food or alcohol, improper chewing, gulping food, smoking, chewing tobacco, and certain food allergies.

Simple remedies, such as antacid medications and peppermint oils like *Pudinhara* and *Amritdhara*, can help alleviate symptoms. Avoiding food for short periods can also assist in recovery. Persistent sneezing and hiccups might be due to allergies. Inhaling fresh air or slowly sipping warm water can provide immediate relief from these symptoms. However, if these symptoms persist, anti - allergic medications are recommended. It is essential to consult with a medical professional before starting any treatment to ensure that it is appropriate for the specific condition.

Gastritis and Gastroenteritis – These conditions involve inflammation of the stomach lining (gastritis) or both the stomach and intestines (gastroenteritis). Gastroenteritis is often caused by viral, bacterial, or amoebic infections, which may be self - limiting or may require antimicrobials. Typical symptoms include acidity, abdominal pain, cramping, excess gas, diarrhea, and belching. Consuming bland foods and avoiding spicy and greasy dishes can help alleviate symptoms. When these symptoms persist, digestive enzymes and antacids might be recommended.

In cases of severe dehydration due to diarrhea, drinking a solution made from lemon, salt, sugar, or an **oral rehydration solution** is beneficial.

However, if the issue is not resolved, hospitalization might be necessary for administering intravenous fluids, electrolytes, glucose, and possibly antibiotics.

Upper Respiratory Tract Infection (URTI) – Infections of the upper respiratory tract manifest symptoms such as a sore throat, irritation, pain in the throat, hoarse voice, cough, cold, and sometimes fever, and are mostly caused by viruses. Conditions like SARS, COVID - 19, and influenza fall under this category.

Preventive measures include avoiding exposure to polluted air, refraining from smoking, keeping away from infected persons, gargling with lukewarm water, and practicing *Neti Kriya* (a nasal cleansing technique).

Drinking a decoction made from cloves, carom seeds, turmeric, black pepper, etc., may provide relief to some extent. However, if the infection progresses from the upper to lower respiratory tract, it can result in pneumonia, a more severe condition affecting the lungs.

Respiratory infections can spread through droplets or become airborne. The recent COVID - 19 pandemic highlighted the importance of wearing masks and practicing social distancing to curb the spread of infection. Interestingly, fever can serve a protective function, potentially inhibiting microbial growth and strengthening the immune response.

Similarly, coughing is the body's way of expelling mucus and phlegm from the lungs and should ideally not be suppressed. Cough suppressants should be prescribed cautiously and only in cases of severe and exhausting cough. However, persistent or severe symptoms, particularly productive coughs, could signal more serious underlying conditions.

Home remedies like turmeric, ginger decoctions, black pepper, carom seeds (*ajwain*), and *Joshanda* can offer relief from minor upper respiratory infections. Over - the - counter products, including lozenges, peppermint balms, analgesics, antipyretics, antihistamines, cough syrups and nebulizing medications can also provide comfort.

Boils and Acne – Acne, commonly referred to as pimples, often appears on the face of teenagers due to hormonal changes during puberty.

Maintaining facial hygiene by washing regularly and refraining from frequently touching the face can help manage acne. Boils, on the other hand, arise from bacterial infections affecting the sweat and sebaceous (oil - producing) glands in the skin. Factors such as malnutrition and poor hygiene increase susceptibility to boils. While the body's natural defenses might clear such infections, maintaining cleanliness is crucial. Topical antiseptic or antibiotic ointments can provide relief when applied to pimples, boils, or other skin infections. Boils around the anal area can potentially develop into painful fistula - in - ano, (abnormal connections between the skin and the anal canal). Individuals with diabetes should seek medical attention promptly to treat skin infections, as they are more prone to complications. Skin lesions with severe itching and a ring - like appearance may indicate fungal infections such as **tinea or ringworm**. Various ointments are available to treat these conditions, but if they prove ineffective, consulting a physician becomes essential.

Hair Loss – Hair health often reflects the body's nutritional status. Lush, long hair in women can signify a well - nourished and healthy body.

Hair loss in women can result from deficiencies in protein, certain vitamins (like the Vitamin B complex, especially Biotin), and minerals. It might also indicate issues with mental health or the quality of sleep. Dandruff is another common cause of hair loss, and various anti - dandruff shampoos are available to address this issue.

Men can experience hair loss even in their prime, leading to **male pattern baldness**. Many over the counter products claim to combat hair loss, but their efficacy is often limited. Solutions like hair patches, wigs, and hair transplants are popular, although transplanted hair can sometimes fall out again. Medications like minoxidil and dutasteride are prescribed to address hair loss, with varying levels of success.

In conclusion, when home remedies or over - the - counter medications do not adequately address bodily ailments, it is vital to consult a qualified physician and heed their advice to ensure well - being. Maintaining health requires ongoing attention and regular learning.

Chapter 7

Select Your Doctor...and Hospital/Clinic

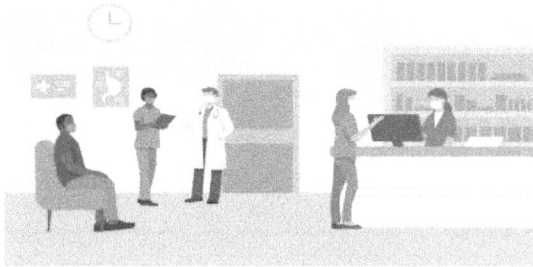

Learning Objectives:

- Recognizing a Good Doctor
- Making the doctor a well wisher
- Knowing about the functioning of a hospital or clinic
- Identifying hospitals and clinics dedicated for quality treatment with affordable and sustainable expenditure

---

In their search for a reputable doctor or hospital for themselves and their loved ones, people often rely on the spread of information about reputable medical practitioners and facilities. Recommendations for reliable doctors or specialists often come from family physicians, acquaintances, well - wishers, neighbors, and other trusted sources. In this digital age, many turn to websites, search engines, and specialized software to find medical professionals. It has become increasingly common to rely on online reviews when evaluating a doctor's expertise.

Additionally, seeking feedback from patients who've previously consulted the physician in question can be valuable. One can also scan newspapers and advertisements for information about healthcare professionals.

Who is a good doctor? Who would be efficient in addressing certain medical concerns? The professional qualifications and experience of a doctor are certainly important. While the methods and practices might vary, meeting a competent doctor is what every patient desires when distressed by some medical issue.

However, it is essential to be wary of quacks who may overstate their capabilities or of an overhyped doctor who engages in untrustworthy and unreliable practices for personal gain. Such quacks masquerading as specialists ultimately damage the cause of humanity. Only those qualified doctors survive and earn respect for those who are transparent and genuine, adhering to the ethics of medicine and human values.

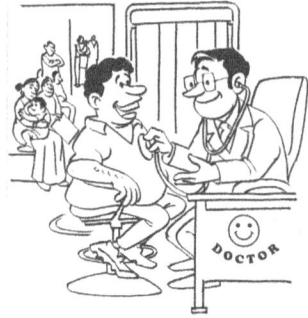

Qualities of a Good Doctor

1. **Effective Communication -** A good doctor is an attentive listener. Competent physicians listen actively to whatever the patient has to say, focusing on understanding the complaints and concerns of the patient to make a good and clear diagnosis. The skill of communication combined with clinical examination also provides effective care to the patient. A good doctor must be aware that their conduct, body language, and the way of examination is what the patients note and accordingly make up their minds about what to say and do in the clinic.

   Furthermore, a commendable doctor effectively communicates in straightforward terms, ensuring that the patient understands and assimilates the recommended treatment or care plan. The doctor's behavior and genuine concern are what the patients grasp at once. Only those patients value the doctor who shows concern for their distress and tries to provide algorithmic diagnostic work - up and effective treatments.

2. **Management Skill -** Maintaining a well - organized practice is what catches the attention of people. Dedication during patient check - ups and caregiving is appreciated by patients and their relatives and friends.

Trust is established when patients feel they have been genuinely listened to and understood. It is crucial for the doctor to prioritize the patient's best interests, ensuring no room for doubt about unnecessary expenses or procedures being incurred by the patient. Patients maintain peace and trust as won by the genuine concern of the doctor.

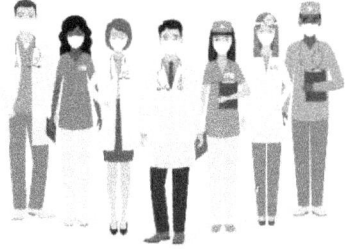

3. **Detective Skill -** An exemplary physician possesses an innate curiosity in ascertaining the disease and how much it is affecting the lifestyle of the patient. A good doctor recognizes that different diseases may present with overlapping symptoms such as fever, headache, sore throat, pain in limbs, and body aches, which may be indicative of common ailments like flu, malaria, typhoid, dengue, COVID - 19, etc.

   To get the right diagnosis the doctor should make an algorithmic diagnostic plan using clinical tools and workup, communicating with the patient about different diagnostic tests, and checking with other medical experts for their views. A good doctor discusses family values and social and economic concerns. Once the final diagnosis is made, the treatment should be initiated.

4. **Working as a Compassionate Guide** – A compassionate doctor not only diagnoses and treats but also guides their patients with optimism and expertise. They facilitate appropriate diagnostic testing and liaise with laboratories to ensure timely and accurate results. At times, they even personally consult with laboratory physicians to convey the finer details of a patient's condition, seeking greater precision in diagnostic tests.

   Unnecessary tests are avoided. The results of the tests are fully utilized to improve clinical decision - making and treatment. A good doctor seeks consultations from other experts when needed, without allowing ego to interfere, ensuring a comprehensive approach to patient management. They are vigilant about the overall well - being of the patient.

5. **Connecting with Patients and Caregivers** – While interacting with patients, skilled doctors strive to understand their socio - cultural background and values. Exceptional physicians are adept at communicating and connecting with patients and caregivers.

    They recognize the emotional turmoil caused by illness and offer advice to alleviate fears and uncertainties. This reflects the doctor's emotional intelligence. Ultimately, good doctors empower their patients and caregivers with knowledge, clarity, confidence, and trust.

6. **Clarity of Vision** – Outstanding and well - regarded physicians cultivate a nurturing environment, establishing a trusting rapport with patients, caregivers, and their medical staff. Their approach to patient management is characterized by kindness, compassion, and a genuine commitment to patient well - being.

7. **Respecting Cultural and Personal Values** – Doctors should recognize the significance of a patient's cultural, personal, and familial background. Their approach to treatment should be holistic, valuing and respecting the perspectives of caregivers and family members.

    Even if the doctor disagrees with a patient's previous treatment or a suggestion from a family member, they should address these differences with respect, not disdain. By bridging minor differences and understanding the patient's unique context, they ensure the highest level of care tailored to the individual's specific needs and values.

8. **Transmitting Education to the Patient** – An exceptional doctor believes in empowering patients and their families through knowledge.

    They take the time to clearly explain the complexities of the disease, ensuring that the patient and caregivers fully understand the situation.

    By addressing questions and outlining the advantages and drawbacks of each treatment option, they enable informed decision - making throughout the healthcare journey. They may also politely inform the patient that while doctors are busy, the family should reach out only when necessary. Providing such information upfront helps to prevent misunderstandings later.

In summary, obtaining a medical degree or excelling in a specific medical field is not what truly defines a doctor.

As we've reiterated, being a doctor means being human first - a caring individual who treats patients with the empathy of a close relative. Those who reach out to a doctor should receive some attention.

However, if a doctor encounters an overly emotional patient or a family that leans too heavily on them, they must diplomatically set boundaries without hurting feelings. At no point should there be negligence or lackluster care, even if the doctor hasn't exchanged pleasantries. A doctor should never be vindictive.

It is important to remember that doctors are not gods, nor should they be seen as such. They are human beings, carrying out a profession and providing a service, using their skills and knowledge to the best of their ability. Patients and their families should also do their part, approaching the doctor with respect and understanding.

Most people are good and recognize that a doctor may be busy or preoccupied. By maintaining a positive attitude and behaving well, families are more likely to receive the best possible attention from their doctor.

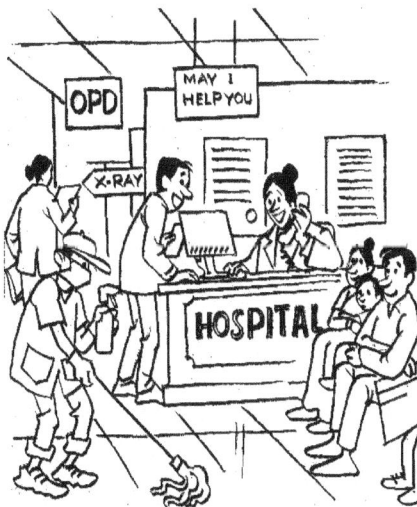

Choosing the right hospital or clinic - Diseases have existed since the dawn of human civilization, presenting a perennial challenge to all living beings. The emphasis on preventing and curing illnesses has grown significantly alongside the overall development of society.

The quality of a society's healthcare system is a crucial indicator of its development. Good healthcare is managed and safeguarded by quality hospitals.

Recognizing this, hospitals were established worldwide to cater to the treatment needs of both residents and visitors.

A top hospital is not defined solely by its grand architecture or luxurious amenities. Rather, it is recognized by its commitment to providing appropriate care to all, ensuring that everyone receives treatment with dignity, at an affordable cost, and without bias or prejudice. The true essence of a commendable hospital lies in its dedication to patient care, where compassion, human values, empathy, and a spirit of camaraderie prevail.

A hospital's merit is primarily assessed by the quality of treatment it offers. Key indicators of a reputable hospital include:

Skilled Leadership – The leader of a good hospital is deeply committed to ensuring the best possible care for all patients. Guided by principles of fairness and equity, the primary focus remains on patient care and well - being.

Clinical Administration and Reception – The administration and **reception** at a hospital or clinic play a pivotal role in shaping the patient's experience and, ultimately, their quality of life. This **frontline** service serves as a lens through which patients and their families perceive the overall quality and ethos of the healthcare establishment. The reception area often becomes the first touchpoint that sets the tone for the entire visit.

It is essential for reception staff to prioritize patients according to their needs. Acutely ill patients, those with pre - scheduled appointments, individuals needing only to share a report, busy professionals, someone needing to catch a train or flight, or a mother who has left a baby behind - all should be triaged with sensitivity and concern. Reception personnel must be adept at handling and managing complaints from disappointed patients and caregivers who feel they are not being attended to in the proper order. A sense of humor can be a valuable tool for breaking the ice and easing tension. The presence of senior consultants intermittently visiting the waiting area can have a significant impact. This personal touch, through casual interactions, brief conversations, and attentive listening, can greatly alleviate the anxieties of patients waiting to be seen. Simple gestures, such as offering tea, coffee, or biscuits, can also be helpful. Empathy demonstrated by reception staff can transform the patient's experience and shape their opinion of the hospital.

In this way, institutions like hospitals create a harmonious, patient - centric environment that fosters understanding and trust. Equally, patients must be aware of the multifaceted roles doctors play, juggling outpatient services, surgeries, administrative duties, teaching commitments, and more.

Coordination – Effective coordination is crucial for the seamless operation of a top - tier hospital. After a doctor sees a patient, subsequent steps - such as laboratory tests, dressings, injections, X - rays, payments, and more - must be managed efficiently to ensure optimal patient care. Patients, particularly those from villages or remote areas who may feel overwhelmed by large hospitals, can benefit greatly from a chaperone service.

Without skilled coordination, the hospital's operations can become disorganized, leading to confusion and inefficiencies. Synchronizing the various functions of different departments and ensuring swift patient care is the hallmark of a well - run hospital. Any disruptions or lapses in coordination can detract from the hospital's overall specialized care

Specialty Hospital/Laboratory – When laboratory and radiological tests are conducted outside the hospital or clinic, patients may incur additional expenses for travel and spend extra time on these tasks. It might be worthwhile for the hospital to facilitate travel and appointments for these outsourced tests. However, many modern specialized hospitals now offer comprehensive care, including necessary tests, all within the same premises.

In large hospitals, there may be queues for diagnostic tests and long waiting lists. To expedite clinical decision - making, certain tests can be conducted with the help of a technician directly in the outpatient clinic or the doctor's office - this is known as a **"point - of - care test."**

For example, conducting routine tests such as hemoglobin, blood sugar, or pregnancy testing in the antenatal clinic itself is an efficient method of care. Some standalone hospitals dedicated to dental or eye care exemplify this model by offering both diagnostic tests and treatments within the same facility. This integrated approach significantly streamlines patient care.

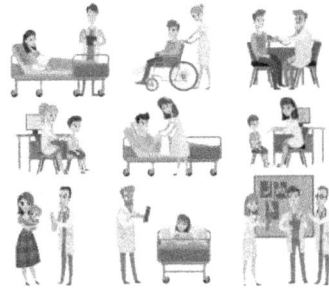

Hygiene & Cleanliness – A hospital's infrastructure should be well - lit and adequately ventilated, creating an environment conducive to healing. A reputable hospital is distinguished by its atmosphere of cleanliness, orderliness, and stringent hygiene standards. Poor cleanliness not only deters patients but can also compromise their health. Organized wards and outpatient departments, with operations running seamlessly, enhance patients' trust in the hospital's services. Adhering to high standards of hygiene is crucial in preventing hospital - acquired infections. All hospital staff, from ward assistants to janitors, should wear **clean uniforms** at all times. Patient amenities such as towels, pillows, and bed sheets should be consistently clean and free from stains, ensuring comfort and dignity for patients. A commendable hospital also ensures an efficient and leak - proof system for the disposal of medical waste. Moreover, the facility must be free from pests like cockroaches, rodents, and mosquitoes to guarantee the safety and well - being of both patients and staff.

Fast Test Technology – A distinguishing feature of a top - tier hospital is its ability to offer instant diagnostic results through advanced equipment and kits. These immediate tests, often referred to as card tests or dry tests, are performed under the direct supervision of specialist doctors. For example, on - the - spot tests like ECGs or Treadmill Tests (TMT) for heart diseases are conducted swiftly, enabling the healthcare team to initiate treatment without unnecessary delays. The availability of such rapid diagnostic tools ensures that patients receive prompt and effective care.

Economic Management – When a serious or acute illness strikes a family, concerns about medical expenses naturally arise. Hospitals invest significantly in high - end infrastructure, professionally trained staff, and timely bill disbursement to ensure that patients receive quality care and comfort. These investments are essential for maintaining the high standards of care provided. It is important for patients and their families to recognize that the systematic expenditure by hospitals is directly linked to the level of care and facilities they receive. Identifying a hospital or clinic with good infrastructure, skilled doctors, and moderate charges in a convenient location can help balance quality care with affordability.

Rate List Transparency – Occasionally, families of patients may express concerns about unexpectedly high hospital bills.

In rare instances, the hospital staff or doctors, being indifferent to the patient's financial situation, may present an inflated bill. To avoid such situations, it is essential for patients and their families to stay informed about billing practices and regularly review their bills during their hospital stay. A transparent breakdown of the hospital bill should be clearly displayed at the billing counter.

Understanding the billing system can help manage expenses more effectively:

Room/Accommodation Charges – Hospitals typically offer various ward categories, ranging from luxurious private wards (equivalent to five - star hotel services) to general wards. Patients can select a ward based on their budget, which significantly affects the overall bill.

Drugs & Disposables – Hospitals should charge patients fairly for medicines, intravenous fluids, syringes, catheters, and other disposables, ideally at or below the maximum retail price, with minimal wastage.

Equipment Usage/Rental Charges – Charges for the use of expensive medical equipment during tests and surgeries, such as laparoscopes or robotic systems, should be transparently included in the bill.

Consultation/Surgeon Fees – Fees for the consulting physician or surgeon may sometimes be adjusted or reduced at the discretion of the treating doctor.

Additional Services – Charges for additional services such as oxygen, nursing care, room heaters, air conditioners, and other amenities should be clearly itemized.

In cases of acute and critical illnesses, hospitals may levy extra charges due to the intensive care services required, which involve significant use of resources and disposables.

Good hospitals maintain transparency by charging patients based on actual expenses incurred. Ensuring that patients and their attendants are fully informed about the breakdown of their bills can help prevent complaints about high charges and promote trust in the healthcare facility.

Personnel – All hospital personnel, including doctors, nurses, ward boys, security staff, laboratory technicians, and clerical staff, should wear their identity cards clearly displaying their name and designation. They should maintain a polite and courteous demeanor, always ready to assist and be helpful.

Teamwork During the Treatment – Good hospitals are renowned in the community for their exemplary teamwork. The specialist doctors and medical staff are committed to providing the highest level of care to patients. Upon admission, the medical staff routinely record the patient's weight and vital signs (temperature, pulse, blood pressure, and respiratory rate). Prompt attention to tasks such as administering injections, intravenous drugs, dressings, wound care, and other critical activities like measuring blood sugar levels is a hallmark of a top hospital.

Priority of the Patient – At times, caregivers may express concerns if their loved ones are not seen by the doctor in the order of their registration. It is important for them to understand that medical professionals often need to prioritize patients based on the severity or urgency of their condition. There may also be other procedural, social, or professional considerations that necessitate out - of - sequence consultations. Doctors often multitask, balancing administrative duties, teaching responsibilities, diagnostic procedures, and direct patient care.

Responsiveness of Medical Staff – Doctors and medical staff should be attentive to patients' needs and concerns. It is essential to communicate clearly when certain requests cannot be fulfilled, explaining the reasons for the decision. The efficiency and promptness with which a doctor manages clinical assessments, testing, and treatment often earn quiet respect and appreciation from patients' families and the broader community. These positive experiences serve as implicit endorsements of the hospital's quality.

Patient Information –The hospital, along with its doctors, strives to keep patients well informed about their condition by educating them to understand the nature of their disease and guiding them to pursue treatment fully. The patient should be able to reach out to their doctors and other staff if necessary. Patients are gradually empowered to undertake long - term treatment for chronic illnesses, including managing sequelae and undergoing rehabilitation.

When disclosing bad news, such as a life - threatening illness like cancer or its sequelae, doctors follow a careful protocol to minimize undue distress and apprehension.

Infrastructural Facilities for Outdoor and Indoor Patients – A good hospital should be well - equipped with facilities that ensure patient comfort and convenience, such as a call bell system for quick internal communication to summon a nurse for administering intravenous infusions, attaching oxygen masks, conducting tests, etc. An efficient fleet of ward boys should be available to assist patients with personal needs, such as passing urine or attending to other calls of nature, ensuring that patients do not feel embarrassed if they become incontinent or soil the hospital bed and linen. Patients should also have access to outdoor areas like courtyards, gardens, and green spaces, with the option to go out in a wheelchair or walk, as appropriate. Additionally, a book trolley or library could enhance the patient's experience during their stay.

Ward Rounds – Ward rounds are conducted by doctors according to a set schedule. It is essential for patients to know both their primary (senior) and assisting (junior) doctors and to understand their respective schedules. During these rounds, doctors perform thorough examinations of the admitted patients almost daily, making crucial decisions about their treatment. To ensure effective and systematic care, patients and their families are encouraged to ask questions during these ward rounds and are advised to refrain from approaching doctors outside of these scheduled times.

Inventory of the Hospital – A good hospital maintains a systematic inventory for each department, ward, and area. Separate inventories are kept for capital equipment like tables and chairs, as well as consumables.

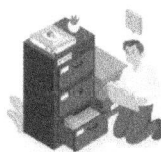

Efficient patient care requires that hospitals consistently stock medicines and essential consumables, such as pots, pans, and catheters. Timely and effective repairs of electrical appliances, medical equipment, and hospital furnishings like fans and air conditioners should be managed by an appropriate maintenance department.

Patient Database – A good hospital maintains a comprehensive database for both outpatient and inpatient records, including patient names, ages, genders, religions, addresses, disease histories, previous illnesses, medications, test reports, and old prescriptions related to the current condition. Specialist doctors rely on this information to provide informed and effective treatment. Nowadays, electronic medical records (EMR) are increasingly popular in the medical field. Patients at a good hospital or clinic can access their data, test reports, and treatment summaries online, including on their mobile devices, from anywhere in the world. Such facilities are expanding rapidly. The value of a hospital is often judged by these parameters, which are recognized worldwide. Recognizing this standard, the Government of India provides recognition to hospitals through the following process:

Recognition of Hospitals and Clinics in India – The National Accreditation Board for Hospital and Health Care Providers (NABH) was established by the Quality Council of India (QCI) in 2005 to accredit hospitals and healthcare providers. The QCI grants recognition to both government and private hospitals after a thorough **inspection** of their administrative procedures and patient care practices. These inspections are based on **600 parameters** set by the QCI, evaluating aspects such as patient registration, admissions, surgeries, and discharge processes. If a hospital fails to meet these standards or does not uphold patient rights and dignity, its accreditation can be revoked. NABH accreditation signifies that a hospital or clinic not only respects patient rights but also maintains the necessary infrastructure, clinical and diagnostic functionality, electronic medical records (preferred), and personnel standards essential for a clinical establishment.

In conclusion, hospitals have evolved alongside the concept of hospitality. While we may not fully understand how the idea of hospitality originated, our generations have long associated it with the act of welcoming and honoring guests in our homes. A hospital, then, is the primary institution where patients are cared for, medically educated, and rehabilitated when they find themselves suddenly deprived of their well - being. Unlike other institutions such as schools, colleges, universities, courts, or playgrounds - each with a specific mission and limitations - hospitals are uniquely imbued with the universal values of humanity.

Chapter 8

Getting the Best Treatment from Your Doctor

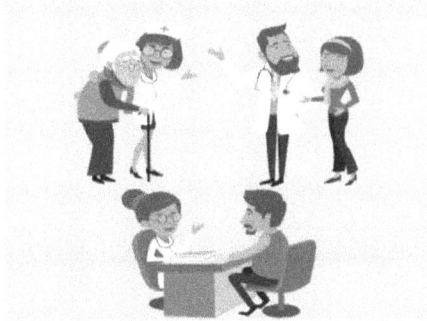

Learning Objectives:

- Replying to queries of the doctor appropriately

- Documenting the symptoms and effects of treatment in a diary, calendar, etc.

To get the best treatment and attention from your doctor, certain skills are necessary. The foremost is to be considerate of the doctor's time and practices before seeking medical advice. The benefits of treatment can be maximized if we are willing to adjust our behavior accordingly.

Here are some tips to help:

1. **Be concise when seeking an appointment**: When illness arises, your initial contact with the doctor should be brief and focused on scheduling an appointment.

2. **Respect the doctor's schedule**: Avoid entering the doctor's chamber unexpectedly; always be mindful of their predetermined schedule.

3. **Punctuality matters**: Strive to arrive at the medical center on time for your appointment.

4. **Follow clinic or hospital protocols**: Ensure your actions do not disturb other patients or medical staff. Adhering to the clinic's guidelines fosters a respectful environment.

5. **Maintain decorum**: Speak softly, minimize conversation, keep your phone silent, wait for your turn according to the appointment sequence, and only sit when invited by the doctor. These behaviors help create a conducive atmosphere for everyone.

6. **Bring the complete medical history**: Carry all relevant medical records, previous test reports, and current medications. Inform the doctor of any allergies to food or drugs. This allows the doctor to understand your past and concurrent illnesses and ensures thorough care.

7. **Present health records for chronic conditions**: If you have chronic conditions like diabetes or high blood pressure, provide a detailed record of your health metrics to the doctor.

8. **Communicate openly**: Answer the doctor's questions honestly and seek clarification on any doubts. Effective communication is key to receiving quality care.

9. **Track your health records**: Keep your health records in a diary or other medium to provide the doctor with necessary information promptly, aiding in appropriate judgment about your treatment progress.

10. **Be transparent about your lifestyle**: Disclose any habits, addictions, or other lifestyle choices. Concealing health information can negatively impact your treatment.

11. **Pay attention during post - consultation**: Listen carefully to the doctor's summary of the diagnosis and treatment plan. Ask for clarification if needed. It's best for one family representative to pose questions, rather than multiple members at different times. In complex cases, doctors may call for family counseling before undertaking

complicated treatments like cancer therapy, transplants, or critical surgeries.

12. **Follow the doctor's advice diligently**: Adhere to the prescribed medication, diet, and any recommended exercises or therapy.

13. **Keep the doctor updated**: Inform the doctor of any changes or developments in your health status.

14. **Express genuine gratitude**: Appreciate the doctor's efforts and maintain a positive attitude. You don't need to say that the doctor is a God for you, but a simple thank you can go a long way.

15. **Ask about follow - up communication**: Inquire if you can consult the doctor via telephone, WhatsApp, email, or other methods for follow - up questions or advice.

We learn from home, school, and community - mostly how to read, write, and speak correctly and politely. These guidelines offer another valuable skill set to help you when seeking treatment from a doctor, whether for yourself or a loved one.

Chapter 9

Making A Diagnosis – History Taking, Communication, Patient Examination and Diagnostic Tests

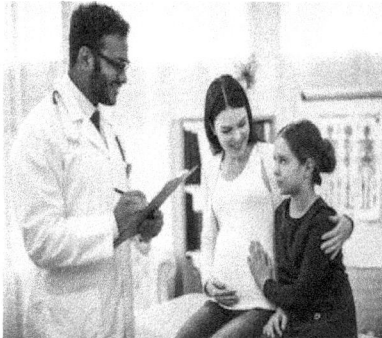

Learning Objectives:

- Understanding how a medical history, personal details and presenting complaints are elicited

- Understanding parts of clinical examination

- Varieties of tests recommended for ascertaining diseases

- Analysis of symptoms vis-a-vis test data and making diagnosis

---

Clinic Practice - A doctor's examination of a healthy person or an individual suffering from any disease is recognized as clinical practice. The doctor diagnoses the disease after gathering a full clinical history and conducting a thorough physical examination of the patient.

Typically, the doctor makes at least a provisional diagnosis or a set of differential or probable diagnoses based on the clinical history and physical examination. Sometimes, the doctor may begin **empirical treatment** even without a firm diagnosis.

Demographic Details of the Patient – The doctor generally asks the patient to provide details such as their name, age, birthplace, current residential address, information about children and family, hobbies, marital and sexual well - being, profession, social and economic status, and any addictions, such as tobacco, alcohol, cannabis, etc. This information complements the diagnostic process.

Presenting Complaints & History of Present Illness – The doctor records the physical and mental **problems causing distress** to the patient, listing the complaints that the patient is concerned about. For instance, a woman may have a lump in her breast but consult the doctor primarily about her acute cough and cold. Similarly, an elderly person suffering from both knee pain and blurry vision due to cataracts will address the knee pain with an orthopedic specialist and the vision issue with an ophthalmologist. The doctor approaches each illness based on the presenting complaint.

The doctor begins by asking **when the patient was last perfectly well** and what the first complaint was, and what other complaints arose in chronological order. The physician then delves deeper into each specific complaint. For example, if the complaint is a headache, the doctor will inquire about its duration, frequency, timing (morning, afternoon, or night), location (front, back, or side of the head), associated symptoms (nausea, intolerance to light and loud sounds), precipitating factors, and any family history of similar headaches. These questions help the physician form an initial impression of the headache's cause.

Similarly, if the complaint is abdominal pain, the doctor asks about the exact location, whether the pain is acute, recurrent, or chronic, its relation to meals, and any associated symptoms such as vomiting, diarrhea, or fever. The doctor may also inquire about related complaints, such as visual disturbances or vomiting, if the primary complaint is a headache. If the primary complaint is fever, the doctor will ask about the duration, pattern (continuous or intermittent), severity (low grade or high grade), and any associated symptoms like cough, sore throat, urinary issues, or jaundice. This process is known as **structured clinical history - taking**.

Medical students learn this structured approach to history - taking and the art of communication with patients presenting with various physical and mental illnesses throughout their studies.

History of Past Illness, Allergies, Other Co - morbidities, and Medications – The doctor may inquire about any significant or major illnesses in the past, including hospitalizations, surgeries, or injuries, even if they are unrelated to the present illness. The doctor will also ask about any known allergies and whether the patient suffers from chronic conditions such as thyroid disorders, rheumatism, cardiovascular disease, diabetes, or high blood pressure.

Such patients often require long - term medication, and it is crucial for the current doctor to be aware of all medications being taken, as they may interact with new prescriptions.

Family History – Some diseases tend to run in families. For instance, if parents have diabetes, there is a higher likelihood of it being passed on to their children. The doctor will document any symptoms of genetic or familial diseases in the patient's record. Additionally, some infectious diseases, like tuberculosis, can be transmitted among family members.

Clinical Examination – Before commencing a formal physical examination, the doctor consciously notes the patient's demeanor, build, behavior, and any obvious signs like skin rashes.

The examination is divided into two parts:

1. General Physical Examination: This involves assessing general findings such as the patient's weight, **vital signs** (pulse, blood pressure, temperature, and respiratory rate), and looking for signs of pallor, jaundice (yellow discoloration of the skin), cyanosis (bluish discoloration), or any swelling. Signs of dehydration are also assessed. Often, a 'head - to - toe' examination is conducted to ensure no findings are overlooked.

2. Systemic Examination: This involves examining different systems of the body - respiratory, cardiovascular, abdominal, nervous, and musculoskeletal (bones and joints). The physician uses various instruments during this examination, including a stethoscope, blood pressure instrument, tongue depressor, hammer, and ophthalmoscope.

When examining specific areas like the abdomen, breasts, or any mass, the doctor typically follows four steps:

1. **Inspection**: The doctor visually examines the area for any changes in the overlying skin, scars, or other abnormalities.

2. **Palpation**: The doctor touches and presses the area, starting with a superficial palpation and then moving to a deeper one. They assess for **tenderness (pain on palpation)**, the size, shape, and consistency of any mass, and whether it moves with respiration (breathing). These findings help identify the organ from which the mass may be arising.

3. **Percussion**: This technique involves tapping a finger of one hand over the other to detect underlying fluid, air, or solid structures.

4. **Auscultation**: The doctor uses a stethoscope to listen for underlying abnormalities in the heart, lungs, or arteries. Variations in the quality of sound detected during auscultation are analyzed to diagnose potential issues.

Office Tests or Point of Care Tests – Measurements of a patient, including **anthropometry** (height, weight, and measurements of the abdomen and hips), may be recorded by the doctor or a trained assistant using small equipment typically kept in the doctor's office. Depending on their specialization, the doctor may have **clinical diagnostic equipment** for point - of - care tests, such as ECG, treadmill tests, ultrasound, ophthalmoscope and endoscopes for inspecting the ear, nose, throat, stomach, large intestine, etc. The availability of point - of - care tests in various hospitals minimizes the need for patients to visit separate facilities, allowing for on - the - spot testing. This enables immediate diagnosis and treatment of common diseases.

Process of Making a Diagnosis – The diagnostic process is often **iterative**, involving repeated history - taking, examinations, and tests. A definitive diagnosis may not always be possible initially, but treatment can still be started **empirically** based on a provisional diagnosis.

After gathering a patient's history and conducting a clinical examination, the doctor typically forms a **provisional diagnosis**, sometimes accompanied by a list of **differential diagnoses**. The doctor then analyzes these potential diagnoses by weighing 'points in favor' and 'points against' each one.

To confirm the provisional diagnosis and progress along the diagnostic pathway, the doctor plans specific diagnostic tests or investigations. These tests may be conducted simultaneously (in parallel) or sequentially (in series), depending on the likelihood of each diagnosis, the cost, and the invasiveness of the test.

Tests can be of several types:

1. Blood Tests – There are numerous tests performed on blood or serum (the liquid part of blood without cells). These include measuring hemoglobin levels, counts of white blood cells and platelets, as well as a wide range of biochemical values like sugar, cholesterol, urea, bilirubin, antibodies for infectious diseases, and tests for thyroid disorders, diabetes, kidney and liver function, and serum electrolytes. The results of many of these blood tests normally vary from time to time and day to day. Several tumor markers, which help in the detection and monitoring of cancers, can also be identified in blood tests.

2. Other Body Fluids – Fluids like urine, pleural fluid, peritoneal fluid, and cerebrospinal fluid are examined to determine the number and type of cells, protein levels, sugar content, chemical composition, and for bacterial culture (growing bacteria on special media). These tests help in diagnosing specific problems.

3. Cytology & Histology – In **Fine Needle Aspiration Cytology** (FNAC), a needle is inserted into tissue or a fluid pocket, and suction is applied to withdraw or aspirate cells from the solid tissue (e.g., lymph nodes) or fluid from the site. These cells are then examined under a microscope to make a diagnosis. A **biopsy** involves removing a small part of the tissue from an organ or lump. The tissue is cut into sections, fixed in paraffin wax, and thin slices are prepared. These slices are then de - waxed, stained, and examined under a microscope - a process known as **histopathology**. **Immunocytochemistry** is a more complex process where the cells or tissues are colored using biological dyes and stains to identify specific components. With advancements in modern medical science, a wide array of tests may be recommended to make an accurate diagnosis

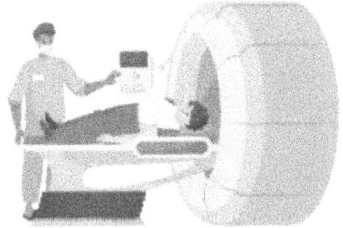

4. Body Organ Imaging – Imaging internal organs is essential for understanding pathology. This is done using X - rays, Computed Tomography (CT scan), Ultrasound, or Magnetic Resonance Imaging (MRI). These techniques produce images of diseases like tuberculosis, liver cancer, gallbladder issues, kidney stones, etc., which can be displayed on screens or printed.

The images created through these methods are digital and consist of pixel images rather than real - time visuals. Specific findings, such as the presence diagnosis of air, tumors, or stones, give characteristic appearances that skilled radiologists can recognize. However, during imaging, certain artifacts - caused by the refraction of rays - may appear as lesions, potentially causing unnecessary concern. It is the radiologist's expertise that allows for the accurate interpretation of these images, distinguishing true pathology from artifacts.

Doctors may advise a range of laboratory tests to reach an accurate diagnosis. After a thorough history and clinical examination, these tests are often performed in a serial - parallel manner. The results of the initial set of tests are reviewed, and if needed, a second series of tests is conducted in parallel. A proficient and skilled doctor aims to provide appropriate treatment with the minimum necessary tests.

In conclusion, this process highlights how doctors function and approach patient problems. The skill of making a diagnosis is painstakingly taught to medical students by their mentors, and doctors often recall anecdotes about their teachers and seniors who excelled in this art. Successfully diagnosing a difficult case brings a profound sense of satisfaction to a doctor.

Often, when a diagnosis is not definitive, the doctor must weigh all options and proceed pragmatically, aiming to start empirical treatment to alleviate the patient's suffering. Diagnosis is the cornerstone that builds the patient's confidence in the doctor. History taking, patient communication, and thorough examination are the primary skills that establish the physician's reliability in the patient's eyes, leading to admiration and trust in the doctor and their team.

Chapter 10

AYUSH – Ayurveda, Yog & Naturopathy, Unani, Siddha, Homeopathy and Other Medical Systems

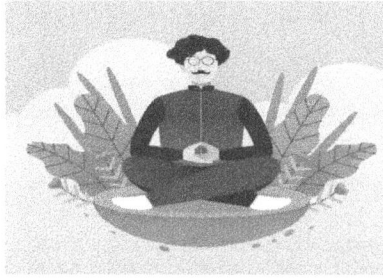

Learning Objectives:

Understanding alternative and complementary systems of medicine

- *Ayurveda* – significance of 4 elements – *dosha, dhatu, mal* and *agni*; balancing the *tri-doshas* (*vata, pitta, kapha*) treating through 8 devices; **Surgery** in ancient India, **Yog** – significance of 8 branches of Ayurveda in curing diseases and restoring health

- **Unani (Islamic) medicine** – the concepts of 7 physiological principles viz; *akran, mizaz, akhlat, aza, arwah, quwa, afaal* and their balance

- **Homeopathic medicine** developed in Germany by Dr. Hahnemann mainly dispensing minimum doses of harmless medicine based on detailed inquiry and symptomatology

---

India has preserved its age - old practice of traditional systems of medicine in the form of *Ayurveda*, *Siddha*, and *Yoga*. Many people in Bharat believe in the efficacy of traditional medicine and continue to practice it.

Naturopathy, also an ancient traditional medicine of this land, nearly died out during the British Raj. However, a blend of Indian and European Naturopathy prevails in government hospitals in India. Similarly, Unani medicine, rooted in Islamic tradition, has its origins in Arab countries, while Homeopathy, a European medicine, has its roots in Germany.

The United Nations, in Article 24, declared that "indigenous peoples have the right to their traditional medicines and maintain their health practices."

In response, the Indian government initiated and promoted *"AYUSH,"* creating a separate Ministry in the Central Government, as well as hospitals and medical colleges dedicated to *AYUSH* practices. The acronym *AYUSH* includes *Ayurveda, Yoga* & *Naturopathy, Unani, Siddha,* and Homeopathy.

Although Homeopathy was not traditionally indigenous to Bharat, a large number of Indians have embraced this form of medicine.

Ancient Indian Medical Systems

Ayurveda Chikitsa **(आयुर्वेद चिकित्सा)** – The term *"Ayurveda"* originates from the Sanskrit words *'ayus'* (आयुस), meaning 'life' or 'longevity,' and *'veda' (वेद)*, meaning 'knowledge.' Thus, etymologically, *Ayurveda* means the 'science of life and longevity.' This ancient system of medicine was developed in the Indian subcontinent over 6,000 years ago and provides a holistic approach to health, emphasizing prevention, wellness, and longevity.

The source of ancient Indian wisdom lies in the foundational texts known as the four *Vedas: Rigveda, Yajurveda, Samaveda, and Atharvaveda* (ऋग्वेद, यजुर्वेद, सामवेद व अथर्ववेद). Composed between 4000 - 6000 BC by Rishi Vyas, these scriptures encapsulate the principles of what is now known as *Sanatan Dharma.* Among these, the *Rigveda* preserves some knowledge of *Ayurveda,* while the *Atharvaveda* is particularly dedicated to the medical systems of that era.

Ashwani Kumar is considered the pioneer of *Ayurveda,* passing down his knowledge to deities and sages like *Indra, Dhanwantri, Nakul, Sehdev, Chyavan, Sushrut, and Charak* (इन्द्र, धन्वंतरी, नकुल, सहदेव, च्यवन, सुश्रुत व चरक), who then propagated and practiced this ancient science.

Four Basic Elements of *Ayurveda*

According to *Ayurveda*, the human body is composed of four fundamental elements (मूल तत्त्व): *dosha, dhatu, mal, and Agni.*

1. **Dosha (दोष)** – *Ayurveda* identifies three primary *doshas: vata, pitta, and kapha.* When these doshas are in balance, termed *"Sam Dosha"* (सम दोष), the body is in a state of complete health.

   An imbalance, or *"Visham Dosha"* (विषम दोष), results in disease. These doshas are not merely body fluids but are vital energies that govern biological activities from which the tissues are formed.

2. **Dhatu (धातु)** – *Ayurveda* describes seven *dhatus* or tissue systems within the body. These are:

   - **Rasa (रस)** – Plasma
   - **Rakta (रक्त)** – Blood
   - **Mamsa (मांस)** – Muscle
   - **Meda (मेद)** – Fat
   - **Asthi (अस्थि)** – Bone
   - **Majja (मज्जा)** – Bone marrow
   - **Shukra (शुक्र)** – Semen or reproductive tissue

3. **Mal (मल)** – These are the body's waste products, which need to be efficiently expelled to maintain health. They include:

   - **Mala (मल)** – Stool
   - **Mutra (मूत्र)** – Urine
   - **Sweda (स्वेद)** – Sweat

Two aspects of waste are recognized: **Mal** is the waste of the body, and **Kitta (कित्त)** is the waste of the seven tissue systems of the body.

4. **Agni (अग्नि)** – Representing the metabolic and digestive fire within the body, Agni governs the process of breaking down ingested food and transforming it into energy. A balanced Agni is crucial for maintaining the body's overall health and vitality.

The presence of organic fire (जैविक अग्नि) is felt in the esophagus, liver, and tissue cells in the form of enzymes.

Thus, health in *Ayurveda* is defined by the equilibrium of these four elements: *dosha, dhatu, mal,* and *Agni.* Conversely, any imbalance among these elements results in illness.

Principle of Dosha in *Ayurveda*

1. *Vata Dosha* (वात दोष):

Residency: Vata resides in empty spaces within the body, such as the stomach, navel, back, thighs, feet, bones, intestines, and colon.

Functions: *Vata* facilitates the circulation of blood, acts as the medium for organ interconnection, and aids in the processing of the seven tissue systems. It is responsible for transferring one *dosha* to another place and for the excretion of stool and other waste. The over - presence of *Vata* is known as *Vata Prakriti* (वात प्रकृति), which refers to the characteristic nature of Vata.

2. *Pitta Dosha* (पित्त दोष):

Residency: *Pitta* resides in locations such as the stomach, small intestine, chest, navel, sweat, lymph, blood, digestive system, and urinary bladder.

Functions: *Pitta,* which is a combination of organic fire and water, controls the functions of hormones and enzymes and plays a role in forming blood, bone, marrow, and waste. It is manifested in wit, courage, and pleasure. The over - presence of *Pitta* is known as *Pitta Prakriti* (पित्त प्रकृति).

It is also known as *Pachak Agni* (पाचक अग्नि - digestive fire). A deficiency in *Pitta* results in weak digestion.

3. *Kapha Dosha* (कफ दोष):

Residency: *Kapha,* which is associated with earth and water elements, maintains stability and structure in the body.

Functions: A deficiency in *Kapha* leads to the accumulation of *Vata* and *Pitta,* which can cause diseases.

Pitta is associated with metabolism (*Chayapachaya* - चयापचय), *Kapha* with anabolism (*Upachaya* - उपचय), and *Vata* with catabolism (*Apachaya* - अपचय). Childhood is characterized by the over - presence of *Kapha*, which governs growth (anabolism). The young stage is dominated by *Pitta*, which controls metabolism. In old age, *Vata* predominates, leading to catabolism. In *Ayurveda*, health is maintained by the balance of the three *doshas* (*Tridosha*) within the body, which aligns with the balance of nature. Diseases are believed to be caused by disruptions in this balance. Factors such as mindless eating, illness - breeding behaviors, neglecting healthy practices, environmental or climatic changes, and non - pragmatic physical activities can lead to illness.

Ashtang Vaidyak (अष्टांग वैद्यक) - *Ayurveda's* Eight Branches

Ayurveda medicine, known as *Ashtang Vaidyak*, is organized into eight specialized branches or *Asht Tantra*, detailed as follows:

1. *Kayachikitsa* (कायचिकित्सा): This branch of *Ayurveda* focuses on **general medicine**, dealing with conditions like fever, ulcers, epilepsy, leprosy, dysentery, and diarrhea. It primarily uses medicinal therapies to treat these ailments.

2. *Shalyatantra* (शल्यतंत्र): Shalyatantra is the branch of **surgery** in *Ayurveda*. It involves the surgical treatment of conditions such as ulcers, piles, and fistulas using tools like razors, knives, and cauterization equipment. The *Kshar Sutra* technique, described in *Ayurveda*, is also employed by modern medical practitioners.

3. *Shalakyatantra* (शालक्यतंत्र): This tantra specializes in the treatment of diseases and conditions of the mouth.

4. *Kaumarabhritya* (कौमार्यभृत्य): This branch focuses on **pediatric and obstetric care**, addressing the health needs of children, pregnant women, and issues related to childbirth and abortion.

5. *Agadtantra* (अगदतंत्र): Agadtantra deals with the treatment of various types of **poisoning**. It uses antidotes to counteract conditions such as food poisoning, snake bites, insect stings, and more. In this context, *"Gada"* means disease, and *"Agada"* refers to agents that rid the body of these diseases.

6. ***Bhootvidya* (भूतविद्या)**: *Bhootvidya* addresses mental disorders and conditions believed to be caused by afflictions from evil spirits. This branch of *Ayurveda* treats psychiatric problems attributed to the curse of deities (देव), demons (दानव), ancestors (पित्र), celestial beings (गंधर्व), spirits (प्रेत), serpents (सर्प), etc.

7. ***Rasayantantra* (रसायनतंत्र)**: Rasayantantra focuses on geriatrics, using chemical medicines to treat diseases related to aging.

8. ***Vajikaran* (वाजीकरण)**: *Vajikaran* emphasizes reproductive health, treating conditions such as ***alpa - shukra*** (अल्पशुक्र) or ***kshina - shukra*** (क्षीणशुक्र), which refer to issues with sperm quality. This tantra aims to improve the quality of sperm and ovum to ensure healthy progeny.

In these eight branches, *Ayurveda* offers comprehensive care, addressing both physical and mental well - being across various stages and conditions of life.

Therapy and Treatment in Ayurveda

Diagnosis in *Ayurveda* involves a comprehensive assessment using multiple methods: pulse examination, urine and stool analysis, tongue observation, visual inspection of the eyes, palpation, and auscultation. Based on the diagnosis, treatment is prescribed under one of the eight *tantras*. *Ayurvedic* remedies predominantly derive from plants and herbs, emphasizing a holistic approach to health.

Ayurveda doesn't just focus on medication but also emphasizes the importance of a balanced diet, moderation in behavior, and abstinence. Medicines and surgical interventions are employed to restore balance in the *tridosha*, facilitating the elimination of accumulated waste and toxins through processes like vomiting or excretion. Laxatives are prescribed to relieve constipation, while specific treatments are provided to stimulate appetite and enhance digestion. Nasal drops are used to relieve nasal congestion.

Ayurveda advocates **holistic** health practices. Light exercises, including *Pranayama* and Asanas, sunbathing, and exposure to fresh morning air, are recommended to boost immunity and overall well - being. Techniques like concentration exercises, meditation, and mental balance practices are advised for psychiatric and emotional challenges.

Recognizing the potential and heritage of *AYUSH*, particularly *Ayurveda*, and the Government of India has ardently promoted it. Several national institutions dedicated to traditional medicine have been established, such as the *Rashtriya Ayurveda Vidyapeetha* (राष्ट्रीय आयुर्वेद विद्यापीठ) in New Delhi, the *Rashtriya Ayurveda Sansthan* (राष्ट्रीय आयुर्वेद संस्थान) in Jaipur, and the *Ayurveda* Post - graduate Education and Research Institute in Jamnagar, Gujarat. Additionally, new All India Institutes of Medical Sciences (AIIMS) have been tasked with integrating *AYUSH* into their programs.

Many leading pharmaceutical companies are now focusing on preparing remedies from herbs, plants, and other natural sources. Some treatments, like **mint extract** for intestinal colic relief, have even been adopted by modern medicine. However, it is crucial to note that these herbal remedies are not always rigorously evaluated.

Yog - Pranayam Chikitsa

Pranayama is one of the eight limbs (*ashtanga*) of Yog. However, it is often mistakenly equated with Yog itself. Many people practicing *Pranayama* daily may claim they are practicing Yog, but these two terms are not synonymous. *Yog* is a comprehensive lifestyle science designed to build the capacity for achieving good health and overall well - being. *Pranayama* (प्रणायाम) is the fourth limb of *Yog* and focuses on respiratory exercises, or breath control, performed in various dimensions.

It is essential to understand that practicing *Pranayama* without knowledge of *Asanas* (physical postures) cannot provide the full benefits anticipated by Patanjali and the contemporary proponents of Yog. *Asana* (आसन) is the third limb of *Yog*, and *Asanas* and *Pranayama* are complementary to each other.

Yog, with its various limbs (*ang*), has been immensely popular in India since ancient times and is held in high esteem globally. This science is considered a panacea for several physical and mental illnesses. The life structure of *Bharatiya* (Indian) people has traditionally evolved around a balanced diet, physical exercises, abstinence, fasting, and meditation. The great sage *Patanjali* is credited with structuring the life of *Bharatvarsha* around the science called *Yog*.

Eight Limbs of Yog:

1. *Yam* (यम) – Emphasizes non - violence, truth, honesty, celibacy, and non - accumulation (abstinence).

2. *Niyam* (नियम) – Focuses on hygiene, contentment, perseverance, austerity, self - study, and concentration on God.

3. *Asana* (आसन) – Involves physical exercises performed in various postures.

4. *Pranayama* (प्रणायाम) – Centers on breath control, creating a balance in respiratory dimensions, and involves the gradual cessation of breathing, including the discontinuation of inhaling and exhaling.

5. *Pratyahar* (प्रत्याहार) – Refers to the withdrawal of sense and motor organs from worldly objects. Attachment to worldly objects is seen as an obstacle to achieving wellness through Yog.

6. *Dharana* (धारण) – Involves concentrating on non - worldly, sublime objects to maintain mental equilibrium, offering relief from agony and distress.

7. *Dhyan* (ध्यान) – Involves developing the flow of consciousness towards creativity.

8. *Samadhi* (समाधि) – The state of deep meditation where one immerses in a state of vacuum or nothingness.

By practicing Yog in all its eight components, it is believed that one achieves the circulation of oxygenated blood throughout the body, develops abstinence from sensual infatuation, and attains mental equilibrium and peace. This process strengthens immunity, wards off mental stress, and helps realize oneness with the Absolute Reality.

Thus, if *Asanas* (आसन) and *Pranayama* (प्रणायाम) are performed according to the principles of abstinence, the states of *Dhyan* (ध्यान) and *Samadhi* (समाधि) are spontaneously achieved.

While the detailed description of all *Asanas* is beyond the scope of this book, a few illustrations of some *Asanas* like *Siddhasana*, *Padmasana*, *Bhadrasana*, *Swastikasana*, and *Vishramkarak Asana* are provided below:

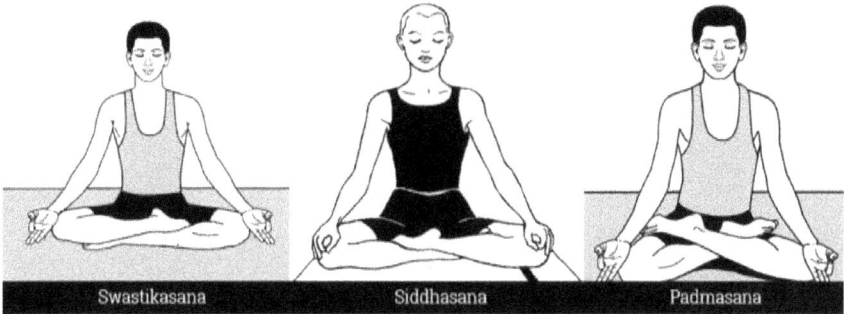

Swastikasana   Siddhasana   Padmasana

Mental stress can be restrained if the above *Asanas* are practiced with proper hygiene. To achieve true happiness, all eight limbs of *Yog* should be practiced regularly. The last three limbs - *Dharana*, *Dhyana*, and *Samadhi* - must be practiced with dedication and in solitude. Incorporating *Yog* into daily life requires training from a skilled preceptor and studying books on the subject. Deep breathing through the nose forms the foundation of Yog practice.

It is advised to wait 20 - 30 minutes after performing *Yog* before bathing or eating. Regular practice of *Yog* maintains and restores the health of the nervous, skeletal, respiratory, and cardiac systems. *Yog* also effectively treats lifestyle diseases such as obesity, high blood pressure, and diabetes, maintains breathing equilibrium, and addresses many women's health issues.

The definition of *Yog* can be understood through the following *Shlok* (श्लोक):

योगः चित्तवृत्तिनिरोधः, योगः समाधिश्च।

योग चित्त की वृत्ति का निरोध एवं योग समाधि है,

योग लय है सांसारिक व्यक्ति का पूर्ण चेतना अर्थात् परम सत्ता से।

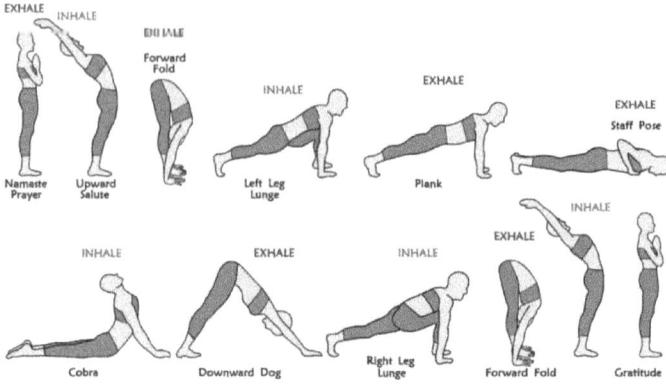

Illustration *Surya namaskar* poses

This verse elucidates that *Yog* is the cessation of mental fluctuations and the unification of the self with Absolute Consciousness, which is the Absolute Reality and Truth. Our sages have defined *Yog* in various ways, all aiming at the complete physical, mental, and spiritual wellness of human beings. Various schools of *Yog* in *Bharat* have developed since time immemorial. Some of these include *Laya Yog* (लय योग), *Hatha Yog* (हठ योग), *Karma Yog* (कर्म योग), *Bhakti Yog* (भक्ति योग), *Gyan Yog* (ज्ञान योग), and *Sankhya Yog* (सांख्य योग), among others. Those interested in detailed information about these different schools of *Yog* are encouraged to consult specific books dedicated to the various aspects of *Yog*.

Yog has been extensively studied in relation to various ailments, in collaboration between practitioners of modern medicine and those of traditional practices. **Numerous randomized clinical trials have been conducted, demonstrating the benefits of *Yog* and *Pranayama* as complementary therapy in conditions such as bronchial asthma, weak muscles, high blood pressure, anxiety, depression, paraplegia (neurological weakness of lower limbs), sleep disorders, and chronic respiratory disorders**, alongside the best supportive treatments.

Unani (Islamic) Medicine – Following the decline of medical knowledge in Greece and Rome, Islamic medicine began to develop in the Islamic countries of Middle and South Asia. This system, often ambiguously referred to as *Unani* medicine (*Unan* is a Greek word - *Yunan* in Hindi), actually evolved from the Arabic - Persian tradition.

In Islamic medicine, the human body is divided into seven components:

1. *Arkan* (अरकान) - Elements: The body is composed of four elements - air, earth, fire, and water.

2. *Mizaj* - (मिजाज) - Temperament: Refers to the mood or temperament of an individual.

3. *Akhlat* (अखलात) - Body Fluids: The body is thought to have four primary humors.

4. *Aza* (अजा) - Organs: These are the basis of health assessments.

5. *Arwah* (अरवाह) - Soul: This refers to the vital force animating various organs of the body.

6. *Quwa* (कुवा) - Strength: Includes *Quwa Tabiyah* (कुवा तबियाह) or natural strength, *Quwa Nafasniyah* (कुवा नफसियाह) or mental strength, and *Quwa Haiwaniyah* (कुवा हैवानियाह) or heart strength.

7. *Afal* (अफआल) - Function: Refers to the functions of the body's organs.

The balance of these components represents a state of health, while their imbalance or disequilibrium results in illness or disease.

The four types of *Akhlat* (अखलात), or humors, are described as follows:

Phlegm - Associated with laziness.

Blood - Linked to optimism.

Yellow bile - Causes irritation.

Black bile - Related to sadness.

The balance of these humours indicates good health, while their imbalance leads to illness or disease. The concept of *Quwwat - e - mudabbira - e - badan* (कुव्वत–ए–मुदब्बिरा–ए–बदन) represents good health. Treatment proceeds after the diagnosis of the disease, focusing on the following principles:

Izalae sabab (इजाल–ए–सबब) - Prevention of the cause of disease.

Tadeele akhlat (तदील–ए–अखलात) - Standardization or balance of the humors.

Tadeele aza (तदील–ए–अजा) - Restoring the normal functioning of tissues and organs.

Illaj bil tadbir (इलाज . बिल . तदबीर) - This refers to regimental therapy, such as cupping therapy, where the toxins of the body are excreted. Treatment is administered using various methods, including perfumes made from plants, bloodletting, Islamic or Turkish baths, and *dalak* (दलक) massage. Diagnosis is made based on the symptoms and mood swings of the patient. To strengthen the patient's immunity, treatment is prescribed through four modalities:

Ilaj - bil - gija (इलाज–बिल–गिजा) - Food moderation and abstinence.

Ilaj - bil - dawa (इलाज–बिल–दवा) - Treatment through medicines.

Ilaj - bil - yad (इलाज–बिल–यद) - Surgical treatment of diseases.

Ilaj - bil - tadbir (इलाज–बिल–तदबीर) - Regimental therapy.

The holistic treatment of disease in this system is referred to as *Tibb* (तिब). For example, the treatment approach is based on *Asbab - e - satta - zaruriya* (असबाब–ए–सत्ता–जरूरिया) – treatment is administered through six modalities:

Hawa - e - muhit (हवा–ए–मुहित) - Taking in fresh air.

Makool - wa - mashroob (माकूल–व–मशरूब) - Consuming food and drink.

Harkat - wa - sukoon - e - jismani
(हरकत–वा–सुकून–ए–जिस्मानी) - Physical activity and rest.

Harkat - wa - sukoon - e - nafsani
(हरकत–वा–सुकून–ए–नफसानी) - Psychological treatment.

Naum - wa - yaqzah (नौम–वा–यक्जा) - Sleep and wakefulness.

Istifragh - wa - initibas (इस्तिफरा–वा–इनीतिबास) - Excreting waste and toxins from the body.

Siddha Chikitsa – This traditional system of medicine was developed by

Agastya Muni in the Tamil language in the land of Tamil Nadu, approximately dating back to the 10th century BC. This medical system was further refined by the *9 Naths* (नाथ) and *84 Siddhas* (सिद्ध) of northern India and the 18 *Siddhas* of southern India, who received their knowledge from *Lord Shiva* (शिव) and *Parvati* (पार्वती). The *Siddha* school of medicine believes that the human body is a replica of the universe ("As is the microcosm, so is the macrocosm"). For example, the universe, its food, and medicine all evolve from the five elements: earth, water, fire, air, and sky (vacuum). Diseases are cured by medicines made from ingredients extracted from these elements in appropriate ratios.

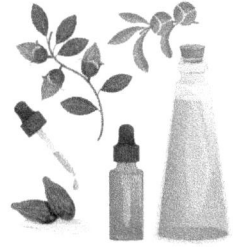

The human body, according to *Siddha* medicine, is composed of the following:

Plasma (सरम) - The basic element from which the body is created.

Blood (चेन्नीर) - The element that nourishes the entire body.

Muscle (ऊन) - The basic element that forms the shape of the body.

Tissue (कोलजुप्पू) - The element that facilitates joint function through lubrication.

Bone (एम्बू) - The basic element that maintains the posture of the body.

Veins (मुलई) - The element that connects the various organs of the body.

Semen (सुकिला) - The element responsible for reproduction.

Diagnosis by Testing – In *Siddha* medicine, the diagnosis of the disease is made based on various diagnostic methods, including the examination of the pulse (नाडी), urine (नीर), stool (मलन), tongue (ना), eyes (कण), touch (तोडल), color (वर्णम), as well as auscultation and palpation (कुरल). Treatment is then undertaken based on the diagnosis.

Pharmacology – *Siddha* doctors were skilled alchemists and poly - pharmacists. They employed various processes such as calcination, sublimation, distillation, fusion, fermentation, boiling, dissolving, precipitation, concentration, and coagulation to prepare medicines. These processes involved burning or smoldering metals, liquefying metals, and refining gold.

They also prepared medicines by fixing sulfur, vermilion, and arsenic. In the realm of chemical medicine, they utilized compounds known as *Uppu* (उप्पू), which included water - soluble inorganic salts.

Additionally, they prepared medicines from the vapors of gold, silver, copper, tin, lead, iron, and insoluble chemicals like sulfur.

Thus, *Siddha* practitioners created a wide range of organic, inorganic, and herbal medicines.

Treatment Process in Siddha – The *Siddha* system believes that the body's state adapts to changes in diet and physical activity, and that disease is caused by stress within the body. For example, the imbalance between the ratios of *Vatam*, *Pitam*, and *Kapham* (वातम:पित्म:कफम) can lead to disease.

They treated diseases with medicines prepared through three main approaches:

1. *Dev Maruthavam* (देव मुरूथुवम) – Medicines prepared from metals and minerals.

2. *Manida Maruthavam* (मनिदा मुरूथुवम) – Medicines prepared from herbs.

3. *Asur Maruthavam* (असुर मुरूथुवम) – Surgical procedures using indigenous methods like bloodletting and incision.

Siddha practitioners treat a variety of diseases, including psoriasis, genital and reproductive diseases, urinary tract infections, menstrual disorders, gastrointestinal and liver diseases, anemia during and after pregnancy, diarrhea, arthritis, and allergies. The *Siddha* system emphasized the systematic treatment of diseases through the principles of *Pathiyam* (पथ्यिम) and *Apathiyam* (अपथ्यिम) – determining what to eat and what to avoid.

Additionally, practices such as *Pranayama*, *Asanas*, and *Yoga* were taught in *Siddha* medicine to help maintain a disease - free body.

Homeopathy – Friedrich Samuel Hahnemann of Germany (1755– 1843 AD, MD Allopath) is credited with the development of homeopathy.

The central principles of homeopathy include:

"Like Cures Like" – The concept that if a substance causes certain symptoms, it can also help to remove those symptoms. A diluted dose of any medicine in homeopathy is believed to stimulate the body's immune system and vital force, thus aiding in the cure of many acute or chronic diseases.

Dilution and Succussion – A second key principle involves the process of dilution and shaking, known as succussion. Solid substances are prepared through trituration and liquid substances are potentiated through succussion, which is believed to increase the medicine's effectiveness.

Single Medicine – Homeopathy often relies on a single medicine to cure a range of diseases, tailoring the treatment specifically to the individual's symptoms.

Individualization and Holistic Treatment – Treatment in homeopathy addresses the patient's physical, mental, and emotional states. For instance, different homeopathic medicines might be used to treat different symptoms of asthma in various patients.

Miasm (Genesis of Diseases) – Hahnemann proposed that diseases are caused by miasms, which are polluted air, vapors, and decaying organic matter. These miasms are thought to be the cause of many diseases like cholera, black fever, malaria, plague, and various epidemics. Miasms are also associated with conditions such as psoriasis (itchy patches on the skin), scabies (a contagious skin disease), sycosis (a viral infection on the scalp), and syphilis (an infection resulting from unsafe sex).

Drug Proving in Homeopathy – The potency of homeopathic medicine is determined on the scale of decimal, centesimal, and 50 millesimal potencies. Homeopathic medicines are prepared in forms such as tincture, trituration, and dilution. Some tinctures are extracted from snake venom or from the liquid material of plants and herbs, which are then mixed with an appropriate quantity of ether or glycerin. Additionally, homeopathic medicines are made from the trituration or dilution of substances like sulfur, mercury, arsenic, zinc, tin, gold, silver, and phosphorus. However, an analysis of 110 homeopathy trials and 110 matched conventional - medicine trials published in "The Lancet" in 2005 concluded that "**the clinical effects of homeopathy were due to a placebo effect."**

According to the study, homeopathic treatments were no more effective than dummy pills, whereas modern medicines were shown to be effective. Despite this, the debate between modern medicine and homeopathy continues, especially in India, which is one of the world's largest markets for homeopathy. India boasts 51 homeopathic universities, 195 homeopathic medical colleges, and 27 state councils, which train thousands of homeopaths each year.

Other Medical Systems of the World

Chinese Medicine – Ancient Chinese medicine, which dates back to around 2700 BC, is rooted in the belief that Yang (the male principle) and Yin (the female principle) are the two fundamental forces governing health and disease. The balance or imbalance of these forces determines the state of health or illness. Chinese medicine emphasizes strengthening the body's immunity to maintain good health. For instance, the prevention of smallpox was attempted through variolation, a method where a small quantity of liquid from an infected individual was inoculated into a healthy person by scratching the skin.

The traditional medical system of China is documented in two significant texts: the *Compendium of Materia Medica* and *Huangdi Neijing*. These books explore various therapies, including medicines made from plants, roots, herbs, minerals, and more. Common therapies in Chinese medicine include acupuncture, cupping therapy, *gua sha*, acupuncture - moxibustion (where a needle prick is treated by burning), *tuina* (a type of massage), and *die - da* (bone - setting practices).

Mesopotamian Medicine – This medical system developed in the region near the Persian Gulf, encompassing ancient civilizations such as Sumeria, Babylonia, and Assyria, approximately 6000 years ago. The medicines in this region were derived from plants, roots, and herbs. Treatments often involved the chanting of mantras to invoke supernatural forces believed to heal the patient. Surgical practices were also employed.

Additionally, Mesopotamian medicine involved various ritualistic practices such as necromancy (contacting the dead), geomancy (interpreting earth's patterns, such as blowing mud from the palm or fist into the air), and animal sacrifice to invoke divine powers. Dreams and spirits were interpreted as omens, guiding the treatment process based on these interpretations. The *Code of Hammurabi*, an ancient legal text, prescribed rigorous physical and mental punishments for inappropriate or misleading treatments.

Injuries were treated by cleaning and dressing wounds with antiseptic substances like alcohol, honey, and myrrh. Handwashing with beer and lukewarm water was a common practice to prevent infections. Dental diseases were treated with herbal remedies or by extraction.

Egyptian Medicine – The Egyptian system of medicine, which existed around 525 BC, is renowned for its non - invasive surgical techniques, bone healing, dental medicine, and pharmacopeia. Egyptian doctors were particularly skilled in the preservation of dead bodies through mummification, demonstrating their advanced knowledge of internal organ cavities. They were adept at extracting internal organs through incisions in the back or, in the case of the brain, through the nostrils and the thin bones of the skull. Although they understood the arterial (vascular) and cardiac (heart) systems, they did not have a complete knowledge of blood circulation. Instead, they believed in bodily channels through which wind, water, and blood circulated, with disease resulting from blockages in these channels. Laxatives like *Julab* (tqykc) were used to treat such conditions.

During surgeries, Egyptian physicians employed instruments like knives, drills, tongs, scissors, blades, and saws. These tools facilitated procedures such as male circumcision and other types of surgeries. Prosthetics were also developed to replace limbs, toes, and even eyeballs. Medicines were prepared from turpentine oil, tannic acid, minerals, and herbs, proving effective in treating various ailments such as intestinal worms, eye diseases, diabetes, arthritis, polio, brain strokes, and paralysis. Bloodletting was another method used to treat certain diseases.

Greek Medicine – Greek medicine is a traditional, local, holistic, and integrative medical system that evolved into what is now known as allopathy.

Dating back to the 12th century BC, this system was rooted in the principles of purity, chastity, and hygiene. The son of the god Apollo, Aesculapius, is recognized as the father of Greek medicine. His daughters, Hygeia (goddess of hygiene), Iaso (goddess of recuperation from illness), Aceso (goddess of the healing process), Aegle (goddess of good health), and Panacea (goddess of universal remedy), each symbolize different aspects of health.

The snake wrapped around the rod of Aesculapius remains a symbol of modern medicine. Hippocrates, a pivotal figure in Greek medicine, contributed significantly to its development. His essays, compiled in the treatise *Corpus Hippocraticum*, challenged the notion that diseases were divine punishments. Instead, he argued that diseases arose from imbalances in nature. Hippocrates introduced the concepts of endemic and epidemic diseases and emphasized the importance of prognosis - the prediction of a disease's future course - alongside diagnosis. This laid the foundation for ethical clinical practice. Greek medicine, much like the *Tridosha* principle in *Ayurveda*, believed that the body's health depended on the balance of four humors: phlegm, yellow bile, blood, and black bile, which were derived from the four elements - earth, water, fire, and air. An imbalance in these humors was thought to lead to illness. Hippocrates advocated for the treatment of patients in hygienic conditions, free of infection, and with honesty and sincerity.

He was particularly skilled in diagnosing lung diseases, including lung cancer and heart disease, using signs such as the clubbing of fingers, which indicates chronic low oxygen levels. His expertise in proctoscopy and the use of rectal speculums allowed him to treat piles effectively, laying the groundwork for modern endoscopy. He also drained pus from the chest using a lead pipe, a precursor to modern thoracic surgery. The Hippocratic Oath, which emphasizes ethics in medical practice, continues to be administered to medical students upon completion of their studies, underscoring the enduring relevance of his teachings.

Roman Medicine – The decline of Greek civilization around the first century BC paved the way for the development of Roman medicine.

During this period, the Romans made significant advancements in public health, constructing roads, sewers, and water distribution systems that improved hygiene and helped prevent the spread of infectious diseases like malaria.

The Roman civilization is credited with establishing a public health system and creating specialist hospitals that operated within a more scientific framework. Galen, a disciple of Hippocrates, played a key role in Roman medicine by applying his knowledge of anatomy and physiology to the treatment of diseases.

Naturopathy – Naturopathy was first advocated by Thomas Allinson in 1880 and later by John Scheel in 1895. It is based on the principles of hygienic medicine, promoting a natural diet and exercise as key components of health. Naturopathy emphasizes the use of phytomedicine (herbal medicine) for treating diseases. Benedict Lust, a German - born American, is recognized as the father of modern - day naturopathy, while Sebastian Kneipp popularized the therapeutic benefits of water treatments. In India, Dr. Prakash Baranwal is known for his contributions to the promotion of yoga, acupressure, and naturopathy.

Today, naturopathy is widely recognized and has gained popularity even within modern medicine. Although it is considered alternative medicine and not entirely evidence - based (EBM), naturopaths describe it as a self - healing and non - invasive approach to treatment. Naturopathy incorporates elements of vitalism, which suggests that life cannot be explained solely by physical or chemical processes, and public health theory, which posits that diseases can be treated through ethnomedicine. Naturopathy operates on the belief that "the treatment of diseases is based on the body's strength to fight infections." Various natural treatment modalities are combined, including water therapy, sun exposure, mud therapy, yoga, acupuncture, acupressure, and homeopathy. Treatment is typically symptom - based, with an emphasis on consuming natural foods, fresh fruits, and lightly cooked vegetables.

Modalities of Treatment –

1. Mud Therapy: Applying mud to the skin is believed to absorb toxins from the body and help excrete them. Mud baths are used to treat conditions such as constipation, nerve weakness, tension headaches, high blood pressure, and obesity, while also imparting a glow to the skin.

2. Enema Therapy: Enemas prepared from pure water, lemon water, or lemon decoctions are administered through the rectum, urinary tract, reproductive system, or ulcers, providing relief from various conditions.

3. Hydrotherapy: This includes treatments such as hip baths, sitz baths (immersion of the anus and genitals in medicated solutions), spinal baths, steam baths, and wet sheet wraps. Sun therapy, fasting, and other natural treatments are also used to relieve acute diseases.

Principles of Naturopathy – Naturopaths believe that nature is the best healer, emphasizing that moderation and abstinence in food consumption can naturally cure diseases. Naturopathy is often referred to as both personal and social medicine. However, it is essential to clarify that the principles of Naturopathy, as outlined in *Ayurveda*, *Siddha*, and *Yoga*, are more qualitative and effective. Modern medicine also recognizes the importance of lifestyle changes in the treatment of many diseases. Doctors today are well aware of the factors that contribute to illness and often advise patients to avoid air and water pollution, limit the consumption of processed and refined foods, engage in adequate exercise, and practice moderation and abstinence alongside taking prescribed medications.

In conclusion, it is common for individuals and scholars to highlight the shortcomings of certain medical systems while attempting to establish the superiority of one over another. However, this often overlooks the unique strengths of each system and the historical and environmental contexts in which they were developed. Every medical system has its own role, producing both beneficial and side effects depending on the environment in which a person lives. This text has aimed to illustrate the basic principles of various medical systems and the different strengths of the *AYUSH* systems - *Ayurveda*, *Yoga*, *Unani*, *Siddha*, and Homeopathy.

While many other traditional medical systems have faded and been replaced by modern scientific medicine, Naturopathy has persisted and been incorporated into modern medical practice.

Chapter 11

Modern Scientific Medicine Vs Allopathy

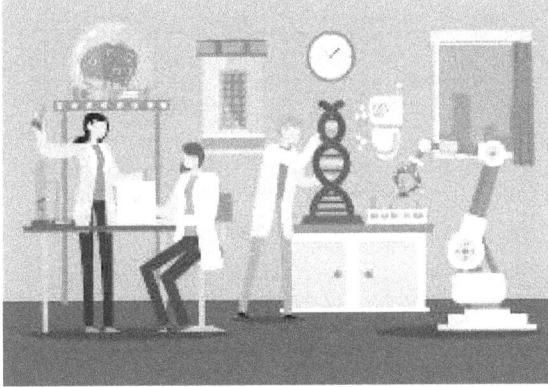

Learning Objectives:

- Evolution of modern medical science based on strong scientific principles during the Renaissance period 16th - 18th century
- Rapid progress of modern medicine during 19th-20th centuries
- How, with the beginning of 20th-century modern medicine paved the way for evidence-based clinical practice, laboratory science, and randomized controlled trials

---

The practice of medicine, which was popular in Europe and North America during the 18th and 19th centuries, was labeled "allopathy" by Samuel Hahnemann in 1810 the founder of Homeopathy. After the decline of Greek - Roman medicine in the Middle Ages (500 - 1500 AD), medical treatment often involved practices such as bloodletting, forced purging, induced vomiting, and using shock therapy to induce sweating. These methods, which later influenced mainstream modern medicine, have their roots in Greek and Roman practices. However, after the fall of ancient Rome around 500 AD, there was a significant decline in medical progress.

This period saw little advancement in medical care, and outbreaks of infectious diseases like the bubonic plague (black fever), smallpox, cholera, leprosy, and tuberculosis occurred unchecked, leading to severe epidemics. Rituals and superstitions were widespread, and instead of addressing bodily ailments, the focus often shifted to spiritual glorification. Surgery, when performed, was done without anesthesia. Greek - Roman medical texts were translated into Arabic - Persian, but practical advancements stalled for centuries.

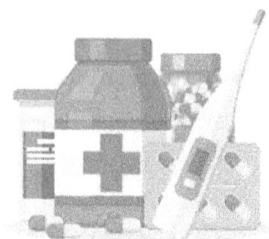

A significant shift in the history of medicine occurred during the Renaissance period (16th - 18th century). This era witnessed a rapid increase in knowledge of anatomy (body structure) and physiology (bodily functions), making the practice of medicine more systematic. Physicians began to adopt a more logical approach to diagnosing and treating diseases, placing vital importance on the principles of diagnosis. The significance of making **differential diagnoses** and **prognosis** (predicting the future outcome of disease) was recognized, leading to the development of clinical medicine as we know it today. Essential steps such as gathering demographic and clinical history, performing physical examinations, planning investigations, making a diagnosis, and advising treatment became standard practice.

This period marked a revolution in medical science, with a series of groundbreaking discoveries following one after another. For instance, the theory of blood circulation was proposed by **William Harvey** in 1628 AD, based on thorough observations from human body dissections. The invention of the microscope by the Dutch father - son, Hans and Zacharias Janssen, in 1585 further propelled medical research and discovery.

The discovery that all living beings are composed of microscopic units came to light in the 1660s. British scientist Robert Hooke was the first to coin the term "cells" when he examined a thin slice of cork under a microscope and observed honeycomb - like structures. Another pivotal discovery was the identification of microbes, or microscopic organisms, which were recognized as the cause of infectious diseases in humans and animals.

Antonie van Leeuwenhoek, known as the Father of Microbiology, made significant improvements to the microscope around 1670 AD and described protozoa and bacteria in his treatise "The Unseen World." It is now well - established that a vast array of different classes of microorganisms is responsible for various infectious diseases.

The antimicrobial properties of certain plants were recognized by Indian and Chinese herbalists long before the advent of modern science.

In the early 1900s, German scientist Paul Ehrlich embarked on a quest to synthesize a "magic bullet" - a compound capable of killing infectious microbes without harming the patient. He succeeded in discovering a drug to treat syphilis. Later, in 1928, Alexander Fleming discovered the antibacterial properties of the mold *Penicillium*, leading to the development of penicillin, the first antibiotic. This discovery marked the beginning of the concept of asepsis and antisepsis in medical practice, which significantly increased the number of surgical operations.

However, it soon became evident that microbes could develop resistance to these agents if they were not used judiciously. **Antimicrobial resistance** has become a significant challenge today, posing a serious threat to public health.

Cancer was first recognized in the 17th century and was initially believed to be related to the lymphatic system. However, German pathologist Johannes Müller later demonstrated that cancer is not composed of lymph but of cells. His student, Rudolf Virchow, further elucidated that cancer cells originate from other cells.

During this period, British surgeon Percivall Pott discovered an environmental cause of cancer in 1775. He observed that small children who were used as chimney sweeps often developed scrotal cancer due to the soot particles left on their scrotal skin.

In the past, there was no effective remedy for pain, leaving individuals to endure suffering during incurable diseases like cancer or surgical procedures. A significant breakthrough occurred in modern medical science when German scientist Friedrich Sertürner introduced morphine, the most effective painkiller still used today to relieve severe pain.

Paracetamol and quinine were also introduced a few years later, further revolutionizing pain management.

The 19th century was a crucial period of rapid scientific advances in modern medical science. The discovery of **general anesthesia** in 1846 was a groundbreaking development, relieving patients from the unbearable pain of surgery and revolutionizing surgical practices. This advancement opened the gateway for more complex surgical procedures. The discovery of several microbes responsible for infections led to the rapid development of newer antiseptics and disinfectants. Alongside, methods and types of anesthesia and surgery evolved rapidly.

The study of cadaveric anatomy progressed significantly. Research and development entered a new phase with the introduction of pathologic anatomy by Giovanni Battista Morgagni (1682 - 1771 AD), who linked diseases to specific organs. Andreas Vesalius (1514 - 1564 AD) conducted a detailed analysis of human anatomy, and Ambroise Paré (1510 - 1590 AD), a surgeon in the French Army, developed cosmetic approaches in surgical practices, promoting surgery as both a science and an art.

In England, surgery advanced in multiple directions, largely due to the influence of the Royal College of Surgeons. The Barber - Surgeons Company was granted a charter to confer the title of Fellow of the Royal College of Surgeons (FRCS) after hands - on training, study in anatomy, surgical pathology, and surgery, followed by rigorous assessment by a board of examiners. Surgeons awarded the FRCS are addressed as "Mister" rather than "Doctor," a tradition that persists today.

The Royal College of Surgeons was established in London, followed by similar colleges in Scotland - Edinburgh and Glasgow - as well as in British colonies such as Ireland, Australia, Canada, Ceylon, and Thailand. Simultaneously, surgery was developing with equal fervor in America, Europe, and India, leading to the establishment of master's programs for teaching, hands - on training, assessment, and accreditation in surgery. Over time, several specialized branches of surgery emerged, including orthopedics and ear, nose, and throat (ENT) surgery. Public health practices, known since the Middle Ages, included the quarantine of leprosy victims and efforts to improve sanitation following the 14th - century plague epidemic.

The recognition that poor sanitation led to epidemics prompted the passage of the Public Health Act in Britain in 1848, followed by similar legislation in other European countries.

The act aimed to protect the public from the spread of communicable diseases. In 1854, English epidemiologist John Snow worked on a cholera epidemic in London, demonstrating that the primary source of infection was contaminated water. He is now remembered as the "father of public health." Rapid advances in scientific knowledge about the factors causing disease led to significant changes in public health practices.

The first vaccine, developed by Edward Jenner in 1796, was against smallpox. About 90 years later, Louis Pasteur discovered another vaccine, this time against rabies. To date, vaccines have been developed against approximately 35 diseases, with ongoing research to create new ones.

Major contagious diseases have been contained by implementing public health norms and safeguarding the environment against viral and bacterial invasion. The World Health Organization (WHO), formed in 1946 - 47 after World War II, monitors, inspects, and surveys global health, paying particular attention to atmospheric and climatic changes.

X - rays were discovered in 1895, and the following year their use as an imaging technique was introduced into modern medicine. Later, ionizing radiation was adopted as a form of therapy against cancer, marking another significant advancement in medical science.

A large number of modern medicines, both synthetic and biologically derived, including medicaments, ointments, and injections, were discovered in the first half of the 20th century. Simultaneously, the 19th and 20th centuries witnessed continuous and rapid refinements in medical science, leading to the widespread adoption of modern medicine across many countries. This period also saw the establishment of numerous medical schools and colleges offering degrees in Bachelor of Medicine and Bachelor of Surgery. Notably, the Grant Medical College was established in Mumbai in 1845, and the Lady Lyall Medical School in Agra followed in 1854.

Thomas Sydenham (1624–1689 AD), born in London, was a pioneering figure in medicine who identified the symptoms of diseases such as scarlet fever, malaria, diarrhea, dysentery, and cholera, along with their appropriate treatments. Often regarded as the first epidemiologist, Sydenham made significant contributions to the field of epidemiology, which greatly enriched modern medical science by enabling the treatment of many prevailing diseases.

He was also the first to recognize the importance of differential diagnosis, laying the foundation for the development of clinical practice. **Clinical Epidemiology** was later introduced as a new basic science by John Paul in 1938.

The discovery of insulin, thyroid hormones, and other molecular components of the human body marked significant advancements in modern medicine. The breakthrough **discovery of the structure of DNA,** or deoxyribonucleic acid, in 1953 by James Watson and Francis Crick, who described it as a double helix or twisted - ladder structure, was a milestone in medical history. This discovery accelerated the development of modern molecular biology and deepened the understanding of protein synthesis driven by genetic factors. By the end of the millennium, scientists had successfully deciphered the **human genetic code**, leading to the ability to sequence the entire human genome, which is now instrumental in identifying diseases caused by genetic mutations.

Clinical epidemiology also evolved significantly over the last century and has become the cornerstone of **Evidence - Based Medicine (EBM).**

The 21st century is witnessing an era of advanced, multi - specialty, and multi - efficacious drugs, developed through rigorous research methods, including **randomized controlled trials.** The development of a new drug can take 10 - 15 years, during which it must be proven safe and effective before being released to the market. These newly developed drugs are thoroughly evaluated against the parameters of EBM and must pass approval by national drug regulatory authorities before reaching the public.

In conclusion, Modern or Scientific Medicine has evolved from the European American system of medicine, historically referred to as allopathy as practiced in the 18th and 19th centuries. However, the field has advanced significantly since then, and **the term "allopathy" is no longer used in most countries.**

Modern medicine has embraced the principles of pure sciences such as physics, chemistry, and mathematics, which have influenced the development of life sciences, the theory of evolution, surgical treatments, pharmacology, and biostatistics. Modern medicine is **dynamic, continuously upgrading itself** through research and the adoption of new technologies.

It addresses both preventive and curative aspects, considering individual, community, family, and public health dimensions. It upholds human values and ethics, emphasizes the health of women, children, and the elderly, and **supports the rehabilitation rights** of differently abled individuals.

Modern medicine is **inclusive**, integrating scientifically proven elements from other medical systems. For instance, it has incorporated the concept that 'the body heals itself,' along with several tenets from naturopathy and *Ayurveda*. Importantly, modern medicine **recognizes its limitations** and candidly acknowledges areas where science has yet to reach a full understanding, such as the unknown causation of certain diseases and the lack of satisfactory cures for others.

Modern medicine **continues to specialize**, with practitioners unhesitant to refer patients to specialists when necessary. This **openness to collaboration and continuous improvement** is why modern medicine is widely accepted by the general public. Other systems of medicine can align with modern medicine by adopting scientific methods and engaging in rigorous research.

Chapter 12

Technology in Modern Medicine, Internet, Google, WhatsApp, Artificial Intelligence and ChatGPT

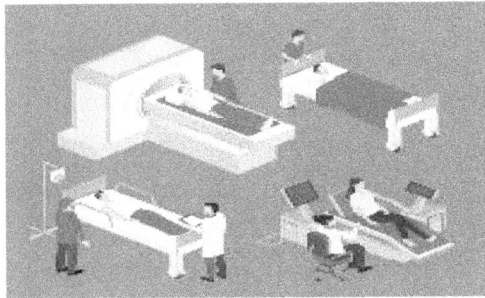

Learning Objectives:

- Understand the difference between knowledge, science and technology
- The contribution of technology in surgery – Minimally invasive surgery, laser and robotic surgery
- Current new technologies in diagnostics and therapeutics - software technologies and artificial intelligence (AI)
- Learning health practices from Internet, Google......
- Communicating with the Doctor through WhatsApp

Knowledge, science, and technology are integral parts of our lives, yet we often overlook the distinctions between them. Understanding these differences can clarify their unique roles:

- **Knowledge** is the information we gather through sensory experiences - seeing, hearing, smelling, touching, or feeling - and through study and training. It encompasses facts, concepts, and skills acquired over time.

- **Science** is the **systematic verification of knowledge** through evidence and scientific experimentation, establishing new standards, theories, and laws. It is knowledge that has been rigorously tested and validated.

- **Technology** is the practical application of scientific knowledge, especially in industry. It is the tool through which scientific understanding is translated into tangible products and processes that solve **real - world problems**. For instance, knowledge in physics, chemistry, biology, economics, and mathematics has led to the development of technologies like transistors, mobile phones, motors, and airplanes, all of which have significantly improved human life.

Medical science is one field profoundly impacted by technology. For example, advancements in organic chemistry, biochemistry and pharmaceutical chemistry, have paved the way for the development of synthetic medicines. Pharmacology, the science of drugs, involves drug preparation, modification, discovery, trials, and the determination of appropriate dosages and administration routes. Pharmaceuticals such as tablets, ointments, and injections, which are prescribed to patients, must receive formal approval from respective drug regulatory authorities in each country.

Just as elements like hydrogen, oxygen, and sulfur combine in specific valencies to form compounds like water (H_2O) and sulphuric acid (H_2SO_4), pharmacologists combine different salts in varying valencies to create medicines.

These drugs, designed to treat conditions such as bacterial infections, malaria, filariasis, and hypertension, undergo years of trials before being approved for use.

Medical technology plays a crucial role in both the prevention of diseases and the treatment of patients. Advances in technology have made it possible to diagnose autoimmune diseases, cancer, and genetic disorders more efficiently, enabling more targeted treatments with fewer side effects. There is no field of medicine left untouched by technology, which continues to evolve and improve patient care. The discussion below gives just a few examples of such technological advances.

Fiber Optic Endoscopy – Physicians frequently need to examine the interior of human body cavities, such as the stomach, peritoneal cavity, and bronchi. Traditional methods were limited because light travels in a straight line, and light bulbs used in earlier endoscopes would become extremely hot, risking tissue burns. Older generation endoscopes, which were straight, metallic, and equipped with wired bulbs at their tips, could only probe short distances and generated significant heat. The advent of fiber - optic endoscopy revolutionized this field.

These modern endoscopes can be maneuvered through body orifices like the mouth and anus, thanks to their steerable tips and cold light sources, which do not heat up and damage tissues. For example, a colonoscope is used to examine the large intestine, an endoscope is employed to inspect the esophagus, stomach, and duodenum, and a cystoscope allows visualization of the urinary bladder.Endoscopes are also vital for obtaining tissue samples from internal organs, where cytology and histopathology confirm diagnoses.

Additionally, they are used in procedures to stop bleeding from blood vessels through techniques like coagulation and embolization. Cardiologists and vascular surgeons often use endo - vascular procedures to enhance blood circulation in blood vessels. Endoscopes equipped with ultrasound devices can image internal body structures, and they are also used to place stents to bypass blockages.

Technology in Surgery – Medical technology has greatly enhanced surgical precision. For instance, in cases of brain hemorrhage or bleeding from the intestines, lungs, or liver, bleeding can be effectively controlled. The process of stopping bleeding is known as **hemostasis** or sealant surgery. This is achieved by accurately locating the bleeding site and using techniques like embolization or coiling to stop it.

Modern advancements also include the use of **endo - staplers**, which allow for the stapling of intestines and other organs through an endoscope, providing a less invasive alternative to traditional sutures.

Additionally, specialized tools such as **diathermy devices** and ultrasonic harmonic sealers are employed in surgeries to minimize bleeding and improve outcomes.

Laser Energy in Medical Treatment – Laser, an acronym for Light Amplification by Stimulated Emission of Radiation, is based on Einstein's quantum theory of radiation. The first laser was produced by Maiman in 1960 using ruby as the lasing medium. Today, various types of lasers, such as Diode and Nd: YAG lasers, are available for a wide range of medical applications. These **include treatments for skin conditions like hemangiomas, port - wine stains, small scars, pimples, and varicose veins.** The carbon dioxide laser, for instance, can cut through tissues with the precision of a scalpel.

In ophthalmology, lasers play a critical role in correcting severe refractive errors, allowing patients to forgo thick glasses through procedures like laser - assisted in - situ keratomileusis (LASIK). Red or green lasers are used to correct certain defects in the retina, the most sensitive layer of the eye. The monochromaticity, brilliance, coherence, and collimated unidirectional properties of lasers make them invaluable in precision surgical procedures.

Anesthesia in Surgery - Anesthesia is essential for performing painless surgical procedures. Depending on the nature of the surgery, it can be administered locally, regionally, or generally. Regional anesthesia, such as spinal or epidural anesthesia, is commonly used for abdominal and lower limb surgeries. Anesthetic agents injected in the neck can block nerves to the upper arm, providing regional anesthesia for surgeries on the upper extremities. Remarkably, some brain surgeries can now be performed under local anesthesia.

For major surgeries involving the heart, lungs, or abdomen, general anesthesia is administered. This involves intravenous anesthetic agents and inhaled anesthetics delivered through a tube placed in the trachea (windpipe). To facilitate surgery within the chest or abdomen, muscle relaxant drugs are administered to relax tissues and muscles, temporarily halting the patient's ability to breathe independently. During general anesthesia, the patient's respiration is supported by a bellow device called an **Ambu bag** or an automated ventilator - all managed through a comprehensive system known as **Boyle's apparatus**.

Tremendous advancements in anesthesiology, pain medicine, anesthetic drugs, and bloodless surgery have made complex procedures like heart, lung, and liver transplants relatively safe over the past two decades.

Microsurgery – Microsurgery involves the meticulous repair of tissue defects, often following the resection of cancer - affected areas.

This is achieved by transplanting or repositioning suitable tissue from one part of the body to another. The donor tissue, along with its small blood vessels, is harvested and then anastomosed (joined) to blood vessels at the recipient site using extremely fine suturing materials. This highly specialized technique, performed under a microscope or with magnified vision, is known as **microvascular surgery**. Reimplantation of severed hands and fingers following accidents is another application of this technique.

Laparoscopic Surgery and Early Recovery – A laparoscope, a type of endoscope, is commonly used in abdominal surgeries, enabling procedures to be performed through small incisions rather than large cuts in the abdominal wall. This technique is known as **minimally invasive or laparoscopic surgery**. In the chest cavity, a similar procedure is called Video - Assisted Thoracoscopic Surgery (VATS).

General surgery experienced a significant transformation in the 1990s with the advent of laparoscopic techniques. In 1882, Carl Langenbuch from Germany performed the first cholecystectomy, a gallbladder removal surgery. Almost 100 years later, in 1985, Dr. Erich Mühe, also from Germany, performed the first laparoscopic cholecystectomy. Although the laparoscope had been around for over two decades before these procedures, the French surgeons popularized and refined the technique, ushering in the era of minimally invasive surgery.

Laparoscopic surgery, with its minimally invasive approach, revolutionized tissue recovery post - surgery. Surgeons honed their precision surgery skills, and multi   dimensional surgical procedures have emerged over the last three decades. The laparoscope, equipped with a 5 - 10 mm tip and a high - resolution digital camera, is inserted into the abdomen through small incisions in the abdominal wall.

The camera provides a color, high - definition view of the internal organs, including the stomach, intestines, liver, and gallbladder, on a large screen in front of the operating surgeon. This laparo - vision or endo - vision, combined with **magnified micro - vision,** allows surgeons to perform highly precise procedures.

To create enough space for surgical maneuvers, the abdominal wall is lifted using **carbon dioxide (CO2) insufflation**, enhancing the visibility of the internal organs and their nerve and blood supply. Laparoscopic surgery typically involves minimal cutting and tissue damage, resulting in less blood loss, reduced postoperative pain, and faster patient recovery.

Consequently, patients are often discharged from the hospital much sooner than with traditional open surgery. This period also marked the advent of **Early Recovery After Surgery (ERAS)** protocols. Previously, surgery often pushed the body into a catabolic state, leading to prolonged recovery, significant inflammatory and metabolic responses, and various side effects. However, general surgeons began focusing on gentler tissue handling, minimizing damage to the operated organ, and avoiding collateral harm by using finer instruments in open surgery. The use of energy sources such as diathermy, harmonic vessel sealers, and lasers further reduced blood loss.

Attention to patient nutrition became crucial, as did early mobilization, proper wound care, intensive respiratory exercises post - operation, effective pain relief, and early resumption of food intake or parenteral nutrition. These practices were all aimed at promoting early recovery after surgery. Additionally, significant investments were made in preventing postoperative infections through high - tech modular operating and post - operation areas, laminar flow systems, aseptic techniques, and the minimal use of antibiotics.

Robotic Surgery – Robotic surgery is renowned for its exceptional precision and the ability to operate with ease in various **difficult - to - reach areas** of the human body. Surgical robots are equipped with multiple laparoscopes, cameras, sensors, and a variety of operating tools. After administering adequate anesthesia and inflating the abdominal cavity, these camera, and tool - equipped laparoscopes are inserted into the target area of the body.

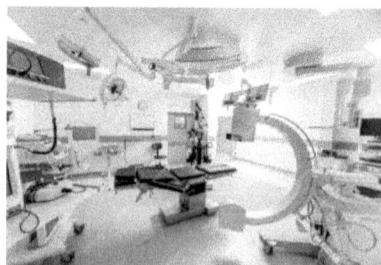

An operator assists by making small incisions through the skin and abdominal wall to insert the camera, scopes, and instruments, which are all connected to a console unit.

The console, typically located in the same room about 4 - 5 meters away from the patient, is where the operating surgeon sits on a multifunctional mobile stool. Once the cameras start transmitting images of the surgical area, the surgeon performs the surgery using finger ports and pedals on the console unit. The surgeon controls the movements of the laparoscopes and instruments while viewing the endo - vision and enlarged images – micro - vision.

It is important to note that robotic surgery is not autonomous; the unique instrumentation of the robot allows for more precise and accurate surgeries, particularly in areas that are difficult to access. This technique is now commonly used for prostate gland surgeries in men, as the gland is situated deep within the pelvis, making it difficult to reach.

Polymerase Chain Reaction (PCR) – PCR is a relatively new laboratory technique that rapidly replicates (amplifies) specific segments of DNA to produce millions to billions of copies, which are then studied in greater detail. This technique is widely used in the diagnosis of infections caused by bacteria, viruses, and other pathogens, as well as in mutation detection, sequencing, genotyping, cloning, microarrays, forensics, and paternity testing.

During the COVID - 19 pandemic, PCR was used to test throat swabs for the presence of the coronavirus. Similarly, tuberculosis bacteria can be detected in pus, body fluids, and tissue using this technique.

Gene Sequencing and Gene Mutation – Detailed knowledge of genetic sequences allows scientists to understand and establish the causality of genetic diseases, leading to the development of new targeted treatments.

Gene sequencing involves determining the sequence of nucleotides in a segment of DNA. The original technique, known as **Sanger sequencing**, sequences a single DNA fragment at a time. In contrast, **Next Generation Sequencing (NGS)** is a massively parallel process that sequences millions of fragments simultaneously in a single run. The key difference between Sanger sequencing and NGS is the sequencing volume. NGS has revolutionized genomic research, allowing an entire human genome to be sequenced within a single day. NGS also has the power to detect novel or rare variants through deep sequencing.

When only the exons (protein - coding regions) are sequenced, it is called whole exome sequencing, which covers about 85% of the genome.

This method is used when a disorder is suspected to be genetic but is not clinically recognizable, or when the patient's symptoms are consistent with a wide range of genetic disorders. By understanding the precise genetic defect, new targeted treatments can be discovered. Patients suffering from genetic diseases due to a recognized disorder of gene sequencing or gene mutation can then be treated if a suitable drug is available.

Pharmacogenomics – The science of pharmacogenomics, which explores how a person's genetic makeup influences their response to drugs, represents a new frontier in personalized medicine. The long - term goal is to enable doctors to select the most appropriate drugs and doses for each individual, leading to **personalized medicine, precision medicine, or targeted therapy.** Different medications may be prescribed for similar diseases caused by different gene mutations. For example, in epilepsy caused by the SCN1A mutation, certain drugs like phenytoin should be avoided, while in cases with SCN2A and SCN8A mutations, high - dose phenytoin may be effective. In pharmacogenomics, the preparation, testing, and trials of medications are conducted using advanced technologies.

Gene Editing – Clustered Regularly Interspaced Short Palindromic Repeats (CRISPR) – Gene editing technology, exemplified by CRISPR, leverages the concept of palindromic sequences - series of numbers or characters that read the same forwards and backwards, such as 121, 242, 383, madam, radar, and civic. This technology has been adapted for gene sequencing and editing, allowing the alteration of specific genetic sequences that cause disease. Gene editing can be used to treat conditions like cancer, HIV - AIDS and rheumatism that result from gene mutations by repairing the mutated genes through precise editing and sequencing.

Health Wearables – Over recent decades, wearable electronic health devices have become increasingly common. The earliest example of this technology is the **cardiac pacemaker**, implanted in the chest to provide the necessary electrical stimulus to the heart when it fails to do so naturally. Today, technologies have advanced so that a doctor can view a patient's ECG in real - time through a mobile app, even from a distance. Health wearables are designed to continuously monitor biological signals with minimal discomfort to the user. They are useful for tracking various health metrics, much like how step counting is tracked by mobile phones.

For example, wearable devices can continuously monitor blood pressure, cardiac activity, ECG, sleep patterns, and blood glucose levels via mobile software. Smartwatches have integrated many of these functions. **Continuous glucose monitoring (CGM)** involves placing a micro - fiber chip under the skin, typically on the upper arm, which provides round - the - clock blood sugar readings on the user's mobile phone. This technology is particularly beneficial for diabetes management and reversal programs, allowing patients to go about their daily activities while keeping track of their glucose levels.

Wireless Brain Sensors – A bio - resorbable device implanted into the brain is showing promise in treating mental health conditions such as depression, psychosis, neurosis, and schizophrenia. Deep brain stimulation (DBS), another advanced neurosurgical procedure, involves implanting electrodes and using electrical stimulation to treat movement disorders associated with Parkinson's disease, essential tremor, dystonia, and other neurological conditions. Numerous other wearables are under development, aimed at assisting individuals with physical challenges, blindness, cerebral palsy, brain atrophy, and various other conditions.

3D Printing – This versatile technology is revolutionizing the medical field by enabling the creation of three - dimensional images and models from computer data. These 3D - printed models are instrumental in diagnosing chronic and acute conditions of the joints, bones, and bone marrow. Technology is particularly beneficial for visualizing and planning surgeries related to the liver, brain, bones, jaws, teeth, tumors, and more. In addition to its diagnostic applications, 3D printing is also being used to create multipurpose pills, where medications can be customized and printed with precise ingredients tailored to the patient's needs.

Artificial Organs – For patients with organ failure, where transplantation is not feasible, wearable artificial organs offer a promising alternative. Technologies like the Wearable Artificial Kidney (WAK) and Implantable Artificial Kidney (IAK) are under development to provide long - term, effective kidney function.

These innovations aim to create accessible, safe, and cost - effective solutions that significantly improve the quality of life (QoL) for patients.

Another cutting - edge technique in biological research is auto - implantation, where artificial organs or tissues can regenerate within the body. For instance, burnt skin might be regenerated using bio - printing, and damaged internal organs such as blood vessels, ovaries, and pancreas could potentially be replaced and naturally integrated into the body's system over time.

Virtual Reality and Simulation – Virtual reality (VR) technology, widely used for virtual tours of natural scenery, museums, and university campuses, is now making significant strides in medical training and treatment.

High - fidelity simulation, a subset of VR, allows for advanced diagnostic and treatment capabilities through telemedicine, enabling doctors to examine patients remotely via computer screens. This technology is also invaluable in demonstrating complex procedures such as hazardous brain surgeries or skilled robotic surgeries.

High - fidelity simulation labs are becoming increasingly popular for training medical professionals in micro - vascular surgery, endoscopic surgery, laparoscopic surgery, and robotic surgery, reducing the need for live or deceased animals in surgical education.

Use of Technology in Ophthalmology – The human eye is a remarkably precise organ, and advancements in technology have significantly enhanced the treatment of various eye diseases. High - precision ophthalmic instruments now enable procedures like corneal laser surgery, where an extremely thin slice is cut on the cornea to **correct high - degree refractive errors**, eliminating the need for thick glasses. Technologies such as phacoemulsification allow the removal of hard, opaque cataract lenses through small incisions, followed by the implantation of **foldable intraocular lenses**.

These innovations have revolutionized cataract surgery, making it less invasive and more effective. Additionally, complex retinal surgeries are now performed using cutting - edge technology, ensuring better outcomes for patients with retinal disorders.

Biomimetics – Biomimetics, also known as biomimicry, is an interdisciplinary field that combines principles of engineering, chemistry, and biology to mimic natural processes and solve human problems.

Derived from the Greek word meaning "imitation of life," biomimetics emphasizes learning from nature's designs rather than extracting elements from the natural world. This science is applied in developing synthetic and biological materials that can function within the body for extended periods without adverse effects. For example, stainless steel plates and screws have long been used to fix bone fractures, but more tissue - friendly and durable materials like titanium are now preferred.

In ophthalmology, biomimetic approaches have led to the development of artificial lenses for cataract surgery. Beyond the eye, biomimetics is also responsible for innovations like **cochlear implants, artificial joints (such as knees and hips), heart valves** made from metal and biological materials, and **dental implants** integrated into jawbones. This emerging industry is rapidly evolving, providing safer and more effective solutions that emulate the functions of natural organs and tissues.

World Wide Web – Internet, Google, WhatsApp

The rapid expansion of internet technology has revolutionized access to information, bringing both benefits and challenges. Society is now flooded with vast amounts of data, some of which is highly useful, while others can be misleading. Search engines like Google have become a constant resource, providing information at the click of a button. For those anxious about their health, it's tempting to seek answers online by entering symptoms or test results into these platforms. However, this can sometimes lead to friction with medical professionals. A doctor may express frustration if a patient starts quoting information from the internet, suggesting that they might as well seek treatment from "Dr. Google."

It is important to remember that while search engines and digital platforms deliver information, they do not offer professional advice. The old English saying, "A little knowledge is a dangerous thing," aptly describes the risks of relying solely on internet searches. Without proper medical training, individuals can easily misinterpret the information they find online, leading to unnecessary worry or incorrect self - diagnosis.

For instance, my niece recently looked up the side effects of steroids prescribed to her mother for an allergy. She read that steroids can cause puffiness and immediately assumed that her mother's facial swelling was due to the medication.

However, doctors understand that while steroids can cause puffiness, this side effect does not occur within a few hours.

In her mother's case, the swelling was due to the allergy itself, not the steroids. Misinterpretations like these are common when lay people rely on **"half - baked" information** from the internet. While it's reasonable to seek information, attempting to apply it without professional guidance can lead to harmful consequences. Ultimately, following the advice of a qualified doctor is the safest path to proper treatment.

For medical professionals, the internet is an invaluable resource - a treasure trove of information available 24/7. It provides access to written content, images, and videos, often making it more versatile than traditional books and journals. As the saying goes, **"A picture is worth a thousand words,"** and similarly, **a video can convey as many as a thousand images.**

Having internet access in an outpatient department (OPD) or during ward rounds can be incredibly useful for quickly checking drug dosages, potential side effects, or other clinical details.

India has experienced a "mobile revolution," with approximately 88% of households now possessing smartphones and internet connectivity.

This shift is particularly notable in rural areas, where mobile phones have become the norm. In many cases, purchasing a mobile phone is a top priority when funds are available, reflecting the central role that mobile technology now plays in daily life.

WhatsApp as a Communication Tool in Healthcare

WhatsApp is a widely used mobile application, almost universally present on smartphones in India. It serves as an **effective communication tool** between doctors and patients, particularly for those in distant or remote areas. Patients can use WhatsApp to send **questions, images, and videos** to their doctors, who can then review and respond **when convenient.**

This method not only saves patients a trip to the clinic but also allows the doctor to respond thoughtfully rather than being interrupted by an unexpected phone call during a busy time. Additionally, WhatsApp messages are saved automatically, providing a record of the communication, which can be useful for both the patient and the doctor.

Artificial Intelligence (AI) is a rapidly advancing field that is increasingly finding applications across various domains, including medicine. AI refers to the use of computers to simulate human intelligence and critical thinking. AI is already being applied in fields such as education, banking, finance, supply chains, retail, e - commerce, manufacturing, and healthcare.

The COVID - 19 pandemic accelerated the adoption of AI, with AI - enabled technologies being used to design algorithms for monitoring and analyzing patient data.

In the medical field, AI has the potential for extensive applications. These include disease diagnosis, end - to - end drug discovery, improving communication between physicians and patients, transcribing prescriptions and other medical documents, and even remotely treating patients.

AI - powered systems can often perform tasks more efficiently than humans, and the use of precise algorithms can yield results comparable to those of human experts in medical sciences. It is anticipated that AI will eventually take over certain roles within the medical field, revolutionizing the landscape of medical science.

AI in medicine will play significant roles in resolving complex algorithms, enhancing analytics, and improving physical detections, ultimately contributing to more accurate and efficient healthcare delivery.

AI in Medicine: Key Applications

- **Early Detection and Diagnosis**: Machine learning models can analyze data from medical devices, tests, or patient - reported symptoms to identify potential risks for diseases or complications. This early detection capability allows doctors to intervene sooner, improving patient outcomes.

- **Clinical Decision Support**: AI - powered tools assist healthcare practitioners in designing personalized treatment plans. By analyzing vast amounts of medical data, including Big Data, AI can detect patterns that might be missed by humans, leading to more effective and tailored patient care.

- **Medical Imaging**: AI is revolutionizing the analysis of medical images such as CT scans, X - rays, and MRIs. For example, AI can identify lesions, such as those in breast cancer, or detect lung abnormalities caused by COVID - 19 through the segmentation of 3D images.

  AI's precision in imaging reduces diagnostic errors, making it as effective as human radiologists in detecting early signs of various conditions

- **Accelerating Drug Development**: AI has the potential to significantly reduce the cost and time associated with developing new drugs. It enhances drug design by analyzing the 3D structures of proteins based on amino acid sequences, and it can identify promising drug combinations. This capability facilitates the discovery of new treatments.

- **24/7 Virtual Assistants**: AI can power virtual assistants that are accessible around the clock. These assistants can answer questions based on a patient's medical history, preferences, and personal needs, providing continuous support and guidance.

- **Improving Clinical Trials**: AI can streamline clinical trials by improving the efficiency of data analysis and speeding up the identification of relevant medical codes linked to patient outcomes. This acceleration can lead to faster trial completion and quicker availability of new treatments.

- **Predicting Health Risks**: AI tools have the potential to predict health risks by analyzing specific biomarkers. For example, by examining the retina, AI can predict the risk of heart attacks, allowing for earlier preventive measures.

ChatGPT: Enhancing Efficiency in Modern Medicine

As outlined in Wikipedia, ChatGPT (Chat Generative Pre - Trained Transformer) is an advanced language model developed by OpenAI, launched in November 2022. This AI - powered tool enables users to refine and direct written content - whether an article, conversation, or detailed write - up - towards a specified length, format, style, level of detail, and language, mimicking human conversation. It is designed to handle routine tasks, thereby freeing up time for more strategic and engaging activities.

For instance, if someone plans a vacation in Thailand, they can simply input the number of days and destination city, and ChatGPT will generate a day - to - day itinerary tailored to their needs. Similarly, doctors who often spend considerable time filling out patient data, writing discharge summaries, completing insurance claim forms, and handling administrative paperwork can significantly simplify their workload using ChatGPT. Modern medical science owes much to the integration of engineering and technology, which continues to advance, refine, and simplify healthcare delivery.

AI and tools like ChatGPT are opening new avenues, enabling future generations to better manage everyday health issues while still relying on physicians and surgeons for complex acute and chronic conditions.

This summary offers just a glimpse into how technological advances, particularly AI, are transforming medical practice. As these technologies evolve, they promise to further enhance efficiency, accuracy, and patient care in the healthcare sector.

Chapter 13

Telemedicine

Learning objectives:

- Getting familiar with the utility of computer-information-technology in telemedicine treatment
- Procuring remote medical care at low cost from home through telemedicine or telehealth

In today's world, information technology has become an integral part of our lives. The widespread use of the internet, computers, and mobile phones has seamlessly integrated into the field of medicine, revolutionizing how healthcare is delivered. Not only has this technology made all forms of medical communication quicker and easier, but it has also made virtual consultations possible through telemedicine. With the ability to transmit images and videos online, telemedicine has added a new dimension to healthcare.

The COVID - 19 pandemic significantly accelerated the adoption of telemedicine worldwide. Telemedicine is particularly useful in cases where the patient does not need to physically visit the doctor, such as when medication doses need adjustment.

It is estimated that **roughly 80% of medical consultations can be effectively conducted online** through telemedicine.

Additionally, telemedicine enhances the likelihood of maintaining thorough records and documentation, reducing the risk of missing vital advice from healthcare providers. The doctor also benefits from having exact documentation of the advice provided during teleconsultations, which increases legal protection for both the patient and the doctor. Moreover, telemedicine offers safety benefits for both patients and healthcare workers, especially in situations where there is a risk of contagious infections.

It is particularly relevant in countries like India, where medical specialists or even basic healthcare services may not be readily available in remote rural areas. Traveling to nearby cities for a medical consultation can be costly in terms of time, effort, and money. A day spent traveling deprives the patient and their family members of a day's earnings and adds unnecessary traffic on roads and a burden on hospitals or clinics. By mainstreaming telemedicine into health systems, we can reduce inequities and barriers to access, making healthcare more inclusive and accessible to all.

Government Initiatives in Telemedicine

Recognizing the importance of telemedicine, the Government of India has launched several telemedicine services to enhance healthcare delivery across the country.

1. **Sanjeevani (2005):** Launched by the Central Government in 2005, Sanjeevani is a hybrid telemedicine software that offers both 'store and forward' and 'real - time' functionalities. This platform was an early step towards integrating telemedicine into India's healthcare system.

2. **Sehat (2015):** In 2015, the Central Government launched Sehat, which expanded telemedicine services to 60,000 Common Service Centers (CSCs) in remote rural areas. These centers, in collaboration with Apollo Hospital, provide specialist consultations using telemedicine tools, making healthcare accessible to underserved regions.

3. **CoNTec (COVID - 19 National Teleconsultation Center):** Established by the All India Institute of Medical Sciences (AIIMS), New Delhi, CoNTec offers 24/7 teleconsultation services with specialist doctors across the country. This initiative was particularly crucial during the COVID - 19 pandemic, providing nationwide access to expert medical advice.

Telemedicine Guidelines and Concerns

Despite these advancements, telemedicine in India faced challenges due to a lack of clear guidelines, creating ambiguity and uncertainty regarding its practice and legitimacy. Until 2019, there were no official guidelines for telemedicine in India.

On 25th March 2020, the Board of Governors in supersession of the Medical Council of India, in partnership with Niti Aayog, released the **Guidelines for the Practice of Telemedicine in India.**

Telemedicine was defined as "the delivery of health care services, where distance is a critical factor, by all health care professionals using information and communication technologies for the exchange of valid information for diagnosis, treatment, and prevention of disease and injuries, research and evaluation, and for the continuing education of health care providers, all in the interests of advancing the health of individuals and their communities."

The guidelines clarified that any registered medical practitioner (RMP) in India is eligible to practice telemedicine.

However, registration was mandatory, and RMPs were required to complete an online program on telemedicine within a specified duration.

Exclusions in the Guidelines:

The guidelines explicitly excluded the following aspects:

1. Specifications for hardware or software, infrastructure building, and maintenance.

2. Data management systems, including standards and interoperability.

3. The use of digital technology to conduct surgical or invasive procedures remotely.

4. Other aspects of telehealth such as research and evaluation and the continuing education of healthcare workers.

5. Consultations outside the jurisdiction of India.

The full guidelines are available at:
https://www.mohfw.gov.in/pdf/Telemedicine.pdf

These guidelines may be amended from time to time, clarifications or advisories issued and drug lists may be modified. The salient points of the guidelines for telemedicine emphasize the following essential principles:

1. **Professional Judgment**: The Registered Medical Practitioner's (RMP) professional judgment is paramount in determining whether telemedicine is appropriate or if an in - person consultation is necessary. The RMP must carefully evaluate the situation to ensure that telemedicine is in the best interest of the patient.

2. **Contextual Consideration**: The RMP should consider the specific context of the patient's condition and the mode of communication (video, audio, or text) being used for the consultation. The quality of care should not be compromised based on the method of communication chosen.

3. **Quick Assessment**: The RMP should make a swift and accurate assessment of whether telemedicine is suitable for the patient's condition. This decision should be based on a holistic view of the patient's situation.

4. **Consistency in Principles**: The core principles of care remain the same regardless of the communication mode used for telemedicine. However, patient management and treatment may vary depending on whether the consultation is conducted via video, audio, or text.

5. **Discretion in Mode of Communication**: The RMP should exercise discretion in selecting the mode of communication based on the type of medical condition. If the patient's condition requires a video consultation or an in - person examination, the RMP should explicitly request it.

6. **Right to Discontinue**: The RMP can decide at any point not to continue with the telemedicine consultation if they feel it is not in the patient's best interest. Similarly, the patient has the right to discontinue the teleconsultation at any stage.

7. **Emergency Intervention**: If the patient's condition necessitates emergency intervention, the RMP should provide advice for first aid, immediate relief, and referral to appropriate care.

These principles ensure that telemedicine consultations are conducted with the same level of care and professionalism as in - person visits, prioritizing the patient's health and well - being.

The steps for a telemedicine consultation are outlined as follows:

1. Identification

a. **Transparency**: Telemedicine consultations should not be anonymous. Both the patient and the Registered Medical Practitioner (RMP) must be aware of each other's identities.

b. **Patient Identification**: The RMP should confirm the patient's identity using details such as name, age, address, email ID, phone number, or any other registered ID.

c. **Age Verification**: For issuing prescriptions, the RMP must explicitly ask the age of the patient. If there is any uncertainty, the RMP should request age proof.

d. **Minor Patients**: If the patient is a minor, teleconsultation is only permitted if an adult is present with the minor. The adult's identity should also be verified.

e. **RMP Identification**: The RMP should provide the patient with their name, qualifications, and registration number from the State Medical Council or Medical Council of India (MCI).

This information should be visible on prescriptions, websites, electronic communications (e.g., WhatsApp, Email), and receipts. The RMP must also ensure that the patient can verify their credentials and contact details.

2. Mode of Telemedicine

a. **Technology Options**: Telemedicine consultations can be conducted using various technologies, including text, audio, and video. Each of these modes has its own strengths, weaknesses, and suitable contexts for delivering proper care.

b. **Flexibility**: During a consultation, it may be necessary to switch from one mode to another depending on the situation.

c. **Real - time vs Asynchronous**: Real - time consultations (e.g., video calls) may be preferable for certain situations, while an asynchronous exchange of information (e.g., email or text messages) might be more appropriate in other cases.

3. **Consent**

a. **Implied Consent**: If the patient initiates the telemedicine consultation, their consent is considered implied.

b. **Explicit Consent**: Explicit patient consent is required if the consultation is initiated by a health worker, another doctor, or a caregiver. This consent can be recorded via email, text, or audio/video message, using simple language.

4. **Record Keeping**: The RMP must document the patient's consent in their records.

5. **Patient Information**

6. **Professional Discretion**: The RMP (Registered Medical Practitioner) uses their professional judgment to determine the type and extent of patient information required, which may include the patient's history, examination findings, investigation reports, and past medical records. This information can be supplemented by conversations with a healthcare worker or provider.

7. **Quick Assessment**: The RMP needs to quickly assess the patient's condition based on the available inputs. If the situation requires emergency care, the RMP should provide immediate first aid advice, relief measures, and guidance for referral. This information can be shared in real - time or later via email or text.

8. **Laboratory/Imaging Tests**: The RMP may advise laboratory or radiological tests. If so, the consultation can be paused and resumed at a later, rescheduled time.

Depending on the assessment, the RMP may recommend a video consultation, examination by another RMP or healthcare worker, or an in - person consultation.

9. **Record Keeping**: The RMP must maintain all relevant patient records, including case history, investigation reports, images, and other documentation as appropriate.

10. **Types of Consultation**

   First Consult: This occurs when:

   - The patient is consulting the RMP for the first time. The patient has not consulted the RMP within the last six.

   - The patient is consulting the RMP for a different health condition than previously discussed.

   - The RMP may have a limited understanding of the patient's condition, especially if the consultation is not via video. If the first consult is via video, the RMP can provide better advice, including the potential prescription of additional medicines.

11. **Follow - Up Consult**: This occurs when:

   - The patient is consulting the same RMP within six months of a previous in - person consultation for the continuation of care for the same health condition.

   - It is not considered a follow - up if there are new symptoms unrelated to the previous condition or if the RMP does not recall the context of the previous treatment and advice.

12. **Patient Management, Counseling, Health Education, and Medications**

13. **Patient Management**: If the condition can be managed via telemedicine, the RMP can proceed with professional judgment to.

14. **Provide Health Education**: This includes health promotion and disease prevention messages related to diet, physical activity, smoking cessation, contagious infections, immunizations, hygiene practices, mosquito control, etc.

15. **Provide Counseling**: This involves specific advice, such as recommending new investigations, dietary restrictions, guidelines for anticancer drugs, proper use of medical devices (e.g., hearing aids), and home physiotherapy to mitigate the underlying condition.

16. **Prescribe Medications**: The RMP can prescribe medicines via telemedicine only if they have gathered sufficient and relevant information about the patient's medical condition and believe that the prescribed medicines are in the patient's best interest. Prescribing medications without an appropriate diagnosis or provisional diagnosis is considered professional misconduct.

17. **Specific Restrictions on Prescribing Medicines via Telemedicine**

    a. **List O**: This list includes medicines that are safe to prescribe through any mode of teleconsultation. These are typically used for common conditions and are often available over the counter (e.g., paracetamol, ORS solutions, cough lozenges). Medicines that may be necessary during public health emergencies also fall under this category.

    b. **List A**: This category includes medicines that can be prescribed during a first consult conducted via video consultation or for refills during follow - up consultations. These are relatively safe medicines with a low potential for abuse.

    c. **List B**: This list contains medications that an RMP can prescribe during a follow - up consultation.

    d. **Prohibited List**: Medicines in this list cannot be prescribed via telemedicine consultations. These include drugs with a high potential for abuse that could harm the patient or society if misused. Examples include medicines listed in Schedule X of the Drugs and Cosmetics Act and Rules or any Narcotic and

Psychotropic substances listed in the Narcotic Drugs and Psychotropic Substances Act, 1985.

18. Issuing a Prescription and Transmission

a.   **Prescription Issuance**: If an RMP prescribes medicines, they must issue the prescription in accordance with the Indian Medical Council (Professional Conduct, Etiquette, and Ethics) Regulations, ensuring that they do not violate the provisions of the Drugs and Cosmetics Act and Rules.

b.   **Transmission of Prescription**: The RMP must provide a photo, scan, digital copy of a signed prescription, or an e - Prescription to the patient via email or any messaging platform. If the RMP transmits the prescription directly to a pharmacy, they must obtain explicit consent from the patient, allowing the patient to choose any pharmacy from which to get the medicines dispensed.

19. Principles of Medical Ethics

a.   **Privacy and Confidentiality**: The RMP must adhere to the principles of medical ethics, including professional norms for protecting patient privacy and confidentiality, as per the Indian Medical Council (IMC) Act.

This includes full compliance with the Indian Medical Council (Professional Conduct, Etiquette, and Ethics) Regulations, 2002, and relevant provisions of the IT Act, data protection and privacy laws, or any applicable rules notified from time to time.

b.   **Binding Obligations**: These principles are binding and must be upheld and practiced by the RMP. However, the RMP will not be held responsible for a breach of confidentiality if there is reasonable evidence to believe that the breach occurred due to a technology failure or by a person other than the RMP.

20. Misconduct in Telemedicine:

When practicing telemedicine, certain actions that compromise patient care or violate ethical standards are strictly prohibited. Some examples of misconduct include:

a. **Insisting on Telemedicine**: RMPs should not insist on telemedicine if the patient prefers or is willing to travel for an in - person consultation.

b. **Misuse of Patient Data**: RMPs are prohibited from misusing patient images or data, especially those that are private or sensitive. For instance, uploading an explicit picture of a patient on social media is strictly forbidden.

c. **Prescribing from the Restricted List**: RMPs are not allowed to use telemedicine to prescribe medicines that are on the restricted list.

d. **Solicitation of Patients**: RMPs are not permitted to solicit patients for telemedicine through advertisements or inducements.

Penalties: Any violation of these rules can lead to penalties as prescribed under the IMC Act, ethics regulations, and other prevailing laws.

21. Documentation:

a. **Record - Keeping**: RMPs must maintain detailed records of telemedicine interactions, including logs of phone calls, emails, chat/text records, and video interactions. Patient records, reports, images, diagnostics, and other data used during the telemedicine consultation must also be retained.

b. **Prescription Records**: If a prescription is issued during the teleconsultation, the RMP is required to maintain this record just as they would for an in - person consultation.

22. Fee for Telemedicine Consultation:

a. **Charging Fees**: RMPs may charge a fee for providing telemedicine consultations.

b. **Receipts/Invoices**: The RMP should issue a receipt or invoice for the fee charged, ensuring transparency and maintaining financial records.

23. Follow - up Consultations:

a. **Definition of Follow - up**: A follow - up consultation occurs when the patient consults with the RMP within six months of a previous in - person consultation, specifically for the continuation of care for the same health condition.

b. **Chronic Diseases**: Follow - ups are particularly relevant for chronic conditions such as asthma, diabetes, hypertension, and epilepsy, where ongoing treatment or medication adjustments may not require an in - person visit.

c. **Contextual Understanding**: Since the RMP and the patient have an established relationship and context from previous consultations, follow - up interactions are more secure and definitive.

24. Emergency Situations:

In telemedicine consultations, particularly during emergency situations, the primary objective should be to ensure that the patient receives in - person care as quickly as possible.

However, in critical moments, the RMP (Registered Medical Practitioner) can play a vital role by offering immediate advice, first aid, and guidance that could potentially save lives.

For example:

a. **Trauma Cases**: In situations involving trauma, the RMP may advise on how to maintain the neck position to prevent spinal injury while waiting for in - person care.

b. **First Aid and Counseling**: The RMP may provide first aid instructions, offer counseling, and facilitate the patient's referral to the nearest healthcare facility.

c. **Mandatory In - Person Interaction**: In all emergency cases, the RMP must advise the patient to seek an in - person consultation with an RMP at the earliest opportunity.

25. Guidelines for Technology Platforms Enabling Telemedicine:

This section specifically pertains to technology platforms, such as mobile apps and websites, that connect patients with RMPs for telemedicine services. These platforms must adhere to the following guidelines:

a. **Verification of RMPs**: Technology platforms must ensure that the RMPs listed on their portal are duly registered with the national medical councils or the respective state medical councils. Due diligence must be conducted before listing any RMP on the platform.

b. **Information Transparency**: The platform must clearly provide the name, qualification, registration number, and contact details of every RMP listed on the platform, ensuring transparency for the users.

c. **Restriction on AI/ML Platforms**: Technology platforms utilizing Artificial Intelligence (AI) or Machine Learning (ML) are prohibited from counseling patients or prescribing medicines. These tasks are solely the responsibility of the RMP, who must directly communicate with the patient.

d. **Support from New Technologies**: While new technologies, such as AI, Internet of Things (IoT), and advanced data science - based decision support systems, can assist the RMP in evaluating, diagnosing, or managing the patient, the final prescription or counseling must be delivered directly by the RMP.

e. **Grievance Redressal**: Technology platforms must have a proper mechanism in place to address any queries or grievances that the end customer may have, ensuring that patients have access to support if needed.

Chapter 14

Infection & Immunity

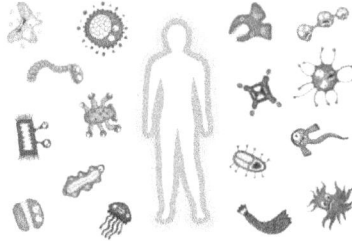

Learning Objectives:

- History of discovery of Infections and micro-organisms - The unseen world
- Types of micro-organisms
- How infections are spread
- How infections are diagnosed
- How infections are treated
- Immunity – innate, active and passive
- The immune system
- Prevention of infection

It is well - recognized today that infections are caused by microscopic organisms. The possibility of their existence was postulated as far back as the 6th century by Jains of India, who called them '*Nigodas*'. They were said to be born in clusters and lived everywhere, including the bodies of animals, plants, and humans. Later, in the 17th century, **Robert Hooke, in 1665,** published a depiction of a microorganism – the fungus Mucor and **Antoni van Leeuwenhoek** observed protozoa and micro - algae microscopically and also described bacteria. Since then, the study of microbes has developed into the whole science of **Microbiology.**

It is now well known that there exists an **'unseen world'** (by the naked eye) of these microbes both within living beings and outside. They abundantly populate the soil, air, water inner linings, and external surfaces of living beings. They exist as single cells or as groups of cells. They have been classified and re - classified. In fact, microbial diversity accounts for most of the biodiversity on Earth. They cause disintegration and decay of animal and plant remains and convert them into simple substances, thus playing an important role in the Earth's ecology. They cause the fermentation of foods and cause bread to rise.

Types of Microorganisms

Microorganisms are divided into seven types: bacteria, archaea, protozoa, rickettsiae, fungi, viruses and multicellular animal parasites (metazoa). Within each type are detailed classifications.

Bacteria: This is a major group of microbes that are **single - celled** and prokaryotic (i.e., they are a primitive type of cell without a nuclear membrane and other cell organelles). They can be pathogenic (disease - causing) or nonpathogenic. Bacteria have a rigid cell wall made of peptidoglycans, a permeable plasma membrane, cytoplasm containing deoxyribose nucleic acid (DNA), ribosomes that synthesize protein, and some may have flagella, pili, and capsules.

They are free living and can survive inside or outside a cell. Bacterial infections can mostly be treated with antibiotic drugs. Examples are tuberculous bacteria, diphtheria bacteria, etc.

Archaea: These are also single celled prokaryotes like bacteria but are only non - pathogenic. Their cell wall differs from bacteria, and they contain a chromosome.

Rickettsiae: These are small rod - shaped intracellular bacteria that typically are found in ticks, lice, fleas, mites, chiggers, and mammals.

Viruses: Viruses are not really cells, but genetic material (DNA or RNA) packaged in a protein coating. They can only reproduce within a host cell.

They are smaller than bacteria. Common cold, rabies, Human Immunodeficiency Virus (HIV/ AIDS), Ebola and COVID - 19 are

Examples of diseases caused by viruses, antiviral treatment is available for some viral infections.

Protozoa: These are single - celled eukaryotes, meaning they have a true nucleus and membranous envelope. They are free - living and larger than bacteria. Protozoa are mostly found in aquatic environments - freshwater or oceans. Protozoa are mostly parasitic, i.e., they live on or in another organism to survive. They may be mobile with the use of flagella or pseudopodia. Examples are amebae, plasmodium (which causes malaria), and Toxoplasma.

Fungi: These are multicellular eukaryotes, which can reproduce both sexually and asexually. They can be both saprophytic (i.e. obtain nourishment from dead material) or parasitic. Examples are yeast, mucormycosis etc. They can be treated with antifungals.

Metazoa: These are multicellular, sexually reproducing organisms with body differentiated into tissues and organs. They are often visible with the naked eye. They may exist as parasites. Examples are round worms, tape worm etc.

Spread of infections – Microorganisms can spread in various ways

1.   Through food and water (**fecal - oral** route). e.g., typhoid, polio

2.   **Fomites -** inanimate objects like a handkerchief, door handles, e.g., respiratory viruses

3.   **Close personal contac**t, e.g., pneumonia

4.   **Air borne** – e.g. tuberculosis

5.   **Droplets** thrown into the surroundings while coughing, sneezing, or talking – COVID - 19, measles, etc.

6.   **Vectors** (usually insects – mosquitos and other arthropods), e.g., Malaria, dengue

7.   **Sexual intercourse,** e.g., HIV/ AIDS

8.   **Blood transfusions**, e.g., HIV, AIDS, hepatitis B

Incubation period – This is the time that may elapse between the infectious agent being introduced in the body and the first symptom of disease.

Diagnosis of Infections: The clinical symptoms of infection may point to a particular organism, but there is a lot of overlap. **Microscopy** may be helpful in recognizing the organism. **Culture** methods are used in which the sample is taken from the patient and inoculated on a growth medium, allowed to grow, and then identified. **Serology** means the detection of **antibodies** produced by the host against the specific infection.

This can be utilized for establishing the diagnosis. Sometimes, **antigens** on the surface of the microbe can be identified. More recently, the **Polymerase Chain Reaction** (PCR) technology has been utilized to identify the specific DNA and RNA (genetic material) of the organism. Multiplex PCR is now being used to multiple possible pathogens in a single reaction. Occasionally, imaging (X - rays, CT, or MRI scans) can be used to suggest a specific diagnosis.

Treatment of Infections: This has been one of the most significant advances in medical science in the last century. The first **antibiotic** used was Penicillin, discovered by Sir Alexander Fleming in 1928. Since then, more and more antibiotics have come into the market. Antibiotics act by killing bacteria or stopping them from multiplying. They can destroy bacteria's cell walls or DNA, which are vital for their survival, prevent the production of essential bacterial proteins, or interfere with bacterial reproduction. Antibiotics can be given through the mouth, intramuscular, intravenously, or topically. Similarly, antiviral, antifungal, and other antimicrobial drugs are being used.

However, antibiotics have to be used very judiciously as more and more bacteria are becoming resistant to them. In fact, **antibiotic resistance** is becoming a major problem worldwide.

Immunity: Simply put, immunity means the power to resist infection or illness. Humans have three types of immunity - innate, adaptive, and passive. The body has a complex network of cells, tissues, and organs that make up the **immune system.**

The immune system includes white blood cells and organs and tissues of the lymph system, such as the thymus, spleen, tonsils, lymph nodes, lymph vessels, and bone marrow.

Innate immunity: All humans are born with innate (or natural) immunity, a type of general protection, which is the body's first line of defense against harmful substances or agents. It is **nonspecific** present from birth and lasts throughout life. Elements of innate immunity include i) physical barriers – like skin, mucus membranes, stomach acid, etc. which prevent harmful substances or organisms from entering the body and ii) cells – like white blood cells (WBC) respond quickly to infection reach the site and mount an inflammatory response.

WBC produce cytokines to kill microbes. iii) proteins – like C reactive protein, interferon, and complement iv) Receptors – toll - like receptors and cell receptors initiate a signaling system. Innate immunity **acts very soon** – in minutes to hours.

Adaptive or active immunity: This is a delayed but very **specialized** response to a pathogenic infection. It works in tandem with players from the innate immune system. Once the body is exposed to an antigen, substance, or organism, it develops 'memory'. Now, when the body is re - exposed to the same antigen or organism, it mounts a quick, **specific** immune response to the offending agent.

This is done by

(i)   specific **antibody** production by B lymphocytes (a type of WBC) and,

(ii)   specifically primed T lymphocytes – **cell - mediated immunity**. This is the principle of action of **vaccines.**

Another type of immunity is **passive** when specific antibodies are provided from outside.

Prevention of Infections

Infections can be prevented in many ways. Firstly, it is important to understand how the infection spreads and therefore protect oneself.

For example, good personal and hand hygiene prevents fecal - oral route of infection, wearing a mask may prevent air borne and droplet infections and control of vectors would protect from vector borne infections like dengue.

Antiseptics & Disinfectants: These are chemical compounds (also called biocides) that kill or inhibit bacteria, viruses, and fungi. They are widely used to control infections. While antiseptics are used to kill organisms on the skin, disinfectants are used to kill germs on non - living surfaces and are generally in a more concentrated form. Examples of disinfectants are alcohol, formaldehyde, glutaraldehyde, chlorine and chlorine compounds, hydrogen peroxide, phenol, etc., used on non - living surfaces.

Examples of antiseptics are chlorine, iodine, and alcohol compounds used in proprietary preparations like Savlon, Dettol, Betadine, and sanitizers. Such substances should be used carefully as they may be flammable, and some may lead to an explosion if mixed.

Other ways of disinfection are cleansing, heating, boiling, sterilization, pasteurization, ultraviolet radiation, flushing, etc.

Vaccines: These are an important means of preventing specific infections. Vaccines are made of biological material. The first vaccine was tried by Dr. Edward Jenner, who found out that people infected with cowpox were immune to smallpox. Vaccines use the knowledge that if a host is exposed to antigenic material from a microorganism, **immune memory** is stimulated.

Now, when the same host is exposed to actual infection by the same agent, the body mounts a much stronger immune response and controls the infection.

Today, vaccines exist against a host of bacterial and viral infections, and more and more are being developed. Vaccines may be made from living but weakened (non - invasive) organisms or from dead (inactivated) organisms.

Newer technology like recombinant vaccines, conjugated vaccines, and mRNA vaccines is being used. The **Global Alliance for Vaccines and Immunization (GAVI)** is an initiative to increase equity in immunization between rich and poor countries of the world.

Autoimmunity – Sometimes the immune system actually attacks the body's own tissues and causes harm. Many diseases like rheumatic heart disease, systemic lupus erythematosus, dermatomyositis etc. are examples of autoimmune disorders. This topic is discussed in more detail under 'Rheumatism and rheumatic disorders'.

In conclusion, infections occur when harmful pathogens, such as bacteria, viruses, or fungi, enter and multiply within the body. The immune system, comprising white blood cells, antibodies, and other defenses, resists and fights off these invaders. A healthy immune system recognizes and eliminates pathogens, protecting against infection.

Factors like vaccination, nutrition, hygiene, and lifestyle habits strengthen immunity. Weakened immunity, due to age, underlying conditions, or certain treatments with immune - suppressive agents, increases infection risk. Effective immunity relies on **adaptive responses** (antibodies and T - cells), **innate barriers** (skin, mucous membranes), **immunization** (vaccines), **and healthy lifestyle choices (balanced diet, exercise, sleep, and a safe environment with quality air, water, food, sound,** and friendly people). Understanding infections and immunity empowers prevention and treatment strategies.

Chapter 15

Spurious Medicines, Expired, Scheduled & Generic Drugs

Learning Objectives:

- Identification of non-original drugs viz; counterfeit, fake, spurious drugs
- Provision of penalty for unauthorized production and sale of spurious drugs
- Expired drugs
- Essential drugs & scheduled drugs
- Branded and generic drugs

India is hailed as the '**pharmacy of the world**' as it has a booming pharmaceutical industry producing quality drugs at affordable prices. Over 100 years, India has emerged as a leading country in quickly adapting to innovative drug production to meet global health crises – as we saw the role played by India during the outbreak of pandemic of Covid - 19.

Drugs and medicines which can be procured without a doctor's prescription are called **Over the Counter (OTC)** medicines. However, like other low and middle - income countries (LMICs) many pharmacological companies are producing non - original/non - standard drugs and selling them in the market by hook or by crook.. There are many types of such medicines - fake drugs, counterfeit drugs and duplicate drugs, forged drugs and spurious drugs.

1. As in other countries, India has a National Regulatory Authority - the **Central Drug Standard Control Organization** (CDSCO) - which sets the rules and standards for the production and sale of medicines within the country. Pharmaceutical companies are licensed by CDSCO, although the regulations and licensing methods vary from country to country.

Medicines are produced in batches, with each package required to display a batch number. It is the responsibility of the licensing authority to conduct random checks on a few samples from each batch of medicines manufactured. The term "spurious medicine" is an umbrella term used to describe various types of non - standard drugs.

2. A product that does not contain the desired quantity of salt or compound, i.e., the absence of the active ingredient or its required amount, makes the drug entirely or partially "fake" and ineffective. For example, a drug claiming to contain paracetamol might only contain a few milligrams of harmless glucose powder without the actual active compound.

3. A fraudulent pharmaceutical manufacturer may replace high - quality salts with lower - quality, cheaper ones during drug production. This is often done by altering the types, valency, or chemical structure of the salts. The packaging and name of the product may closely resemble the drug prescribed by a physician or a standard - approved drug, allowing it to be sold under the guise of the original prescribed medicine. Such drugs are often substandard and have not undergone the rigorous quality checks required. As a result, consumers are deceived because the efficacy of the drug is not guaranteed. The packaging and labeling of these medicines are usually inferior. For instance, the spelling on the wrapper may be subtly altered to resemble popular "over the counter" items.

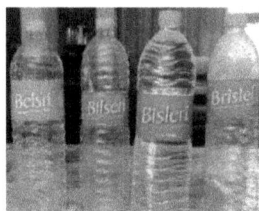

For example, "Crocin," "Disprin," or "Benadryl cough syrup" might be sold as "Crocxin," "Dicprin," or "Banradryl." If one carefully examines and compares the labels, the difference becomes apparent. The fraudulent manufacturer gains short - term profits from such practices. Imitation or forgery is always punishable by law. In some cases, the product may contain the actual active ingredient, but the labels merely resemble the original medicine. Such drugs are often referred to as "imitated" or "duplicate" medicines. Consumers are advised to verify the authenticity of the product with their physician. This practice is not only common in the marketing of medicines but also in cosmetics, fashion, and other consumer items. Only a few consumers are able to detect these counterfeits.

4. When a manufacturer duplicates a popular and frequently sold brand without possessing the necessary license and copyright for that brand and sells the product in the market looking almost identical to the standardized brand, it is considered fraud. This practice is deceptive, and even if the content and ingredients are equal in quality, quantity, and efficacy, it is not an ethically justifiable market practice. Additionally, these products are not tested by drug control authorities, allowing them to enter the market through illegitimate means.

5. If a patient consumes spurious drugs, they may experience unexplained side effects or allergic reactions. Medicines, in addition to the active ingredient, also contain preservatives and fillers.

    Proper manufacturing, handling, packaging, and transportation of medicine must always be adhered to. Certain doses are carefully calculated to account for residuals during the transfer of medicine from vials to syringes. Extra measures are taken to compensate for diminished potency during the shelf life of the product. These stringent checks and balances are integral to good manufacturing and selling practices. However, fraudulent manufacturers often evade these ethical standards, using various shortcuts to earn significant profits.

Essential Drug List – the World Health Organization (WHO) issues recommendations on the essential drugs every two years. National experts deliberate on this and finalize the list for their country.

Regulations on Life - saving Drugs – The erroneous or wrongful use of certain life - saving drugs, such as those used for heart attacks, heart failure, or shock, can be life - threatening. According to directives from the WHO, these life - saving drugs are strictly permitted to be sold only with a prescription. They are prohibited from being sold in retail as individual tablets by cutting the wrapper. If such medicines are sold this way, without their full name, strength, and identification clearly visible, they may be wrongly administered to the patient. Legal actions may be taken against the piecemeal sale of such drugs.

Scheduled Drugs - The Drugs and Cosmetics Rules (India), 1945 classify drugs under several schedules and outline the guidelines for their storage, display, prescription, and sale.

For example, Schedule G drugs are hormonal preparations, and scheduler X drugs are addictive substances. Besides, about 70 drugs and fixed dose combinations are banned in India, the latest addition to this list being anti - cough preparations for children under 5 - year - old.

Expired Drugs – If the expiry date on the drug wrapper has passed, the drug typically will not become harmful if used - at least if the color of the pills or syrup has not changed. However, the potency of such medicines may be reduced due to poor storage, making them less effective. Expired injectables and life - saving drugs should not be used under any circumstances.

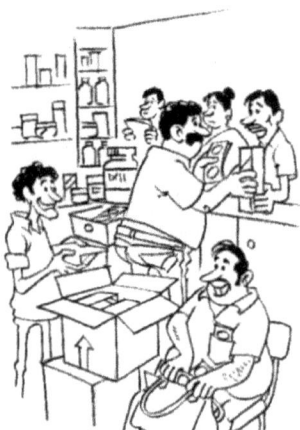

Generic Medicines – A generic drug is a medication created to have the same quality, safety, dosage, strength, intended use, form, route of administration, effects, and side effects as branded drugs. According to the FDA, generic drugs are just as effective as their branded counterparts. Generic drugs typically cost 30% - 80% less than branded drugs. Large pharmaceutical companies spend many years in research and development of new drugs and getting them approved by regulatory authorities.

Randomized clinical trials of new drugs are extremely expensive to conduct. Similarly, big pharmaceutical companies purchase copyrights for medicines produced by pharmaceutical scientists and drug designers. They hold the patent for the manufacture and sale of these drugs for a finite number of years (17 years in the U.S.). In most cases, generic products become available after the patent protections afforded to the drug's original developer expire. Before this time, the invented branded drugs cannot be made, used, distributed, imported, or sold by others without the patent owner's consent.

After the patent period expires, the drug formula may be used by other companies. The manufacture of the drug no longer requires preclinical/clinical trials and repeat testing in animals, which is time -

consuming, because the branded versions have already been tested and approved for efficacy and safety. Once the patent period ends, the non - branded generic versions enter the market, leading to competition that typically lowers prices for both the original branded drugs and their generic equivalents. The manufacturers of generic drugs do not have to undergo clinical or market studies and simply conduct a laboratory test of the genuine ingredients.

The generic drug must have the same active ingredients and in the same amount as the original or branded version. However, the other ingredients in the pill, such as fillers (inactive substances used to fill pills or capsules for easier handling), can differ. The appearance of generic drugs may vary with different manufacturers, but this should not or does not affect the effectiveness or safety of the drugs. Similarly, changes in the fillers do not impact the drug's effectiveness. Some doctors are hesitant to rely on the efficacy of generic drugs and refrain from prescribing them, but this concern is often unfounded. Frequently, the same drugs, with nearly identical formulas, are manufactured using innovative processes and undergo nominal testing for chemical and pharmacological similarity.

When prescribing, doctors typically use the name of the salt, not the brand. For instance, a doctor might prescribe Cefixime instead of a brand name like Mahacef or Taxim O. Generic medicines usually do not come as mixtures of two salts or in combination with other drugs. Generic drugs are available at a lower cost - typically 30 - 80% cheaper than branded versions - thereby reducing drug expenditures. However, there are critical factors that must be safeguarded, such as the purity, potency, stability, and release of the drug inside the body.

In 2008, the Government of India, through the Department of Pharmaceuticals, launched a new initiative called 'Jan Aushadhi' or 'medicines for people.' This program makes unbranded quality medicines available to the poor at reasonable prices through government - supported retail outlets. The *'Jan Aushadhi Kendras'* sell only generic - name medicines to the extent possible.

Trust in generic medicines evolves over time, and the efficacy of these medicines is proven when modern medical practitioners readily prescribe them, and patients show sustained response and satisfaction.

The National Medical Commission (NMC) recently issued guidelines requiring doctors to prescribe only generic medicines. However, several medical associations have expressed concerns, and the requirement for all doctors to prescribe only generic medicines is currently under review.

Modern medicines undergo stringent good manufacturing practices. The ingredients of these medicines have been tested and verified by large randomized clinical trials. When more than one pharmaceutical company produces the same medicine, the ingredients must be exactly similar and equivalent. To ensure safe delivery to the end user, security packaging and hologram identification are also used.

However, such manufacturing practices may not always be followed in traditional medicines. In traditional medicines, there is no standardized parameter for testing or validating the ingredients of the drugs, and the same preparation from two manufacturers may not be equivalent.

In conclusion, fraudulent practices are common in the production and marketing of many products we use daily, and medicines are no exception. Just as we verify and validate other consumer goods, we must learn how to identify effective medicines. We can seek assistance from our consulting physicians and knowledgeable friends to ensure the authenticity of the medicines we purchase.

It is important to demand a detailed bill or receipt when buying medicines so that, in the case of counterfeit or spurious drugs, we can file a complaint. All citizens should report such incidents to the appropriate authorities to seek redressal and ensure that violators are punished.

Chapter 16

Evidence - Based Medicine & Randomized Trials

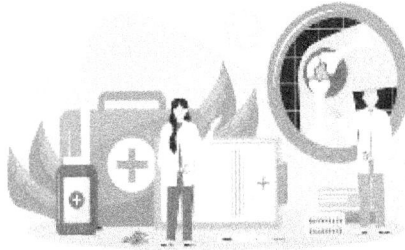

Learning Objectives:

- Need for medical treatment based on scientific evidence
- Efficiency and efficacy of medicines developed after **randomized controlled trials**
- Evidence-based diagnosis, clinic practice, cafeteria approach treatment
- Utility of evidence produced by Laboratory Tests
- Concept of risk factors and prognostic factors

In earlier times, doctors relied on their own intuition and exploration of diseases to carry out treatment. This approach, known as the subjective method, involves understanding symptoms and diseases based on personal judgment. However, this method had its limitations, as **biases** could influence the inquiry. In contrast, modern medicine is grounded in scientific evidence, validated through rigorous experimentation.

In the late 19th century, the values and priorities of patients began to be considered more critically in the diagnosis and treatment of diseases.

Pioneers such as **Dr. David Sackett** and **Dr. Gordon Guyatt** are renowned for their contributions to clinical research methodology. As the era of Renaissance and modern discoveries unfolded, medical professionals began conducting research to create objective evidence supporting the efficacy of treatments. This shift marked a significant move towards basing clinical practice on solid scientific evidence.

Today, modern physicians strive to base their diagnoses and treatments on the **best available evidence**, a practice known as evidence - based medicine (**EBM**). EBM involves using objective, scientifically validated evidence to guide patient care. The application of EBM in treatment is clarified through several key variables, ensuring that patient care adheres to the highest standards of scientific rigor.

1	Best evidence of effectiveness through clinical trials and consensus thereof	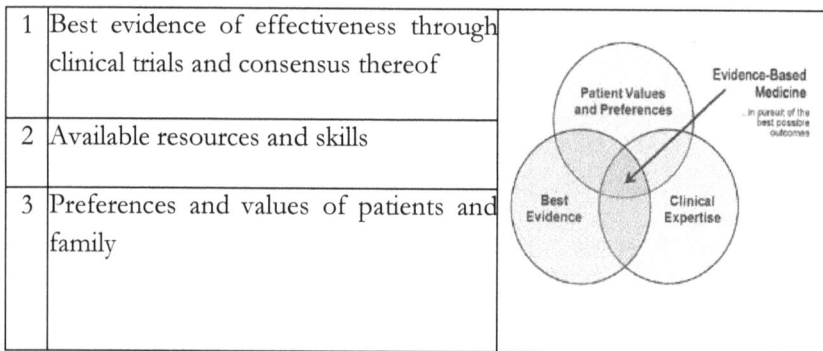
2	Available resources and skills	
3	Preferences and values of patients and family	

Sometimes, in the absence of sufficient evidence, empirical treatment may be recommended based on a physician's experience and the resources available.

Drug Research & Development

When a new drug is discovered whether by chance or through deliberate efforts by a chemist or pharmaceutical researcher, it undergoes a thorough examination to determine its suitability as a pharmaceutical product.

This process includes studying the drug's **pharmacokinetics** - its dosage, route of administration, and eventual clearance (excretion) from the body. This initial step is conducted in a laboratory setting by chemists or pharmaceutical scientists.

Following this, the drug enters the preclinical research phase, where it is tested on laboratory animals to evaluate its safety and efficacy.

For a new drug to be applicable to human use, its effectiveness and safety must be demonstrated through clinical trials involving human subjects. After successful testing in laboratory animals, the drug progresses to clinical trials, where its use in humans is carefully monitored and evaluated. This transition from laboratory research to practical application in patient care is often referred to as "from bench to bedside."

There are 4 phases of human Clinical Trials:

- **Phase 1**: First testing in humans, primarily to test **safety**. A drug is given to a small number of volunteers who are closely monitored for any side effects,

- **Phase 2**: Testing in a small number of patients to assess safety, monitor how a drug is metabolized, and to gather initial data on efficacy and doses,

- **Phase 3**: A large trial in patients to test efficacy and safety. This is the stage of a **randomized controlled clinical trial (RCT)**. Pivotal phase 3 trials (or registered trials) provide the key data on **efficacy** in submissions for regulatory approval,

- **Phase 4:** Studies undertaken after a drug has been licensed (post marketing) to gather further safety, efficacy, **or effectiveness data** in routine clinical use.

Decades may pass before a single molecule is proven safe and effective enough to be prescribed as a pharmaceutical drug. This lengthy process underscores the importance of upholding ethical standards and ensuring that no harm comes to any human or animal during research and development.

Methodology of Randomized Controlled Trials (RCTs)

In modern medicine, drugs are approved for market use only after they have successfully passed the rigorous testing process of randomized controlled trials (RCTs).

Human trials are inherently complex, and the efficacy of a drug is always assessed by **comparison with a control group**.

The control group receives a **placebo** - a 'dummy' substance that resembles the drug in appearance but lacks the active ingredient.

To avoid **subjective bias**, where the researcher's expectations could influence the outcomes, it is essential that the researchers remain unaware of whether the participants are receiving the actual drug or a placebo. This is particularly crucial because the **researcher's biases could lead to a perceived or exaggerated effect**. Additionally, differences among participants could skew results either in favor of or against the drug's efficacy.

To address these challenges, the **process of randomization** is employed. Participants are randomly assigned to one of two groups, known as "arms" - the intervention group and the control group. The intervention group receives the drug, while the control group either receives no treatment or a placebo. The assignment to each group is determined by a random number table, ensuring that the **researcher has no control over which participant receives the drug or placebo.**

Participants are closely monitored, and outcomes are meticulously documented. The results from the intervention group are then compared statistically with those from the control group. In some trials, both the researchers and participants are **blinded** to whether they are receiving the drug or placebo - a process known as **double - blinding**. This additional layer of blinding, often managed by a third party, further reduces bias. Trials that incorporate this approach are referred to as randomized, double - blind, placebo - controlled trials.

While almost all forms of therapy can be tested through RCTs, blinding may not be feasible in all cases. For example, large - scale treatment strategies or vaccination programs are often tested through Field Trials, where the outcome of events is measured in broader community settings.

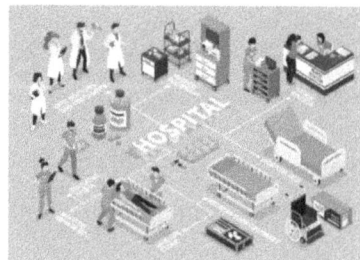

During the trial period, drugs are rigorously tested for all types of side effects, and any adverse effects must be meticulously recorded and compared. The Randomized Controlled Trial (RCT) is considered the "**Gold Standard**" for assessing the efficacy of a treatment. Such trials represent the highest form of scientific evidence in clinical research, offering a robust methodology through which drugs and treatments are audited and evaluated by third parties or specialists without bias, prejudice, or predisposition.

A newly developed drug or a variant of an existing drug group is also tested through RCTs to determine its efficacy, equivalence, or superiority over existing molecules. Simultaneously, the drug's safety profile and side effects are documented. Conducting RCTs has become a specialization in itself, with dedicated courses available for learning how to properly conduct these trials. Experts are often hired to oversee large - scale randomized controlled clinical trials or field trials.

Despite the rigorous standards set by RCTs, some experienced and skilled doctors refute the utility and efficacy of Evidence - Based Medicine (EBM). These practitioners argue, often based on fallacious logic, that the compilation of evidence is time - consuming and unnecessary.

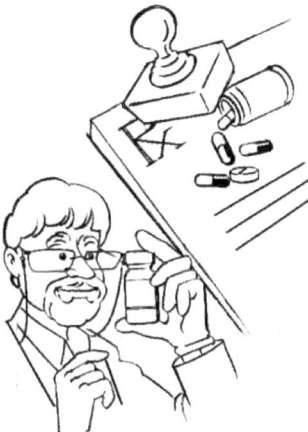

In contrast to the stringent requirements of modern scientific methods, "old wives' remedies" or home remedies are often recommended based on anecdotes or stories passed down through generations.

These remedies are frequently accepted as effective simply because improvement occurred **after** their use. However, it is important to recognize that time is often the greatest healer, and many chronic diseases have a relapsing and remitting course. RCTs address these types of confounding factors by incorporating a control group for comparison.

Sometimes, drugs developed for a specific disease through randomized trials may need to be repurposed for efficacy in other conditions.

In such cases, the drug must undergo RCTs once again, with clinical reports from doctors necessary for further validation. The effectiveness of any drug is further confirmed through long - term usage after it enters the market. This ongoing evaluation process is known as a **Phase 4 Trial**, which monitors the drug's performance in society. Occasionally, licenses for emergency use are granted, as happened with various vaccines during the coronavirus pandemic.

In summary, the rigorous scientific process that each modern (scientific) medicine undergoes before approval is extensive. It often requires several years - if not decades - to bring a drug from initial discovery to market, ensuring that its validity and safety are well - established.

Evidence - Based Treatment in Surgery

Surgical procedures and the adoption of new surgical equipment often cannot undergo the same meticulous scrutiny as randomized controlled trials (RCTs) due to the practical and ethical challenges involved. The efficacy of new surgical technologies and procedures is typically established gradually within the professional community, as older - generation surgeons may not be as skilled in using them. Data and outcomes from new surgical procedures become more widely accepted after extensive use and peer review. Initially, these procedures gain evidence of efficacy through case - series analyses, and randomized trials comparing old and new surgical methods, if feasible, may be conducted later.

Take, for example, the introduction of robotic surgery for common procedures like gallbladder removal (cholecystectomy), hernia repair, and uterus removal (hysterectomy). Robotic surgery, while innovative, is expensive and was initially adopted by certain enthusiasts without substantial primary data or large case series. In some instances, start - up technologies gain popularity even without RCTs or extensive published data. Robotic surgery has shown clear superiority in prostate cancer treatment, but it is time and future trials that ultimately establish the utility of new technologies across various aspects. There is a saying, "*You get the treatment at the door you enter...*" This means that a visit to an Ayurvedic doctor will likely result in Ayurvedic medicines being prescribed, while a modern doctor may recommend investigations and prescribe contemporary medications.

Consider a cardiac patient diagnosed with coronary artery disease. A cardiologist might recommend treatment with several drugs and a restricted lifestyle, while a cardiac surgeon might suggest surgery to improve the patient's quality of life through specific surgical interventions. In such cases, there is often no clear evidence as to which treatment is more effective or justifiable. Two equally qualified and reputed physicians may offer different opinions, each based on their assessment and experiences, leaving the patient confused by the opposing viewpoints.

Published evidence from RCTs may be interpreted differently by physicians, who might tailor the information to support what they believe is the most appropriate intervention. Financial considerations also play a role. Some doctors may present the patient with a range of options - a "**menu**" or "**cafeteria approach**" to treatment. Similarly, in breast cancer treatment, a woman may be given the choice between undergoing a mastectomy (complete breast removal) or opting for breast conservation surgery followed by radiotherapy. While the latter offers the advantage of preserving the breast, it typically involves a more prolonged and costly treatment process. In such cases, the decision may depend on how much value the woman places on cosmetic outcomes, her financial situation, and her personal values regarding breast restoration.

In summary, while evidence - based medicine remains the gold standard, surgical decisions often require a blend of clinical evidence, physician experience, patient values, and practical considerations. As surgical technology evolves, so too does the need for ongoing research and trials to guide best practices and ensure that patients receive the most effective and appropriate care.

Evidence Generated by Tests

In clinical practice, alongside history - taking and physical examination, various tests are conducted to diagnose and monitor diseases. These include laboratory tests on blood and other body fluids, as well as advanced imaging modalities like X - rays, ultrasound, echocardiography, CT scans, MRI, and PET scans. Additional tests assess electrical activity, such as ECG and EEG, while others involve microscopic examination of biopsied tissues (histology).

The diagnostic accuracy of new tests - measured by their **sensitivity, specificity, positive and negative predictive values, and likelihood ratios** - are emerging parameters that help determine the utility of these diagnostic tools.

Disease Causation

For many diseases, the exact cause remains unknown. Modern medicine acknowledges this and actively seeks to understand the origins of illnesses. It is well recognized that most diseases result from a **complex interplay of factors**, making them **multifactorial**. Diseases may have both genetic and environmental causes, and these contributing factors are termed '**risk factors.**' Modern clinical research employs scientific procedures and epidemiological methods to gather evidence about disease causation. The strength of association between various predisposing risk factors and disease occurrence is then calculated through statistical analysis.

Prognosis

The natural course of a disease provides insight into its likely 'future outcome.' Various factors, known as **prognostic factors**, influence disease prognosis. The strength of association between these factors and disease outcomes can be clarified through clinical research. Additionally, certain proteins, or 'markers,' can be tested in the blood to help diagnose, monitor treatment, and predict outcomes. These are referred to as biomarkers and, in the case of cancers, tumor markers.

Utility of Evidence - Based Medicine in the Development of Traditional Medical Systems

The effectiveness of traditional medical systems such as *Ayurveda*, Yoga, Siddha, Homeopathy, and Naturopathy can be validated if these systems also undergo the rigorous testing of randomized controlled trials (RCTs). The Government of India is actively promoting these traditional systems and aims to integrate their medicines into mainstream healthcare. To support this initiative, institutes like the *Ayurveda* Education and Research Institute in Jamnagar, Gujarat, and the *Ayurveda* National Research Institute in Jaipur, Rajasthan, have been established.

The *AYUSH* Ministry has issued directives for testing both traditional and new *AYUSH* drugs using evidence - based methodologies, an initiative supported by the World Health Organization (WHO). Consequently, it is now mandatory for *AYUSH* drugs to undergo RCTs. However, conducting randomized trials is challenging - they are labor - intensive procedures involving third - party auditing of adverse side effects, blinding of participating doctors and patients, data monitoring committees, and peer review before publishing results. These trials are expensive and time - consuming, often taking years to complete for a single agent.

Unfortunately, the term **'evidence - based medicine'** has been co - opted by some *AYUSH* manufacturers to advertise their products, even when these products may not have undergone RCTs and may not adhere to good manufacturing, packaging, and transportation practices.

In conclusion, the randomized controlled trial is the **gold standard** scientific technique that has proven invaluable in safeguarding human health against fatal diseases. Today, public health, social medicine, and community medicine are practiced worldwide based on evidence - based scientific knowledge. Medical ethics dictate that practitioners should base their treatment on the principles of evidence - based medicine. If a patient does not benefit, they should at least be spared from harm. Implementing evidence - based medicine in its true sense ensures that all patients receive quality treatment.

Chapter 17

Burden of Diseases, Causes of Death, Triple Burden and DALYs

Triple burden – Incidents of Death

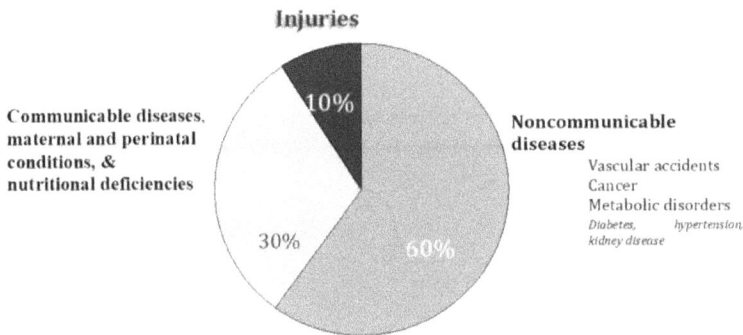

Injuries

Communicable diseases, maternal and perinatal conditions, & nutritional deficiencies

10%

30%

60%

Noncommunicable diseases
Vascular accidents
Cancer
Metabolic disorders
Diabetes,   hypertension,
kidney disease

Learning Objectives:

- Understanding 'burden' of disease
- 3 groups of diseases – the 'triple burden' and reasons for their occurrence
- Occurrence of disease – sporadic, endemic, epidemic and pandemic
- Global Burden of Diseases (GBD) and DALY
- Epidemiologic transition

At the turn of the 20th century, before and during the First World War, outbreaks of communicable diseases such as plague, influenza, and the Spanish flu devastated society, causing widespread suffering.

The subsequent world wars brought further irreparable loss, with millions of young lives lost or disabled.

The horrors of cruelty and genocide, particularly against Jews, reached their peak during this time. The climax of this destruction was the atomic bombings of Hiroshima and Nagasaki, which left lasting scars on humanity.

During this period, life expectancy across the globe was low, and death rates were high.

After the end of the Second World War, the major nations of the world called for introspection and "healing." This led to the formation of the United Nations Organization (UNO) in 1948. One of the key achievements of the UNO was the **Universal Declaration of Human Rights in 1948,** which upheld the dignity of every human being.

Human development was placed at the forefront of global priorities. Over time, with advancements in science and medicine, there has been a steady increase in life expectancy worldwide. In India, for instance, life expectancy at birth rose from 32 years in 1947 to 70 years in 2022.

However, the situation still varies significantly across countries depending on their level of development.

In public health, understanding "What are people dying from?" is crucial. This knowledge allows for a focus on the most significant causes of death, enabling the development of strategies to save lives. Diseases are generally categorized into two major groups: communicable and non - communicable.

Communicable diseases are those that can be transmitted from one person to another, often referred to as infectious illnesses. These diseases are caused by infectious agents or microscopic organisms, such as bacteria, viruses, protozoa, metazoa, rickettsiae, and fungi, which are abundant in our environment and in infected individuals.

Examples of communicable diseases include tuberculosis, malaria, plague, smallpox, chickenpox, measles, pneumonia, diarrhea, HIV/AIDS, the common cold, and COVID - 19. These infectious agents can be spread through various means, including contaminated food, water, droplets, air, hands, fomites (inanimate objects that can carry infection), sexual contact, animals, and insects or arthropods. During medieval times, these diseases were the major cause of untimely death.

However, in the 20th century, humanity found cures for many of these diseases through the development of antimicrobials, vaccination, and improved sanitation. While there has been a global reduction in these diseases, they continue to pose challenges in Low and Middle - Income Countries (LMICs).

Non - communicable diseases (NCDs), on the other hand, are those that do not spread from person to person. The major NCDs include cardiovascular diseases, cancer, chronic lung or respiratory disorders, mental health issues, diabetes, and kidney disorders. Cardiovascular diseases, primarily caused by the deposition of **atherosclerotic plaques** in the arteries of the heart and brain, lead to heart attacks and strokes, respectively. Atherosclerosis is a process that typically progresses with age but is accelerated by factors such as an unhealthy (sedentary) lifestyle, poor diet, diabetes, obesity, and high blood pressure. Cancer, often regarded as a scourge of modern times, is increasing both in actual cases and in recognition due to better diagnostics. It is characterized by the uncontrolled growth of cells and can originate from any tissue in the body. While the causes and risk factors for some cancers, such as lung, breast, blood, mouth, cervix, and prostate cancers, are known, the causes remain unknown for the majority of cancers. Early detection and treatment can make many cancers curable.

Top 10 global causes of death and disability in 2019

1. Cardiovascular or heart disease – 16%

2. Stroke 11%

3. Chronic obstructive pulmonary disease - 6%

4. Lower respiratory infections

5. Neonatal conditions - birth asphyxia, birth trauma, neonatal sepsis and infections, and preterm birth complications – reduced but still important

6. Trachea, bronchus, lung cancers

7. Alzheimer's disease and other dementias – have come into the top 10

8. Diarrheal diseases – This has greatly reduced in the last 2 decades

9. Diabetes mellitus – has come into the top 10 in the last decade

10. Kidney diseases

It is seen that seven of the ten leading causes of deaths in 2019 at the global level were noncommunicable diseases. These seven causes accounted for 44% of all deaths or 80% of the top 10. However, all noncommunicable diseases together accounted for 74% of deaths globally in 2019 and 80% in developed countries.

The burden of a given disease or health problem in a society, country, or region is its **impact** on the population. This impact is measured using indicators such as morbidity, mortality, and financial cost.

The Global Burden of Disease (GBD) Study, initiated in 1990 under the leadership of Dr. Christopher Murray from the USA, aimed to assess the rates of mortality and disability from major diseases, injuries, and risk factors across different regions worldwide. This comprehensive study involved collaboration among over 3,600 researchers from 145 countries. The 2003 results highlighted significant disparities in the causes of untimely death and disability across various regions, with Sub - Saharan Africa and the Indian subcontinent bearing the highest burden of disease.

The study introduced the concept of **Disability - Adjusted Life Years (DALY)**, emphasizing that individuals may survive mortality but continue to live with a disability. The impact of the disease is thus a combination of morbidity and mortality. The impact of mortality is measured as Years of Life Lost (**YLL**), calculated as the difference between life expectancy and the average age of death due to a particular disease.

The impact of morbidity is measured as Years Lived with Disability (**YLD**), which is calculated as the number of new cases multiplied by the disability weight (**DW**) and the average number of years lived with the disease before death or remission. The disability weight is assigned to each disease or disability as a fraction of complete health.

The formula for DALY is: **DALY = YLL + YLD**

The study identified the major causes of disease burden, now categorized into three groups known as the '**triple burden**.' Understanding these causes of death and disability is crucial for implementing preventive measures, improving healthcare, allocating resources effectively, and developing relevant technologies to save lives and minimize disability.

The pattern of diseases varies significantly across different nations, depending on their level of development.

Group 1: Communicable Diseases, Nutritional Disorders, and Reproductive and Child Health Disorders

Group 1 encompasses communicable (infectious) diseases as well as disorders related to nutrition, reproduction, and child health. While disorders of nutrition, reproduction, and child health are not communicable diseases, they are included in this group because they are **largely preventable** and closely tied to the health infrastructure and services of a country. Despite ongoing global efforts to combat communicable diseases, they continue to pose significant challenges, particularly in low and middle - income countries (**LMICs**).

When any disease or event occurs randomly without any specific pattern, it is said to be **sporadic**. When it remains present in a specific locale throughout the year, affecting a small portion of the population, it is referred to as **endemic**. If an infectious or communicable disease begins affecting over 4% of the population, it is classified as an **epidemic**.

However, when such a disease transcends national borders and spreads across multiple countries, it is termed a **pandemic,** as happened with Coronavirus.

In some developing countries in Asia and Africa, 60% to 70% of deaths are attributed to communicable diseases. Neonates and infants worldwide often succumb to pneumonia, diarrhea, measles, and malnutrition.

According to a 2008 report published by the World Health Organization (**WHO**), 32% of all deaths globally, or approximately 13 million deaths, were caused by diseases in this group. The spread of communicable diseases can be mitigated through preventive measures such as mass vaccination programs, ensuring the availability of clean drinking water, safe waste disposal, maintaining hygiene in food and eating habits, and reducing the environmental pollution. Additionally, good nutrition plays a crucial role in preventing deaths due to infection, as malnutrition exacerbates the mortality due to infectious diseases.

In contrast, developed countries in America and Europe have significantly reduced deaths caused by infections, nutritional disorders, and inadequate maternal and child healthcare. These reductions have been achieved through poverty alleviation, excellent healthcare services, robust healthcare infrastructure, and widespread health education.

Group 2: Noncommunicable Diseases (NCDs)

As already stated, noncommunicable diseases (NCDs) include cardiovascular diseases, strokes, cancer, diabetes, and chronic respiratory and mental illnesses. Unlike communicable diseases, NCDs are not spread through infections or contact with others. Instead, they are typically caused by unhealthy behaviors, familial or genetic factors, and environmental exposures. Unlike epidemics, NCDs do not affect entire societies at once, though their prevalence can be high in certain populations. With the control of infectious diseases, NCDs have become the leading causes of death globally, accounting for 30 to 40 million deaths per year.

In modern times, NCDs present a significant threat to global health, imposing a substantial socio - economic burden on both developed and developing countries. In India, NCDs are responsible for 40% to 60% of all deaths, leading to approximately 15 million untimely deaths each year.

Diabetes, a major NCD, has affected large populations worldwide, with the number of people affected projected to increase from 200 million in 2003 to 330 million by 2030.

Cancer is gaining increasing attention in the modern era. Its rise is both real and apparent, as it is now more frequently recognized and diagnosed. Cancer is caused by the uncontrolled growth of cells in specific organs or tissues of the body.

It is primarily due to genetic predisposition, which is occasionally inherited, and environmental factors such as chronic irritation, radiation, and infections like HIV and hepatitis B.

While the causes and risks of some cancers are known, many remain unidentified. Important cancers include those of the lung, breast, blood, mouth, cervix, and prostate. Early detection and treatment can make many cancers curable.

NCDs are largely driven by economic and behavioral factors. For example, a **sedentary lifestyle** devoid of physical exercise and **unhealthy eating habits**, such as consuming refined flour, excessive sugar, sweets, soft drinks, and oily foods, contribute significantly to the occurrence of NCDs.

Urbanization, industrialization, exposure to carcinogenic substances (such as lead, chromium, acids, radium, uranium, and thorium) in industrial workplaces, pollution in water, air, and noise, and substance abuse (including tobacco, alcohol, cannabis, cocaine, and other drugs) among adolescents and youth are also key contributors.

These factors impose a heavy burden on financial resources and hinder all - round development.

According to the World Health Organization (WHO, 2023), NCDs are responsible for 74% of all deaths globally, with 77% of these deaths occurring in low and middle - income countries (LMICs). Cardiovascular diseases account for most NCD deaths, followed by cancers, chronic respiratory diseases, and diabetes (including kidney disease caused by diabetes). These four groups of diseases account for over 80% of all premature NCD deaths.

Group 3: Injuries, Accidents, and Violence

In Group 3, injuries, road traffic accidents, violence, war, homicide, and suicide are included. Among these, road traffic accidents are the most common cause of mortality. During wartime, large numbers of young men lose their lives in a short period. Accidents frequently affect men on the road, but domestic accidents, such as accidental burns suffered by women working in kitchens, are also common. Additionally, industrial accidents, building construction mishaps, agricultural incidents, and sports - related injuries are daily occurrences. Although stringent preventive measures and good practices are mandated in industries and construction sites, better implementation is necessary to prevent accidents and minimize injuries.

In sports, protective gear and adherence to rules are crucial to preventing injuries. Falls are a common mode of injury, with children falling from heights while playing on stairs and terraces and the elderly slipping in bathrooms. Proper fencing on terraces is essential to prevent falls in children.

Accidents in nuclear plants can cause grievous injuries to human and animal populations in contaminated regions, leading to death, respiratory diseases, cancer, and long - term morbidities. Similarly, incidents such as poisonous gas leaks or spills of toxic fluids like acid and oil can affect a large number of human, animal, or marine lives. These situations require stringent regulations and regular drills to prevent and combat such disasters.

Fire accidents are a significant concern both at home and in workplaces. Mandatory fire - fighting infrastructure and readiness in places like airports, industries, and during large gatherings is essential. Firefighting equipment and chemicals are continuously researched, developed, and upgraded.

Public spaces, businesses, hospitals, airports, etc., must follow stringent measures to prevent fire accidents, build escape routes, install on - site firefighting equipment, and conduct regular drills.

Drowning accidents can be prevented by providing anti - drowning gear, trained swimmers, speed boats, and watchtowers. Several accidents also occur due to animal bites, especially for those who travel in wilderness areas. Providing protective gear and training is crucial for their safety.

Smart telecommunication and flying doctors provide resources, help, and evacuation during such disasters. It is noteworthy that while injuries account for only 8 - 12% of the total deaths in society, they predominantly affect young people - those on the roads, fighting in wars, working at construction and industrial sites, young women in kitchens, and those engaging in outdoor activities like picnics and adventure rides.

Over 1.5 lakh people in India are killed yearly in road traffic accidents alone, with 60% of them between 18 - 35 years old. The lives of the younger generation are the treasure of society, and the loss of such precious lives due to accidents is an irreparable cultural and economic loss.

Societies that fail to frame and implement stringent regulations to prevent accidents and injuries suffer greatly, both culturally and economically.

Epidemiologic Transition – In the past, infectious diseases dominated in most countries. But death rates from infectious diseases have fallen quickly in the past 100 years – faster than other causes. Similarly, hunger and famine no longer kill people. Nutritional standards have gone up.

Mother and childcare have reduced maternal and neonatal mortality. This is a shift from one phase to another phase determining the leading causes of death. Now, non - communicable diseases – such as heart diseases, respiratory diseases, mental conditions, and cancers, are the most common causes of death globally. **As a country develops and becomes affluent, the pattern of disease changes.**

The transition took place from group 1 diseases to group 2 and 3 diseases - this is known as 'epidemiologic transition.'

Triple Burden in India: About three - quarters of deaths and DALYs occur in rural areas. More than a third of national DALYs arose from communicable, maternal, perinatal, and nutritional disorders.

Cardiovascular (heart) disease accounts for about 60% of deaths. The prevalence of diabetes and its complications and childhood malnutrition is particularly high in India. Both these contribute to death from other causes. Children in India suffer from a triple burden of malnutrition – undernutrition, overnutrition or obesity, and micronutrient deficiency.

Top causes of deaths in India – GBD 2016

1. **Heart (cardiovascular) disease** – For more than 2 decades, heart disease has remained the leading cause of death In India. Risk factors are metabolic syndrome, unhealthy diets, inactivity, obesity, high blood pressure, and smoking.

2. **Chronic lung disease** – Chronic exposure to **air pollution** has its toll on lung health. Air pollution is a major health problem in cities in India. Various state governments are doing their level best to control this menace.

3. **Diarrhea** – Addition of Rotavirus vaccine to India's universal vaccination program in 2016 to protect children against the leading cause of severe diarrhea in young children, helped lower numbers rapidly. Deaths due to diarrhea are rapidly declining.

4. **Stroke** was ranked as the 6th biggest killer in 2005 and rose to become the 4th in 2016 in India. The risk factors for stroke are the same as heart disease, but stroke is often more disabling because it may cause paralysis

5. **Lower respiratory infections** – These are caused by large number of microbes, including Coronavirus. They are a killer in both young children and the elderly.

6. **Tuberculosis** – India accounts for more than a fourth of new tuberculosis (TB) cases globally. India's national program provides free medicines and treatment to all, but a major obstacle to eradication is that many patients do not complete the treatment.

7. **Neonatal preterm birth** – With 80.8% of India's annual births taking place in health institutions, deaths from premature birth - related complications had dropped since 2005 when it was the 4th cause of death.

8. **Self - harm or suicide** – They are now India's 8th biggest killer, climbing up two places from the 10th leading cause of death in 2005.

9. **Road injuries** – Deaths from road traffic accidents have risen over the last two decades. States that showed the sharpest increase were Kerala, Uttar Pradesh, and Chhattisgarh.

10. **Other neonatal conditions** – Breastfeeding, vaccination against common infections, and neonatal care are helping more babies thrive and survive neonatal infections such as septicemia, birth asphyxia, and birth trauma.

Chapter 18

Health Seeking Behavior

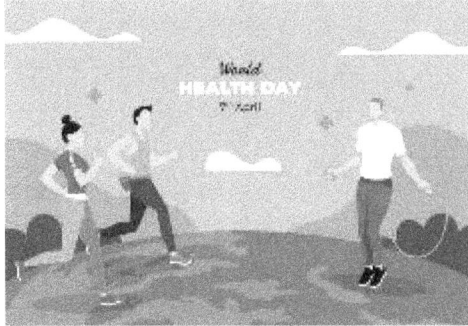

Learning Objectives:

- Meaning of Health Seeking Behavior
- Tenets of Health Seeking Behavior
- Preventing accidents
- Abstaining from substance abuse
- Seeking health care and complying with treatment
- Postulations of health-seeking behavior

While we may know what is good for our health, as humans, we often struggle to adopt the right attitudes and actions to maintain and promote it. Hygiene and health are learned behaviors. One may be born healthy, but staying healthy requires knowledge and wisdom. The foundation of any health system lies in the value system of a society. Without instilling health - related values in the community, we risk developing harmful habits and attitudes, making us more susceptible to diseases.

For example, smoking cigarettes or pipes was once considered a sign of sophistication in the 1950s. Today, however, society has largely rejected this habit, and smokers have to smoke in private.

A health - promoting behavior involves avoiding activities that could harm our well - being, such as smoking. Health norms vary according to religious customs, traditions, and the regional or national environment. Some health - related values are passed down from older generations, serving as a valuable legacy from our ancestors. Conversely, if we fail to recognize and uphold the principles of health - seeking behavior, it is often condemned as "**illness - breeding behavior**" or "**health - risk taking behavior.**" Therefore, it is crucial to identify and embrace behaviors that promote health to ensure a healthier society.

Tenets of Health seeking behavior:

1. **Hygiene** – In all societies and educational institutions, knowledge about personal hygiene and health - promoting habits is disseminated. This includes, for example, brushing teeth, bathing daily, ablution, proper waste disposal, hand washing, cleaning clothes and periodically cutting nails, dressing hair, menstrual hygiene, etc., are taught from childhood. Controlling mosquitoes by all means viz; minimizing open and stagnant water puddles, preventing mosquito bites by using gauze doors, mosquitos - nets, and repellents may prevent diseases like malaria, filaria, dengue, encephalitis, chikungunya, yellow fever, etc. These collective measures improve and strengthen the infrastructure of public health.

2. **Norms of a healthy lifestyle** –A disciplined regular routine is paramount as it maintains health and augments our day - to - day work. Having healthy and sound sleep regularly nourishes the body and mind for everyday agile working. Sleep hygiene is taught as good, disciplined behavior in many households. The adage 'early to bed and early to rise makes a man healthy, wealthy, and wise' is followed by successful people as their lifestyle, as is sticking to a schedule of work, eating, exercising, sleeping, socializing, etc. People leading irregular and disorganized routines may show spurts of success but, in the long term, are seen to succumb to irrationality.

3. **Regular Exercises** – like walking, sports, Yog - Pranayam, etc., are conducive to a healthy life. A sedentary lifestyle results in weight gain and depression—a risk factor for diabetes, high blood pressure, atherosclerosis, heart disease, stroke, and death. Obese people succumb to ill health more easily.

4. **Maintaining Body Weight** – This is important because humans do not have natural control over eating. Our height and structure are largely determined by inheritance, but body weight has to be controlled. Modern medical science prescribes a parameter – Body Mass Index or **BMI, which equals body weight in kilograms divided by height in meters** square or Kg/M2. The normal BMI in adults should be between 18.5 to 24.9. Taking **a healthy diet** with appropriate calories from balanced dietary ingredients is advisable. A balanced diet contains all the necessary seven components protein, fat, carbohydrates, fiber, water, minerals, and vitamins. Fast foods, processed foods, and refined flour are harmful. Natural sugar like **jaggery** rather than white or refined sugar is recommended nowadays. Food enriched with excessive cholesterol and sugars may cause obesity, atherosclerosis, heart attack, etc. Salt intake in excessive quantities causes hypertension (high blood pressure). The normally available salt is mostly sodium and should be consumed frugally as it causes hypertension. To avoid excess sodium intake, potassium - enriched salt may be substituted for sodium salt. Salt in India is **iodine - fortified,** which prevents thyroid disease.

5. **Accident and Injury Prevention** – This should be adopted by each and every citizen. The ardent duty of all parents is to inculcate tenets of safety in children at home, workplace, schools, play fields, and especially on the roads. Children and teenagers should not be encouraged to drive motorized vehicles up until they attain the legal age. In India, cycle helmets and other protective gear should be compulsory for bicycle riders. At the time of purchase of a new automobile, citizens should be ready to spend money to maximize the safety features of the vehicle.

Examples of these are the number of airbags, the ability of the vehicle to take impact and crash without harming the occupant, the brake system, etc. Say 'no to alcohol' when about to drive. Keeping the vehicle tip - top - especially the tyres - is a good investment. Tyre - air pressure should be checked regularly. Five important causes of automobile accidents are – over speeding, napping, tyre burst, alcohol while driving, and rash driving. Children should be seated in special car chairs with seat belts. Restraint in seat belts prevents serious forward fall injury when a sudden brake is applied. Household injury prevention starts with the construction of safe houses with proper fencing on stairs and rooftops.

To prevent the elderly from falling in bathrooms, the installation of grab bars and straight walking without uneven flooring and a well - lit toilet are necessary. Kitchens should have a slab for cooking, and stoves should not be placed on the floor. Industrial regulations and good construction practices should be followed to prevent workplace injuries. Harmful substances and drugs must be kept out of reach of children, preferably in child - safe containers. Knives, scissors, matchboxes, chemicals, etc., must be kept out of the reach of children. Loose electric wiring and defective cooking gas tubing can cause short circuits and gas leakage, etc., leading to furious fire accidents. Thus, you may notice that all around us at home, office, workplace, and on the road and in traffic, there are innumerable safe behaviors that we can adopt. Our house and workplace construction and furnishing should be with all the safeguards to avoid accidents. Similarly, our car should have all the safety features. When external factors beyond our control (**environment**), like bad weather, torrential rain, poor visibility, etc., strike us, our preparedness should be such to minimize the injury and be able to get the best help and treatment.

6. **Unsafe Sex** –Indulging in sex just for impulse or pleasure without following safety measures may cause sexually transmitted diseases. HIV and AIDS are fatal diseases that may be thus guarded against.

7. **Utility of Traditional Wisdom** – Many times, simple household remedies and traditional medicines may ameliorate crises. On the other hand, sticking to traditional remedies for long, when genuine advice from scientific and modern medicine is contrary, may make us miss the bus. It is seen many times that diseases like cancer advance beyond cure because biopsy, surgical treatment, or radiotherapy are refused. Alternative and traditional medicines can bring equivalent relief from symptoms like neck, shoulder, and back - aches, several types of rheumatic disorders, anorectal conditions and many day - to - day common illnesses.

8. **Abstinence from Substance Abuse** – Addictive substances like tobacco, alcohol, and drugs like cannabis, opium, smack, heroin, etc., being detrimental to health are not advised to be indulged in. Continued smoking and tobacco use is a health risk - taking behavior that causes respiratory and cardiac diseases besides cancer. Tobacco kills more people, followed by alcohol and drugs.

The deleterious effects of tobacco take place after 20 to 40 years of continued use, and people continue with the practice of tobacco abuse because the effect (cancer) is remote. Alcohol consumption in high and moderate amounts becomes overtly harmful in 15 - 20 years, whereas drug addiction kills its victim much earlier within 2 to 5 years.

9. **Seeking medical care and treatment** – Early solicitation builds confidence among family members. Neglecting certain symptoms and routine checkups is an illness - breeding behavior. Illness in a family member should be promptly ascertained for its severity and attended to appropriately. It should be a custom to provide professional antepartum and post - partum care to women in the family. This ensures her proper nutrition and safe delivery. Women's health measures like mammogram screening for breast cancer, gynecological examination, and cervical cytology to rule out cancer of the uterus (womb) / cervix should be prioritized. Similarly, the health of the male members by regular cardiac checkups, blood sugar, blood pressure, prostate, etc., should be done from time to time. Safe handling of newborn children and vaccination of children go a long way in reducing child mortality. Such behaviors are protective of the health of our family.

10. **Compliance with treatment** – Complying with a doctor's advice is a crucial aspect of health - seeking behavior. Many people, after experiencing partial relief from symptoms of a chronic disease, mistakenly believe that the treatment has served its purpose and, therefore, discontinue their medication prematurely. This can lead to serious consequences, such as the emergence of drug - resistant tuberculosis, which often results from a failure to complete the prescribed course of treatment. Similarly, patients with chronic conditions like diabetes and hypertension often neglect the importance of adhering to their medication regimen consistently - 24/7, 365 days a year. This lack of adherence can lead to poorly controlled conditions, increasing the risk of severe complications. For instance, uncontrolled high blood pressure may trigger a stroke, while uncontrolled diabetes can result in complications such as gangrene in the toes, eye problems, and kidney failure. Furthermore, untreated metabolic syndrome, which includes obesity, hypertension, diabetes, and dyslipidemia, significantly increases the risk of early death and fatal heart attacks.

Following medical advice to the letter is essential in managing chronic diseases effectively and preventing potentially life - threatening complications. An extreme example of health - seeking behavior is worth noting. For instance, just as we often choose a home near good schools to facilitate our children's education, a couple suffering from severe diabetes and hypertension deliberately bought a house next door to a physician.

They became friends with the physician and his family, which not only saved them money on routine consultations and trips to the hospital but also ensured prompt treatment during a major cardiac event.

This illustrates that health - seeking behavior is key to a happy life, and living a happy life is a testament to a successful one. A person conscious of healthy living will quickly seek remedies in response to any alarming health situation. The knowledge of health - seeking behavior is further enriched by understanding the values embedded in the sociocultural and economic fabric of society.

Someone who prioritizes good health also becomes familiar with various health models, whether they are traditional remedies within the community or formal setups like clinics and hospitals provided by the government.

Every society has certain health belief models (HBM). A person's or a community's health behavior may be influenced by two primary factors:

1. how 'threatening' the outcome of a disease is perceived to be and

2. how effective a particular behavior is judged in reducing that threat.

These two factors largely determine the health behaviors (**Health - Seeking Behavior**) prevalent in a person or community.

With the rise of nuclear families, various theories of human behavior have gained traction in explaining how economic activities, social relations, political actions, and health - related behaviors are shaped. The Theory of Planned Behavior, proposed by the eminent psychologist Icek Ajzen from the USA, has applications in advertising, public relations, consumer finance, sports, and healthcare. He argues that a person's intentions are determined by three factors: attitude, subjective norms, and perceived threats.

Currently, health policy in every country is shaped by considering the significance of the **Human Development Index (HDI).**

In countries like the USA, Great Britain, and Germany, individuals reaching certain age milestones are now required to undergo the **Behavioral Risk Factor Surveillance System (BRFSS).** This initiative encourages people to stay vigilant against the dangerous consequences of heart failure and stroke by getting tested for lifestyle - related diseases such as obesity, diabetes, hypertension, snoring, sleep apnea, and heart conditions.

Individuals are trained to manage their **Body Mass Index (BMI)** and **Metabolic Syndrome**, aiming to lead vigorous and active lives. Similarly, the youth are encouraged to adopt healthy habits to ensure long and safe lives. Thus, hygienic practices and health - promoting behaviors in daily life can only be regulated through wisdom and pragmatic thinking.

In conclusion, health - seeking behavior is a broad subject, where not only medical scientists but also social scientists and psychologists contribute solutions for disease prevention. Individuals learn and are influenced by their associations and experiences in understanding what is beneficial or harmful to them. Trust, sincerity, and consistency in following social norms such as cleanliness, exercise, yoga, *Pranayama*, and sports are crucial.

In India, behaviors that enrich the age - old value systems of our ancestors are undoubtedly considered health - seeking behaviors in all aspects of life.

Chapter 19

Quacks & Unqualified Medical Practitioners

Learning Objectives:

- Who are quacks?
- Why do quacks practice freely in India?
- What are common practices of quacks?
- What is the law regarding quackery?

In Uttar Pradesh, not so long ago, a man was arrested for allegedly injecting 41 people with the HIV virus using a single infected needle. This incident underscores the alarming fact that **'quack doctors'** are able to practice freely in India, often aided by the desperation of poor villagers and the shortage of qualified doctors. This medical scandal came to light when state health workers, during a routine screening, found over 24 HIV - positive cases in just one tehsil in the state. An investigation revealed that an unqualified medical practitioner while assuring cheap treatment, had used a single syringe on multiple poor patients. The incident in Unnao district paints a grim picture of the neglect in healthcare. Unfortunately, such incidents are not uncommon in India.

Healthcare in India is plagued with numerous challenges. On the one hand, state - run public hospitals are under - resourced and overcrowded, while on the other hand, private hospitals are prohibitively expensive for the poor, especially those in rural areas. There is a significant urban - rural divide in terms of equity in healthcare. Even when qualified doctors are available, they rarely choose to settle in rural areas. As of 2018, there was one government doctor for every 10,189 people and one government hospital bed for every 2,046 people, while the World Health Organization recommends 1 doctor per 1,000 populations.

This highlights the severe shortage of qualified doctors, particularly in rural areas, a gap that is often filled by **'quacks'** or *jhola chhap* doctors.

According to the Indian Medical Association, there are over 10 lakh quacks practicing in India. This group includes compounders, assistants to doctors, lab technicians, medical store owners, and *vaidyas*. In Delhi alone, it is reported that some 50,000 quacks practice 'medicine', according to the Delhi Medical Council.

There is a demand for such practitioners in rural areas. A study by the National Institute of Public Finance and Policy (NIPFP) in urban slums of Delhi revealed that in about 80% of cases, a private doctor was approached for treatment. "The most appalling finding, however, is that almost 15% of the patients opted for treatment from an unregistered private practitioner." These practitioners are none other than "**quacks**," locally referred to as *"Bangali daaktar."* They attract a significant number of patients due to their proximity, perceived utility, and low charges.

Since ancient times, quackery has been the promotion of cures, remedies, or medical treatments that have not been proven to be beneficial. Quacks, the vendors of mythical and contrived medicines, were often seen as outright fraudsters who boasted about miracle cures that they know are ineffective.

The word "**quack**" itself dates back to the 17th century, having evolved from the Dutch word **quacksalver**, meaning "**hawker of salve**." Traditionally, it referred to someone who boasted about their salves or ointments. During the Middle Ages, such vendors in Europe and Asia sold fraudulent remedies - types of ointments, balms, and oils - on roadsides, in buses, trains, and residential areas, loudly proclaiming cures for maladies like scars, wrinkles, white spots, stains, black patches, and baldness.

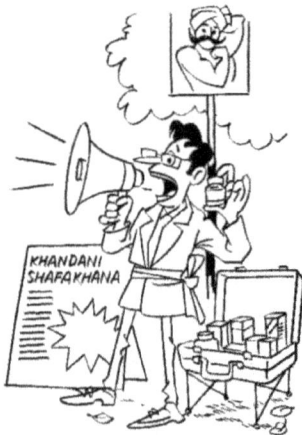

Today, the term "**quack**" is also used to describe **unqualified practitioners.**

178

A small survey conducted in rural and semi - rural areas of the Lucknow district in India, published in 2007, revealed that only 5.7% of medical practitioners held an MBBS degree, while 32% were qualified *AYUSH* practitioners who also dispensed modern medicines. The remaining practitioners were essentially unqualified, with some having only completed high school. A WHO report published in 2016 found that only one in five doctors in rural India are qualified to practice medicine, underscoring the widespread issue of unqualified practitioners. More than half (57.3%) did not have a medical qualification, and almost a third (31.4%) of those calling themselves doctors were educated only up to Class 12.

Practices of Quacks: Although traditionally referred to as *"jhola chhap"* or barefoot doctors, quacks in villages nowadays present a different profile. Many now operate well - furnished clinics and even multi - storied hospitals with operating theatres. They often pose as having degrees or titles such as **"electro - homeopathy"** or **"rural medical practitioner"** (RMP), or GMP. However, if asked to show their credentials, the truth would be revealed.

Many 'quacks' have gained experience by working with qualified doctors as compounders, acquiring a basic knowledge of common ailments and remedies before starting out on their own. They may be skilled in administering injections, intravenous drips, and even performing minor surgeries. They often maintain liaisons with city doctors who advise them on difficult cases. Most of these practitioners dispense drugs in the form of powders in small paper envelopes without disclosing the names of the compounds. Some of these **"envelopes"** may actually contain corticosteroids, a group of strong medicines that can reduce fever but may have several harmful side effects. Other commonly used drugs include antibiotics (whose indiscriminate use can lead to antimicrobial resistance) and pain relievers. These practitioners also often earn through kickbacks from diagnostic establishments.

Why do quacks flourish in India? The reasons why rural India presents a fertile ground for the practice of quacks are not difficult to understand:

The **shortage of qualified doctors** and the availability of quacks present a significant challenge in rural India. As previously mentioned, the number of qualified doctors is far below the required level for our large population.

Even if more qualified doctors were available, they are often reluctant to settle in rural areas due to underdevelopment and safety concerns.

When rural residents need to travel to nearby cities to see a doctor, they lose a day's earnings and incur transportation costs for at least two family members. In contrast, quacks are readily available within the village, thus fulfilling a crucial need.

Ignorance: The rural population, often illiterate, may not distinguish between unqualified practitioners, *AYUSH* doctors, and modern medicine practitioners due to sheer ignorance. The "**doctor**" is accepted at face value.

This contrasts sharply with the situation in Kerala, where a majority of the population is literate. Patients in Kerala typically seek out a postgraduate doctor practicing modern medicine - an MBBS degree alone may not suffice.

Charges: A quack is likely to charge significantly less than a qualified private doctor, making them more accessible to the rural poor.

Behavior: Quacks are generally soft - spoken and approachable, which makes them more relatable and easier to deal with for the rural population compared to government doctors.

What does the law say regarding quackery?

Indian law is unequivocal: unqualified practitioners without medical qualifications must be punished, and their premises disbanded.

Moreover, if a person is qualified in any particular system of medicine (such as *Ayurveda* or Homeopathy), they are legally permitted to practice only within that system.

Practicing in any other system without the proper qualifications renders them a mere 'pretender' or charlatan, subject to punitive measures.

The Clinical Establishment Act of 2010 aims to regulate both the public and private health sectors in India, with a specific focus on unqualified medical practitioners (UMPs) and the eradication of quackery. The legal framework leaves no room for the operation of UMPs.

However, despite clear legal guidelines, the law has seen little success in terms of implementation, highlighting the gap between intention and action.

Although the law is explicit, it is rarely enforced. Offenders, when jailed, often easily secure bail, and while their clinics may be dismantled, they frequently resume operations elsewhere. Health administrators at the sub - national and sub - state levels are often aware of these activities but choose to overlook them due to deficient administrative resources and a lack of political will.

The existence of these self - styled doctors presents a complex issue. Some argue that in the absence of qualified doctors, quacks provide a necessary service and cannot be easily dismissed. One short - term solution may be to update their knowledge with selective training to prevent high - risk practices, such as the indiscriminate use of corticosteroids, injections, and intravenous fluids. Another approach could be to link these practitioners to qualified specialist doctors in cities via telemedicine, redefining their role as 'physician extenders,' nurse practitioners, or another suitable title. In this model, the rural population could consult these practitioners locally, who would then connect them to city specialists for advice on treatment through telemedicine.

The physician extender would then follow up with the patient, minimizing harm while improving access to first - line healthcare. This arrangement could benefit the rural patients, the practitioners, and the city specialists alike. Over time, with development, the improved availability of qualified medical practitioners, and more efficient health services, the need for quacks would naturally diminish.

Chapter 20

Child Health

Learning Objectives:

- Importance of Child Health
- What is different about children?
- Definitions of periods in childhood
- Causes of child mortality
- Preventive pediatrics
- Newborn care, growth monitoring and nutrition
- Basics of Immunization
- Adolescent health – special needs of adolescents

Child Health and Pediatrics: An Essential Branch of Medicine

Pediatrics is a crucial branch of clinical medicine that is intricately linked to preventive medicine. The early years, particularly from birth to age five, are marked by a high risk of mortality and are also vital for the development of lifelong attitudes, customs, and psychological processes.

Children under 18 years of age constitute approximately 472 million people or 33.7% of India's population.

This group is not only vulnerable in terms of health but also represents the future of the nation. Investing in children's health is, therefore, a national priority. The medical specialty dedicated to the health and well - being of children is called Pediatrics.

While the age cutoff for being considered a child has varied over time and across countries, most nations now recognize 18 years as the upper limit for placing individuals under the care of pediatricians.

Why Treat Children Differently?

Are children simply miniature adults? The answer is no, and there are several reasons why they require specialized care.

1. **Different Disease Spectrum**: Children are more commonly affected by congenital (present at birth) and hereditary (inherited but may develop later) disorders, as well as nutritional and infectious diseases. In contrast, adults are more prone to degenerative conditions such as atherosclerosis, coronary artery disease, and hypertension. Although there is some overlap with many adult diseases beginning in childhood and many hereditary and infectious diseases affecting adults, the overall spectrum of illnesses is distinct.

2. **Higher Metabolic Rate**: Children have a much higher metabolic rate than adults, which means their fluid and calorie requirements per kilogram of body weight are higher. Consequently, drug doses, vital parameters like heart rate and respiratory rate, and the proportion of body water are all higher in children.

3. **Growth and Development**: Children are in a continuous state of growth (increase in size) and development (maturation of function). Chronic diseases can significantly affect these processes, and there can also be primary disorders related to growth and development.

4. **Different Response to Illness**: Children tend to deteriorate more rapidly than adults when ill, but they also recover faster. This necessitates careful monitoring and often means that there is a lower threshold for investigation and treatment in pediatric cases, particularly in younger children.

5. **Communication and Examination Challenges**: Young children often cannot communicate their symptoms effectively, requiring physicians to infer much from the child's behavior and the observations of caregivers. Pediatric history must often be taken from the mother or primary caregiver. Examining children can be challenging as it requires establishing rapport, and a complete examination may not always be possible without the child's cooperation. Some clinical signs also differ in young children, adding another layer of complexity to pediatric care.

Pediatrics is a field that not only addresses the unique medical needs of children but also plays a pivotal role in shaping the future of a nation by ensuring the health and well - being of its youngest citizens.

Definitions:

- Embryo: The earliest stage of development in the womb, during which critical body structures and organs form.

- Fetus: The term for the embryo after the 11th week of pregnancy.

- Neonatal Period: The first 28 days after birth.

- Infancy: The period from birth to the end of the first year of life.

- Post - neonatal Period: The time from 1 month to the end of the first year.

- 0 - 5 Years (Under 5): A vulnerable age group due to a higher risk of mortality.

- Adolescence: The period from 10 to 21 years of age.

- Normal Birth Weight: Approximately 3 kg.

- Low Birth Weight (LBW): A birth weight below 2500 grams.

- Very Low Birth Weight (VLBW): Below 1500 grams.

- Extremely Low Birth Weight (ELBW): Below 1000 grams.

- Premature Birth: A baby born before 37 completed weeks of gestation. Premature and low birth weight babies face unique health challenges.

Causes of Death:

It is well known that nearly 90% of all child deaths are preventable. Most commonly, these deaths occur during the neonatal period, with major causes being sepsis (bloodstream infection), pneumonia, low birth weight, and birth asphyxia (lack of oxygen at birth).

After the newborn period, acute respiratory infections and diarrhea remain the leading causes of child mortality. Malnutrition is a significant contributing factor, as it increases the risk of death from other causes. India has the highest rate of child malnutrition globally, even surpassing that of sub - Saharan Africa.

Simple, low - cost interventions can significantly reduce child mortality in low and middle - income countries like India. These interventions include:

1. Antenatal, intrapartum, and neonatal care

2. Early breastfeeding initiation within one hour of birth

3. Exclusive breastfeeding for the first six months of life

4. Appropriate complementary feeding

5. Vaccination

6. Case management of pneumonia and diarrhea

Newborn (Neonatal) Care:

The neonatal period is a critical time with the highest risk of mortality. About two - thirds of all infant deaths and half of all under - five deaths occur during this period, with more than half of these deaths happening within the first week.

Therefore, to reduce infant mortality, it is essential to focus on reducing neonatal mortality.

At birth, the infant is suddenly transitioned from the comfort of the uterus to the external environment, which is significantly harsher. Rapid changes occur, especially in the circulatory and respiratory systems, to adapt to the following needs:

1. Stabilization of breathing and heart function with a spontaneous rhythm

2. Maintenance of body temperature

3. Establishing feeding

If spontaneous breathing does not occur within a minute after birth, the baby must be resuscitated immediately. The delivery room should be equipped with the necessary resuscitation equipment.

Once the baby begins breathing, an initial examination should be conducted in the delivery room to check for any birth injuries, detect congenital malformations (especially those requiring urgent treatment), and assess maturity based on specific parameters. Birth weight should be measured. A second, more comprehensive physical examination and measurement, preferably by a pediatrician, should take place within 24 hours of birth.

Low Birth Weight (LBW) Babies:

In India, approximately 30% of babies are born with low birth weight (LBW). LBW babies fall into three categories:

- **Preterm or Premature Babies:** Born before 37 completed weeks of gestation.

- **Mature Babies with Intrauterine Growth Retardation (IUGR):** These babies, also called **small for gestational age (SGA),** have restricted growth before birth and weigh less than the 10th percentile for their gestational age.

- **Both Preterm and SGA:** Babies who are both premature and have IUGR.

Globally, about 9 - 12% of births are preterm. LBW babies, particularly those in the premature group, face a significantly higher risk of death because almost all of their organ systems are immature and unable to function independently. There is a stark difference in the survival rates of premature babies depending on where they are born, as saving them often requires expensive infrastructure and trained staff. In developing countries, more than 90% of extremely premature babies die, compared to only 10% in high - income countries.

A low - cost method for saving LBW newborns is **Kangaroo Mother Care (KMC)**. This technique involves keeping the tiny infant in close **skin - to - skin contact** with the mother's chest for at least eight hours a day until the infant reaches a weight of around 2 kg.

KMC has been shown to reduce neonatal mortality by 40%, decrease neonatal infection, sepsis, and hypothermia, increase exclusive breastfeeding, promote faster weight gain in the baby, and enhance mother - baby bonding. It has now become a standard care practice in both developed and developing countries.

Infant Feeding: A detailed discussion on infant feeding is beyond the scope of this book, so only the essential aspects will be covered. The ideal food for a baby is human breast milk. No other feeds, not even water, are required until the baby is 6 months old. Under normal conditions, Indian mothers secrete 450 - 600 ml of breast milk daily, containing about 1.1 grams of protein and 70 kcals per 100 ml. Early (within the first hour of birth) breastfeeding should be initiated, and exclusive breastfeeding should be continued for 6 months.

The thick, yellowish milk produced in the first 3 - 4 days is called **colostrum**, which is highly beneficial for the baby. Scientific data suggest that non - breastfed infants in developing countries are 5 - 10 times more likely to die in the first year.

Advantages of breastfeeding include:

(i)   It is hygienic, cheap, and readily available to the baby at the right temperature
(ii)   It fulfills the nutritional needs of the baby in the first few months
(iii)   Due to the presence of antimicrobial factors and antibodies, it protects against infection
(iv)   It is easily digested by both term and preterm babies and is almost completely absorbed and utilized
(v)   It promotes bonding between mother and baby
(vi)   It prevents low calcium and magnesium levels in the baby
(vii)   It protects against obesity in the baby
(viii) It helps in proper spacing of children.

Breastfeeding also offers several advantages to the mother, such as delaying the next pregnancy, lowering rates of breast and ovarian cancer, and improving bone health. Even if direct breastfeeding is not possible, hygienically expressed breast milk can be given.

Expressed breast milk is milk squeezed out of the breast, stored, and fed to the baby by the mother. Breastfeeding should be continued even during illness when the baby may not accept other foods. Even small amounts of breast milk are highly beneficial and should preferably be continued until 2 years of age or longer.

However, breastfeeding alone is insufficient to sustain the infant's growth beyond 6 months of age. Solid foods should be introduced at around 6 months, a process called **complementary feeding**. Start with 3 - 4 feeds per day and build up to 5 - 6 feeds per day by the time the baby reaches 1 year of age. Introduction of solids can begin with *dal, khichdi*, and porridge.

Food should be hygienically prepared after proper hand washing. Initially, only thin, gruel - like foods will be accepted and swallowed, but later, semisolid foods can be given. Foods cooked for the family can be mashed to make them soft and then offered to the baby. Care should be taken to include enough green leafy vegetables and fruit.

Malnutrition: The prevalence of malnutrition in young children in India is the highest in the world. Globally, one - third of malnourished children are Indian, despite India being one - sixth of the world's population. Malnutrition is mostly due to a deficiency of protein and calories.

Chronic malnutrition leads to stunting (low height for age), while acute malnutrition leads to wasting (low weight for height). According to the Government of India's National Family Health Survey 5 (NFHS 5 - 2019 - 21), 36% of children under 5 years of age are stunted, 19% are wasted, 32% are underweight, and 3% are overweight. Important risk factors for malnutrition in children include maternal malnutrition and lack of schooling.

Malnutrition induces an immune deficiency state, making the child more prone to infections, creating a vicious cycle of malnutrition and infection. It is estimated that malnutrition is an underlying cause in 30% of deaths in children under 5 years old in India.

Micronutrients are an essential part of our diet and are needed in minute quantities. They include vitamins and minerals.

Vitamins are of two types:

1. fat - soluble (vitamins A, D, E, and K, which are stored in the body) and

2. water - soluble (B group and vitamin C, which are not stored).

Vitamin A deficiency is the most common cause of preventable blindness in children globally. Vitamin D deficiency is extremely common in India, with a prevalence of 76%. A lack of this nutrient leads to diverse health disorders besides rickets and osteomalacia (weak bones).

Important minerals include iron, calcium, zinc, and iodine. Foods can be fortified with micronutrients; an example is iodine - fortified salt, which has drastically reduced the prevalence of goiter and cretinism. Iron is found in good quantities in green leafy vegetables.

A deficiency of iron, vitamin B12, and folic acid leads to anemia (or low hemoglobin in the blood). Nutritional anemia is extremely common in children under 5 years of age (67%) and women (57%), with a prevalence in men (aged 15 - 49 years) of 25%. Calcium is abundant in milk, dairy products, and leafy greens. Vitamin B12 (cobalamin) is not found in plant foods, so infants should be offered some foods of animal origin as well.

Growth monitoring: Growth and development are essential phenomena in children, yet they are unique to each child. Growth refers to an **increase in size**, while development refers to the **maturation of skills**.

Determinants of growth and development include sex, race, genetic influences, nutrition, disorders of the kidney, endocrine glands, heart, and brain, infections, physical environment, and psychological and economic factors. Growth and development generally follow a predetermined pattern. Developmental **milestones** are age - specific functions achieved at particular ages, such as walking without support or speaking in short sentences of 2 - 3 words. Development is usually assessed in four domains: gross motor, fine motor (hand - eye coordination), language, and social skills. Surveillance of growth and development is an important means of detecting nutritional disorders and other diseases. Growth surveillance involves plotting measurements such as weight, height, and head circumference on growth charts created from the same racial population.

Development is assessed by comparing the milestones achieved by the child with the standard. Monitoring growth and development is a crucial part of child health services, with measurements recorded serially on growth charts.

An important group of developmental disorders in children is **neurodevelopmental disorders**. This term encompasses epilepsy, intellectual disability, impaired vision or hearing, neuromotor deficits, speech and language disorders, attention deficit hyperactivity disorder, and **autism spectrum disorder (ASD).** The latter has become extremely common worldwide in the last two decades, with prevalence in India of 1 in 68, and boys - to - girls ratio of 3:1.

Criteria for ASD include :

(i)   persistent deficits in social communication and interaction,

(ii)   restricted, repetitive patterns of behavior, interests, or activities and,

(iii)   onset before 3 years of age.

Pediatricians should be familiar with early 'red flag' signs of autism. The cause of autism remains unknown for most affected children, though genetic factors are believed to be significant. Over the last 5 - 6 years, a link to high screen time exposure (television, mobile phones, iPads, etc.) in the first two years of life has been observed, though it requires further study. No pharmacological therapy has so far proven beneficial.

Immunization: Immunization refers to the development of specific immunity to an infection by administering a modified infectious agent or its component (antigen). This process leads to the formation of 'memory cells' and the production of antibodies specifically targeting the agent. When the body is later exposed to the actual infection, the immune system mounts a much stronger response, successfully protecting the host.

This is called '**active immunization.' Passive immunization** is also used in certain situations, where antibody preparations are injected directly into exposed individuals, as with rabies immunoglobulin or anti - diphtheria immunoglobulin. Vaccines are available against many infectious diseases, and immunization has been hugely successful in protecting against dangerous infections.

Vaccines may be made from modified live organisms (live attenuated), killed organisms (inactivated), extracted cellular fractions, parts of toxins, etc. Recent advances in vaccine technology include recombinant DNA vaccines, polysaccharide vaccines, conjugate vaccines, chimeric vaccines, and mRNA vaccines. For some infections, several different vaccines are available.

Smallpox has been eradicated globally through vaccination, and polio has been eliminated from nearly all countries, including India. Infections that can be prevented by vaccination are known as **vaccine - preventable diseases**. The Global Alliance for Vaccines and Immunization (GAVI) was launched in 2000 to support the vaccination of eligible children and adults in the world's poorest countries.

Each country has its own immunization schedule based on its needs. The Government of India provides free vaccinations against 12 diseases in children - 11 diseases nationally and one (Japanese encephalitis vaccine) in selected districts. Additionally, the Indian Academy of Pediatrics recommends certain 'optional vaccines,' such as those for chickenpox and hepatitis A.

Adolescent Health: Adolescence is the period of transition between childhood and adulthood, generally considered to be between 10 - 19 years of age.

According to the 2011 census, adolescents comprised 20% of India's total population. During this period, adolescents experience rapid growth, pubertal changes leading to dimorphic body shapes, and the formation of sexual identity. There is also a strong desire for greater independence - personally, emotionally, and financially. The capacity for abstract thinking develops during this time. As a result, this age group faces unique health challenges, including mental and psychological health issues, sexual and reproductive health concerns, nutrition, immunization, and substance abuse. During this transitional phase, education within the family, school, and society plays a critical role in the development of personality and values. To help adolescents reach their full potential, it is the government's responsibility to promote a safe environment, ensure good health and optimal nutrition, foster learning, competence, education, and skills, enhance employability, encourage connectedness and positive values, and create awareness about their contributions to society.

Chapter 21

Women's Health

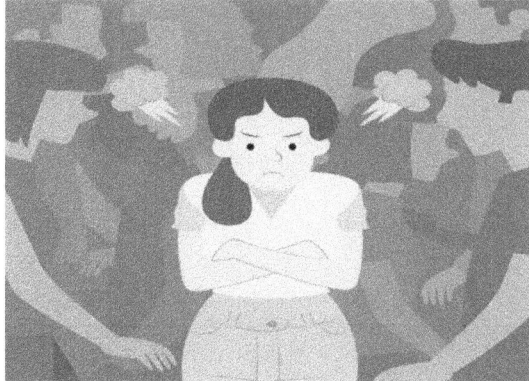

Learning Objectives:

- Brief anatomy and physiology of female reproductive tract

- Common women's health problems in reproductive organs - vaginitis, vaginal discharge, dysmennohrea, menorrhagia, uterine fibroids, polycystic ovarian syndrome (PCOS), premenstrual syndrome (PMS), endometriosis, urinary tract infections (UTIs), incontinence of urine.

Despite feminist movements, many women continue to face social and economic inequality, with specific health concerns related to their bodies requiring special attention. Women's healthcare is crucial, as underscored by the **Beijing Declaration on Women's Health in 1995**, which focused on common health issues affecting women. Today, nearly 500,000 women worldwide die annually from uterine and breast cancer. In developing countries, 220 million women aged 15 to 44 suffer from sexual diseases.

The maternal mortality rate (MMR), which measures the number of maternal deaths per 100,000 live births, reflects the health infrastructure of a country. A century ago, the MMR was 5,000 per 100,000 live births.

In India, special efforts have reduced the MMR from 113 in 2016 to 97 per 100,000 live births in 2018 - 2020. In contrast, developed countries like those in Europe, Australia, and Canada have MMRs ranging between 5 and 10, while in Afghanistan, the rate exceeds 600. Additionally, women's mortality rates continue to rise each year due to HIV/AIDS, human papillomavirus (HPV) infections, and unsafe sexual practices. Women who use tobacco are also at a higher risk of developing lung and oral cancers.

Menstrual Bleeding: The female reproductive system comprises two ovaries and fallopian tubes, one on either side of the pelvis. The **fallopian tubes** lead into the cornuae of the **uterus,** a hollow structure located just behind the urinary bladder. The uterus is lined by the **endometrium**, surrounded by thick muscle tissue known as the **myometrium**, and covered by the peritoneum, referred to as the **perimetrium**. The uterus opens at the **cervix**, which then leads into the **vagina**. Both the endometrium and myometrium are highly sensitive to hormonal changes, allowing the uterus to expand significantly during pregnancy.

From **puberty** to **menopause**, women experience a **menstrual period** approximately once a month, every 21 to 35 days, with the period lasting anywhere from 1 to 7 days. During this, the endometrial lining of the uterus is shed off resulting in menstrual bleeding. These cyclical changes occur due to changes in female hormones - estrogen and progesterone. Around the middle of the cycle, which begins on the first day of menstruation, ovulation occurs, releasing an egg from the ovary.

Common Women's Health Problems (excluding Obstetrics):

Dry Vagina and Painful Sexual Intercourse – Many women experience discomfort in their genital area and may be hesitant to seek medical attention. The female hormone estrogen plays a crucial role in the development and protection of reproductive organs. During and after menopause, a decrease in estrogen levels can lead to vaginal dryness, resulting in vaginal atrophy.

Treatment includes counseling for women, their families, and partners, addressing depression, and managing the underlying causes. In specific cases, estrogen hormone creams or pills applied to the vagina can help increase moisture and alleviate symptoms.

Vaginal Discharge (Leucorrhoea) – Vaginal discharge can result from bacterial, fungal, or **trichomonal** infections. It is characterized by a whitish discharge, itching, redness of the vulva, burning sensation, and pain during urination (dysuria) or intercourse. Diagnosis and treatment are based on vaginal examination and lab reports. It's important to note that itching and redness in the vagina can also be early symptoms of diabetes.

Dysmenorrhea – Pain associated with menstruation, known as dysmenorrhea, is extremely common. It usually manifests as cramping pain in the lower abdomen, lower back pain, and pain radiating down the legs. It may also be accompanied by nausea, vomiting, diarrhea, fatigue, and weakness. Treatment includes rest and hot fomentation. If pain persists, painkillers can be taken.

Menorrhagia – Menorrhagia refers to **heavy or prolonged bleeding during periods** and is a common disorder. The cause is often hormonal. Both ovulatory and anovulatory cycles can result in excessive menstrual loss without any other abnormality, known as **dysfunctional uterine bleeding.** Other causes include uterine problems such as fibroids and adenomyosis. Occasionally, menorrhagia can indicate a coagulation disorder. Severe menorrhagia can lead to iron deficiency anemia. Investigation may involve a pelvic exam, blood counts, ultrasound, Pap test, and endometrial sampling.

Post - Coital Bleeding – Bleeding after intercourse is a serious symptom that **may indicate cervical cancer**.

Bleeding Between Periods – This refers to any vaginal bleeding that occurs outside of a normal period. It may be heavier than a normal period or very light ("spotting"). Causes include inflammation of the vagina, cervix, or uterus, uterine fibroids, endometriosis, polyps, and cancer. Additionally, young women may normally experience slight bleeding during ovulation, typically 10 to 14 days after the onset of their period, due to a temporary drop in estrogen levels. Irregular periods can also occur in girls who have just started menstruating (menarche) and women going through menopause, which can be mistaken for bleeding between periods.

Uterine Fibroids – These **benign tumors** arise from the uterine muscle and are very common, affecting one in five women during their childbearing years. Half of all women have fibroids by age 50.

The cause is unclear, but they are thought to be related to hormones and genetics (they can run in families). Fibroids vary greatly in size, from microscopic to several pounds, and often occur in multiples. They may shrink after menopause. Symptoms include bleeding between periods, menorrhagia, prolonged periods, cramping, and pain during periods, a feeling of fullness in the lower abdomen, and frequent urination. However, fibroids may be asymptomatic. Investigations include pelvic examination, ultrasound, hysteroscopy, magnetic resonance imaging, and biopsy.

Treatments for fibroids are symptomatic, including tranexamic acid to reduce bleeding, iron supplements for anemia, pain relievers, and hormones to reduce heavy bleeding. Definitive treatment may involve surgery, depending on the patient's age and whether future pregnancy is planned.

Polycystic Ovary Syndrome (PCOS) – PCOS is a very common hormonal disorder affecting adolescent girls and women of childbearing age. The exact cause is not fully understood, but it likely involves a combination of genetic and environmental factors. Women with PCOS may experience missed or irregular menstrual periods, may not ovulate regularly, and often have multiple small cysts on their ovaries. Elevated levels of androgens (male hormones) can lead to symptoms such as excess facial hair growth, acne, infertility, and weight gain. Additionally, increased insulin resistance associated with PCOS can predispose women to type - 2 diabetes. Treatment options include birth control pills to regulate menstrual cycles, hormones to improve fertility, diabetes management, and procedures to remove excess hair.

Premenstrual Syndrome (PMS) – Some women experience physical and emotional symptoms a few days before the start of their menstrual cycle, which typically subsides once the period begins. These symptoms may include lower abdominal pain, breast tenderness, swelling, mood swings, swelling in the feet, lower back pain, and general body aches. In some cases, women may also experience anxiety, restlessness, and depression, which can escalate to antisocial and even criminal behavior.

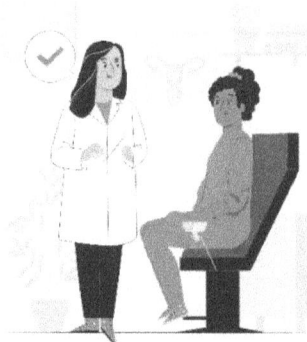

The severity of PMS varies widely among women; while some may have mild symptoms, others may experience severe discomfort. Hormonal changes during the menstrual cycle are believed to contribute to these symptoms.

Endometriosis – Endometriosis occurs when tissue similar to the endometrium (the inner lining of the uterus) grows on other organs, such as the ovaries, fallopian tubes, and tissues around the pelvis. This ectopic tissue is hormonally sensitive and can lead to fibrosis, adhesions, and scar tissue formation. When endometriosis affects the ovaries, it can result in chocolate - colored cysts. The main symptom is painful menstrual cramps, which can range from mild to severe, typically affecting the abdomen, pelvic region, and lower back. Other symptoms include pain during sex, heavy bleeding during periods, light bleeding between periods, painful bowel movements, and infertility. Diagnosis involves a pelvic examination, ultrasound, and MRI, often followed by laparoscopy and biopsy. Treatment options depend on age, severity, and whether pregnancy is planned and may include hormonal drugs (e.g., birth control pills, Danazol, GnRH agonists, Centchroman) or surgical removal of the ectopic tissue.

Urinary Frequency and Urgency – It is normal for an adult to urinate about 1.5 liters a day, but drinking more fluids can result in up to 4 liters of urine. Normal daytime urination frequency is usually 6 to 10 times, and a typical urge to urinate occurs when 300 - 400 ml of urine has collected in the bladder. Severe urgency may occur when the bladder holds more than 500 ml of urine. Urinary frequency and urgency are distinct conditions, though they can occur together. Causes of urinary frequency include urinary tract infections (UTIs), anxiety, stress, diabetes mellitus, diuretic medications, and diuretic drinks. Other causes include abnormal nervous system function, tumors in the pelvis, inflammation of the bladder wall (interstitial cystitis), and bladder overactivity.

Urinary Tract Infection (UTI) – UTIs are more common in women than in men, with approximately 40% of women and 12% of men experiencing a UTI at some point in their lives. The infection can affect various parts of the urinary system, including the kidneys (nephritis), urethra, and bladder (cystitis), with the latter being the most common.

Symptoms include a strong urge to urinate, burning during urination, frequent urination, cloudy urine, blood in the urine, and foul - smelling urine. Nephritis is usually associated with fever. Women are more susceptible to UTIs due to the structure of their urinary tract, and pregnant women are at higher risk. Risk factors include unsafe sexual practices, diabetes, poor hygiene, incomplete bladder emptying, diarrhea, urinary tract obstructions, kidney stones, a dry vagina, a weakened immune system, and excessive antibiotic use. Diagnosis involves a urine culture to determine bacterial sensitivity.

Depending on the severity, further tests such as ultrasound, CT scan, MRI, urodynamic testing, or intravenous pyelography may be required. Treatment typically involves antibiotics, and structural abnormalities of the urinary tract may require surgical intervention.

Urinary Incontinence – Involuntary leakage of urine is known as urinary incontinence, which can manifest in various forms:

Stress Incontinence – This type occurs when urine leaks during activities like coughing, sneezing, laughing, or physical exertion due to weakened pelvic floor muscles. It is typically treated with surgery.

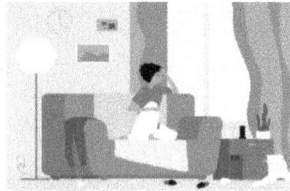

Urge Incontinence or Overactive Bladder – In this condition, the urge to urinate is sudden and intense, often resulting in leakage before reaching the toilet. Medications can help reduce urgency and manage symptoms.

Overflow Incontinence – This condition involves continuous leakage from a full bladder. Causes may include bladder tumors, neurological disorders, or other bladder diseases.

Investigation of Urinary Incontinence – Diagnosis of urinary incontinence may involve urine routine and microscopy, urodynamic studies, pyelogram, cystoscopy, and pelvic or abdominal ultrasound. Treatment focuses on addressing the underlying cause through medications and surgery. Effective medications are available for urge incontinence, and Kegel exercises, which strengthen pelvic floor muscles, can be beneficial. Stress incontinence is usually treated successfully with surgery.

Prolapse of the Uterus – Uterine prolapse occurs when the pelvic floor muscles and connective tissues stretch and weaken, no longer supporting the uterus effectively. This can lead to the uterus descending into the vagina and, in severe cases, protruding out. Uterine prolapse is commonly seen in postmenopausal women, especially those who have had multiple vaginal deliveries.

Contributing factors include being overweight, chronic constipation, chronic cough or bronchitis, and repeated heavy lifting. Mild uterine prolapse typically doesn't require treatment. However, severe prolapse that causes discomfort or disrupts daily life may benefit from intervention. Treatment options include self - care measures like **Kegel exercises** to strengthen pelvic floor muscles, weight loss, and prevent constipation, as well as surgical procedures for more severe cases.

Cancer of the Uterus, Ovaries, and Cervix – Symptoms of these cancers can include abdominal pain, lumps or swelling, and irregular or excessive vaginal bleeding. These conditions are discussed in detail in the chapter on cancer.

Breast Diseases – Women may encounter a range of breast - related issues, including nipple problems and breast cancer. Breast cancer is the leading cause of premature mortality among women worldwide and is covered extensively in a separate chapter dedicated to breast diseases.

Chapter 22

Maternal and Child Health (MCH) Programs, MCH Indicators & Family Planning

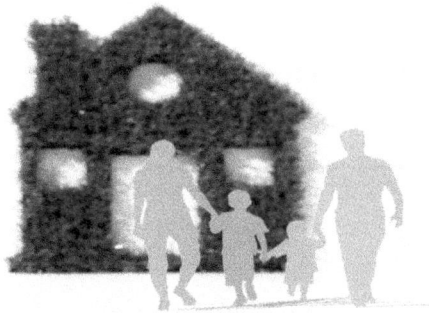

Learning Objectives:

- Maternal & Child Health indicators – a measure of development of the nation
- Significance of Reproductive-Maternal-Neonatal-Child and Adolescent Health (RMNCH+A) Program
- Components of RMNCH+A
- Temporary and permanent methods of Family Planning & Contraception

Women of childbearing age (15 - 44 years) constitute 52.4% of the female population, while children below 15 years of age make up 26.5% of the population. Together, these two groups account for over 57% of the total population in India, making them a significant focus for health services. Consequently, the country has implemented specific health programs for them, known as **Maternal and Child,** which are discussed below.

Maternal and Child Health (MCH) Programs were initiated as early as 1900, recognizing the vulnerability of mothers and children. The Republic of India gave further momentum to these programs after 1950. Over time, MCH has incorporated various initiatives, including primary health care, national family planning, family welfare programs, immunization, child survival, safe maternity, and the elimination of neonatal diseases. By 1996, these programs were well established. The **United Nations Organization (UNO)** defines MCH as the future legacy of a country, emphasizing four key parameters: the health of women during pregnancy, prenatal care, childbirth, and postnatal care. Globally, maternal and child health is considered a priority due to the vulnerability of these groups.

Child mortality under five years of age remains alarmingly high in developing countries, accounting for nearly 50% of all deaths in some regions. This age group is given special attention as a separate health parameter because a significant proportion of these deaths are due to preventable causes. For health care services, the mother and child are treated as one unit. The UNO's objectives stress the importance of the complete well - being of the mother and child, which largely depends on safe pregnancy and childbirth. The World Health Organization (WHO) defines the objective of MCH as "promoting, preventing, therapeutic, and rehabilitation care for mother and child."

In India, the **Pre - Conception and Pre - Natal Diagnostic Techniques (PC - PNDT) Act** was enacted in 1994, making gender determination during pregnancy and female feticide criminal offenses. This act was introduced with the goal of maintaining a balanced sex ratio in the population.

The Government of India launched an ambitious initiative in 1952 known as the **National Family Planning Program** - the first of its kind in the world. The program initially focused on promoting the small family norm. During that time, families in India typically had an average of 4 to 6 children, with some having as many as 8 or 10. However, it was later realized that poor child survival rates were a significant factor contributing to the prevalence of large families. This insight led the government to shift its focus, transforming the **National Family Planning Program** into the **National Family Welfare Program** in 1977.

In parallel, the **World Health Organization (WHO)** launched the **Expanded Program of Immunization** in 1974, which was later renamed the **Universal Immunization Program** in 1985. This program was subsequently integrated into the **Child Survival and Safe Motherhood Program** in 1992. All these initiatives culminated in the comprehensive **Reproductive and Child Health (RCH)** Program in 1997, followed by its second phase, **RCH 2**, in 2005. Over time, the program evolved to include adolescent health, leading to the current **RMNCH+A** initiative, which encompasses **Reproductive, Maternal, Neonatal, Child, and Adolescent Health**.

The development of these programs was rooted in pragmatic thinking and the experience gained gradually over seven decades.

The major objectives were threefold:

    (i)   **Immediate:** to promote the health of mothers and children,

    (ii)   **Intermediate:** to reduce infant and maternal mortality, and

    (iii)   **Ultimate:** to stabilize the population.

The goals of **RMNCH+A** include reducing maternal mortality rate (MMR), infant mortality rate (IMR), and total fertility rate (TFR), increasing couple protection rate, achieving 100% immunization coverage for children, and encouraging breastfeeding along with mother and child nutrition.

The Reproductive, Maternal, Neonatal, Child, and Adolescent Health (RMNCH+A) program has incorporated **eight key components** that encompass all states, districts, tehsils, and rural areas in India:

1. **Reproductive Health**: This program focuses on promoting healthy marital relations, ensuring safe maternity, preventing unintended pregnancies, and the appropriate use of contraceptives. It also includes safe termination of pregnancies, conception and reproductive services, treatment of reproductive tract infections (RTI) and sexually transmitted diseases (STD), referral of pregnant women to hospitals, reproductive health services for adolescent girls, remedial measures for infertility, and screening and treatment for cervical and breast cancers.

2. **Maternal Health**: Pregnancy is a critical phase in a woman's life, beginning with conception. Maternal health services are provided throughout the various stages of maternity, which include the antenatal (prenatal), intranatal, postnatal, and inter - conceptional periods.

   These services aim to ensure the health and well - being of the mother during her reproductive years.

3. **Antenatal Care: Pregnancy tracking** in villages is conducted by Auxiliary Nurse Midwives (ANMs) with the assistance of Accredited Social Health Activists (ASHAs) and Anganwadi workers. **At least four antenatal visits** are arranged to Primary or Community Health Centers. The objectives of antenatal care are to promote and protect the health of the mother and fetus, detect high - risk cases for special attention, anticipate and prevent complications, alleviate anxiety, prepare the mother for childbirth, and provide family planning education. Examinations include weight, blood pressure, gestational age assessment, and if possible, ultrasound. Supplements of calcium, iron, and folic acid are provided, and investigations include urine tests for protein, blood sugar levels, blood group and Rh factor, and tests for syphilis. Two doses of the tetanus toxoid vaccine are administered to protect the newborn against tetanus.

4. **Intranatal Care**: The objectives of care during delivery include ensuring thorough cleanliness and asepsis, delivering the baby with minimal injury to both mother and child, being prepared to handle complications, and providing immediate care for the newborn. The **Janani Suraksha Yojana** promotes institutional deliveries to reduce complications and lower maternal and infant mortality.

5. **Postnatal Care**: The postnatal period extends up to 42 days after delivery. During this time, both mother and baby require care, typically provided in a hospital setting. For the mother, important aspects include preventing complications, promoting a rapid return to optimal health, supporting breastfeeding, providing family planning education, and offering basic health education. For the baby, services include establishing breastfeeding, immunization, identifying congenital malformations, preventing and recognizing infections, and counseling family members on recognizing danger signs such as poor feeding,

lethargy, difficulty breathing, fever, convulsions, cold skin, severe jaundice, and low urinary output.

6. **Care during the Inter - Conceptional Period**: During this period, women should receive nutritional supplements to prevent anemia. If planning a pregnancy, folic acid supplementation is recommended. If pregnancy is not planned, the use of contraceptive methods is advised.

7. **Child Health & Wellness**: Preventive pediatrics includes activities such as home - based neonatal care, growth monitoring, nutritional surveillance, immunization, and regular health check - ups. Under RMNCH+A, the government has established a comprehensive infrastructure for newborn health care at the community level. Every newborn receives a package of **Essential Newborn Care**.

    Facility - based newborn care programs provide appropriate care for sick newborns at different health facilities as needed, including **Newborn Care Corners** at labor rooms or obstetric operation theaters, **Newborn Stabilization Units** at **First Referral Units** or Community Health Centers, and **Special Newborn Care Units (SNCUs)** at District Hospitals.

This also includes home - based management by village - based frontline health workers or ASHAs to prevent neonatal infections or sepsis.

Essential New - born care as prescribed by WHO includes:

- Immediate care at birth (delayed cord clamping, thorough drying, assessment of breathing, skin - to - skin contact, early initiation of breastfeeding)

- Thermal care

- Resuscitation when needed

- Support for breast milk feeding

- Nurturing care

- Infection prevention

- Assessment of health problems

- Recognition and response to danger signs

- Timely and safe referral when needed

India Newborn Action Plan – Launched in 2014 under the **National Health Mission**, this program aims to accelerate the **reduction of neonatal mortality rates to single digits by 2030**. Recognizing that mortality among **low birth weight (LBW)** babies significantly contributes to neonatal deaths, special suites called **Kangaroo Mother Care (KMC)** lounges are being established in districts. For those unable to produce sufficient milk, support is provided through **human milk banks** being established in certain states and districts.

Nutrition – In response to the significant problem of malnutrition in children, the Government of India has implemented various public health programs. These include the **Mid - Day School Meal Program** and the **Integrated Child Development Scheme (ICDS).**

In 2018, the government launched the **Poshan Abhiyaan**, focusing on improving the nutritional wellness of adolescent girls, pregnant women, lactating mothers, and children aged 0 - 6 years.

The broad - spectrum objectives of this initiative are as follows:

- Prevent and reduce stunting in children (0 - 6 years)

- Prevent and reduce under - nutrition (underweight) in children (0 - 6 years)

- Reduce anemia among young children (6 - 59 months)

- Reduce the prevalence of anemia among women and adolescent girls in the age group of 15 - 49 years

- Reduce low birth weight (LBW)

Growth Monitoring: Growth and development are essential yet unique processes in every child. Growth refers to an **increase in size**, while development pertains to the **maturation of skills**. Monitoring growth and development is crucial for detecting nutritional disorders and diseases.

Growth surveillance involves plotting measurements such as weight, height, and head circumference on growth charts developed from the same racial population constructs.

Development is assessed by comparing the milestones achieved by the child with the established standards.

Immunization: The Government of India provides free vaccinations against 12 diseases in children - 11 nationally and one (Japanese encephalitis) sub - nationally. The immunization program involves vaccine manufacturing, safe transport, cold chain maintenance, storage, administration, and post - vaccination surveillance. The **National Immunization Schedule** for India outlines the timelines and vaccines provided to ensure comprehensive protection against these diseases.

Infants At birth	BCG, Intradermal Left upper arm (Against tuberculosis) 0 - dose OPV, two drops, Oral (Against Polio) Hep - B (birth dose, 0.5 mL, Intramuscular, (Against Hepatitis B)
6 weeks	Pentavalent - 1, 0.5 mL, Intramuscular (against Diphtheria, tetanus, pertussis, hepatitis B and H. influenzae infection) OPV - 1, two drops, Oral (Against Polio) *Rotavirus Vaccine, five drops of Rotavac/2.5 ml of Rotasil, Oral (against diarrhea caused by rotavirus) IPV - 1, fractional dose (0.1ml), intradermal (Inactive polio vaccine) PCV - 1, 0.5 ml, intramuscular, (Against pneumococcal infection)
10 weeks	Pentavalent - 2, 0.5 mL, Intramuscular (against Diphtheria, tetanus, pertussis, hepatitis B, and H. influenzae infection) OPV - 2, two drops, Oral (Against Polio) *Rotavirus Vaccine, five drops of Rotavac/2.5 ml of Rotasiil, Oral, (against diarrhea caused by rotavirus)

14 weeks	Pentavalent - 3, 0.5 mL, Intramuscular (against Diphtheria, tetanus, pertussis, hepatitis B and H. influenzae infection) OPV - 3, two drops, Oral (Against Polio) IPV – 2 0.5 ml, fractional dose (0.1ml), (Inactivated polio vaccine) Rotavirus Vaccine, five drops of Rotavac/2.5 ml of Rotasiil, Oral (against diarrhea caused by rotavirus) PCV – 2, 0.5 ml, intramuscular, (Against pneumococcal infection)
9–12 months	MR, 0.5 mL, Subcutaneous (against measles and rubella or German measles) #Japanese Encephalitis (1st Dose), 0.5 mL, Subcutaneous, In select endemic districts only PCV – B, 0.5 ml, intramuscular, (Against pneumococcal infection) IPV, third dose fractional dose (0.1ml), Intra - dermal IPV (Inactivated polio vaccine) Vitamin A first dose, 1 mL (100,000 IU), Oral
Children 16–24 months	DPT booster - 1, 0.5 mL, Intramuscular (Against diphtheria, pertussis, and tetanus) #Japanese encephalitis (second dose), 0.5 mL, Subcutaneous, # In select endemic districts MR (second dose)/MMR* 0.5 mL Subcutaneous [against measles, mumps & rubella (German measles)] *MMR Presently given in Delhi, Goa, Sikkim, and Puducherry Vitamin A - second dose, 2 mL (200,000 IU), Oral #J.E. vaccine Given only in select states, district, and cities that are endemic for the disease
Every 6 months till 5 years of age	Third to ninth dose of Vitamin A, 2 mL (200,000 IU), Oral The 2nd to 9th doses of Vitamin A can be administered to children 1 - 5 years old during biannual rounds, in collaboration with Integrated Child Development Scheme
5–6 years	DPT Booster - 2, 0.5 mL, Intramuscular, Upper arm (against diphtheria, tetanus, and pertussis)

10 years	TD (Tetanus & Diphtheria), 0.5 mL, Intramuscular, Upper arm
16 years	TD (Tetanus & Diphtheria), 0.5 mL, Intramuscular, Upper arm
Pregnant women	TD - 1* (Tetanus & Diphtheria) 0.5 mL Intramuscular Upper arm
4 weeks after TD - 1	TD - 2 (Tetanus & Diphtheria) 0.5 mL Intramuscular Upper arm *If the pregnant woman has received two TD doses in pregnancy within the last 3 years, only one TD - booster is required during the present pregnancy.
Apart from the above, there are other optional vaccines – e.g., chicken pox (Varicella) and Hepatitis A recommended by the Indian Academy of Pediatrics, which can be given at a cost	

Reference: GOI Immunization Handbook for Medical Officers, New Delhi, Department of Health and Family Welfare 2017 GOI, 2023.

(https://twitter.com/MoHFW_INDIA/status/16112353669039104)

Strengthening TD10 and TD16 Vaccine Implementation, Operational Guidelines, and Strategic Plan. Immunization Division, MoHFW, New Delhi.

Adolescent Health – In order to ensure holistic development of the adolescent population of around 25 crore, *Rashtriya Kishor Swasthya Karyakram* (RKSK) was launched in 2014. The Government has the responsibility to ensure that adolescents reach their optimal potential. Accordingly, the Reproductive and Child Health (RCH) program was expanded to RMNCH+ A – Reproductive maternal, newborn, child and adolescent health. The priority interventions for adolescents are information and counseling on adolescent sexual and reproductive health issues (**sex education, menstrual hygiene - provision of hygienic sanitary napkins and their safe disposal,** etc.);

Nutritional supplements (along with weekly supplementation of **iron and folic acid**), preventive health check - ups, **prevention of substance abuse** and non - communicable diseases, **immunization** and **counseling against violence** and injuries.

MCH Indicators – Maternal and child health indicators are a measure of the level of health care services in the overall development of an area, state, **or country**.

One important MCH indicator is the maternal mortality ratio (MMR) – It is defined as the 'total number of female deaths due to complications of pregnancy, childbirth or within 42 days of delivery due to puerperal causes during a given year per 100,000 live births in the same area and year.

India has seen a rapid decline in MMR from 398/100 000 live births in 1997–98 to 99/100 000 (90–108) in 2020 against a **global MMR of 223 (2020).**

MMR = Total no of female deaths due to pregnancy, childbirth, or within 42 days of delivery due to puerperal causes x 100,000

Infant mortality rate (IMR): This is the number of deaths of infants under one year of age per 1,000 live births.

$$\text{IMR} = \frac{\text{Total number of deaths in infants before one year of age}}{\text{Total number of live births in that area \& year}} \; x\; 1000$$

IMR for India in **2023 was 26.619** deaths per 1000 live birth

$$\text{Neonatal mortality rate} = \frac{\text{Total number of deaths below 28 days of age}}{\text{Total number of live births in that area \& year}} \; x\; 1000$$

NMR for India for 2023 was **22 per 1000 live births**

$$\text{Under five mortality rates} = \frac{\text{Total deaths in children under 5 years of age}}{\text{The total number of live births in that area \& year}} \; x\; 1000$$

U5MR for India in 2023 was 35 per 1000 live births

Crude Birth Rate (CBR) = Number of live births per 1,000 population: (Number of live births/Estimated midyear Population) * 1,000

CBR for India is **2.03 (2021)**

Death Rate = Number of deaths per 1000 population (Number of deaths/ Estimated mid - year population) * 1000

Family Planning & Contraceptive Methods: The invention of family planning and contraceptive methods marks a significant milestone in human history, empowering women to control fertility. It can be argued that the women's liberation movement gained momentum with the ability to control birth.

Natural Methods: Many couples successfully maintain small family norms using natural methods throughout their marital life. One such method is coitus interruptus, where ejaculation is prevented from occurring in the vagina, which can be highly effective if practiced correctly. Another natural method is timing intercourse to avoid the female ovulation period, which typically occurs midway through the menstrual cycle. Women who track their menstrual cycles can avoid intercourse during the fertile window.

Contraceptive Devices: India was one of the earliest countries to officially adopt family planning as a national program in 1950. Contraceptives enable women to make choices about their lives and live according to their preferences. Men are now equally encouraged to use effective contraceptives to promote and conserve maternal health. The use of contraception can prevent genital tract infections and sexually transmitted diseases like syphilis, gonorrhea, herpes, and AIDS and help preserve women's health. Optimal use of contraceptive devices also reduces the need for abortions.

The Ideal Contraceptive: The ideal contraceptive should be safe, effective, reversible, easy to use, efficient, affordable, and free from side effects. Pregnancy can be avoided through various methods, but not every method is suitable for everyone. Couples should select the most appropriate contraceptive using a "cafeteria approach" from the following "menu" of contraceptives.

1. Temporary Contraceptive Methods

a. **Barrier Method – Condom** is a barrier method that prevents the fusion of sperm and egg. Condoms made of latex rubber and attractive designs and colors are easily available in the market and are popular throughout the world. Male condoms are used without many social, cultural, or religious barriers. They, in addition, prevent infections and sexually transmitted diseases.

The male condom is a good, convenient, suitable, and agreeable barrier; it may be made even more effective if **spermicidal jelly** is applied by the female during intercourse. This is called the 'joint method of contraception.' The male condom, when used alone, has an efficacy of up to 90 - 95% and up to 99% when used with spermicidal jelly.

b. **Intra - uterine Device (IUD)** – This device is implanted in the uterus of women and prevents the fusion of sperm and egg. In earlier times, a 'T' shaped loop made of plastic was implanted in the uterus, but nowadays, various medicated IUDs and drug - eluting **IUDs** called **Copper - T** are available. A medical examination by the specialist is necessary whenever any problem arises, as well as at appropriate intervals. **Copper - T** is effective for at least 5 years and may be replaced as needed. It can be inserted easily into a woman's womb and also removed within a few minutes. It is generally inserted by a gynecologist or family planning worker. This is an excellent spacing device between 2 successive births. IUD is highly efficient, with a 97% success rate, and the use of another method, like a condom or spermicidal jelly, is not required.

Whenever the couple wants another baby, this device is removed easily. **Side effects of IUDs** – IUDs are generally tolerated well. However, some women may complain of **pelvic pain**, which may be psychological also.

Rarely, IUD may migrate from the uterus and cause uterine perforation. Rarely, an **ectopic pregnancy** may occur while wearing an IUD. In an ectopic pregnancy, the fertilized egg gets attached outside the uterus cavity - in the fallopian tube, abdominal cavity, cervix, or ovaries due to which the fetus may grow at some other place. Ectopic pregnancies, when diagnosed, have to be terminated by a qualified obstetrician.

c. **Hormonal Contraceptive** – Hormonal contraceptives are available mostly as pills, injections, and subcutaneous implants.

Currently contraceptive pills are the most commonly used method of birth control both by married and unmarried couples throughout the world. These also have 95 - 97% efficacy. Most hormone contraceptives are used or implanted in the female partner.

Male hormone contraceptives have been a matter of research. Recently a convenient, efficacious male hormonal contraceptive may temporarily retard, or block sperm production is being claimed – Its phase III and market trials are ongoing.

d. Hormonal pills commonly known as **Oral Contraceptive Pills (OCPs)** or colloquially 'pills' are of many types and can be administered on a daily basis, 1 - 21 days after the menstrual period, on a once - a - week basis or post - coitally an 'emergency pill.' These pills can be taken in privacy by women and are used both to avoid pregnancy by unmarried women and by married women for spacing between children. Various pills have different salts and concentrations of the two female hormones estrogen and progesterone. The ratio of estrogen hormone was higher in older generation pills which was somewhat harmful. The new generation pills prepared with a currently determined ratio of both the hormones are highly successful and mostly harmless without any side effect.

However, in some societies the side effects of contraceptive pills are overstated. The pills containing both estrogen and progesterone are called **combined pills** – these pills are advised to be taken continuously for 21 days starting with the first day of the period.

If forgotten to be taken on a day, it is advised to ingest 2 pills the next day. After stopping the course after 21 days the woman gets **breakthrough bleeding.** Contraceptives pills are also used for regulating menstrual cycle. Another very effective contraceptive pill devoid of serious side effects developed by Central Drug Research Institute, Lucknow, India is called **Centchroman or Saheli or Ormeloxifene** which is to be taken once a week only.

This contraceptive is equally effective, inexpensive and devoid of side effects. It has been officially adopted by the Ministry of Health & Family Welfare (MoHFW), Government of India for contraception.

OCPs are beneficial for women because they help in regulating menstrual cycle. Users suffer less from iron deficiency anemia, loss of bone density, ovarian cysts, endometrial cancer, ovary epithelial, colorectal and breast cancer. Now the new generations of pills are free of side effects like thrombo -embolism, heart attack, brain stroke etc. That these pills on continuous use may increase weight, cause breast cancer or other cancer are misconceptions.

Apart from pills, **contraceptive hormone injections** of different periods (trimonthly, bimonthly or monthly) are also available. Trimonthly hormone injections are **DMPA/Depo - Provera** and bimonthly hormone injections are **net - en/norethisterone enantate**. Combined injectable contraceptives (CICs) which are monthly hormone injections, may be taken only on medical advice. Now, synthetic hormone injections are also prepared with appropriate ratio of both hormones. These should only be taken on doctor's advice.

Post - coital Contraception Pills – In the event of contraceptives not being used before coitus, conception can also be prevented by taking hormone tablets known as **morning after pills** within 72 hours of intercourse.
This is also called **emergency contraceptive pills**, are quite effective and available in the market.

Termination of Pregnancy – In the event of not using contraception during coitus or the contraception being unsuccessful, termination of pregnancy may be necessary.

The **Medical Termination of Pregnancy (MTP)** Act was notified in 1971, and women resorted to termination of pregnancy, citing various reasons. It allows the woman to exercise her choice. Termination of pregnancy is less in vogue in recent years because of better knowledge and use of contraceptive methods.

Abortion in a few countries like Ireland is prohibited. New laws on abortion have also been passed in the United States of America, and certain states prohibit it. Successful abortion may be brought about by using hormone tablets on the advice of the doctor. Using abortion pills irrationally on the advice of chemists, quacks, and the internet may be harmful to health.

2. Permanent Contraceptive Methods involve surgical procedures – vasectomy in men and tubectomy in women.

a. **Male Sterilization or Vasectomy** – This is a highly efficient permanent method of sterilization, which some men happily opt for. Vasectomy can be done in primary health centers (PHC), local medical camps, or big hospitals after giving local anesthesia. Only one or two small incisions or skin punctures on the male scrotum are required through which the 'vas deferens' are delivered and severed. Its reversal is also possible with a varied success rate of 50 - 80%, and it is done by trained surgeons or plastic / micro - vascular surgeons who can join 2 - 3 mm tubes. Men avoid vasectomy due to being misguided that the procedure would result in a lack of sexual pleasure and impotence, which is actually more a myth than fact.

b. **Female Sterilization or Tubectomy** – In this, the fallopian tubes are surgically blocked, clipped by a ring, or partly cut and removed. This will prevent transmission of the ovum into the uterine cavity. This type of surgery is very effective and may be reversed if required. Tubectomy is more commonly adopted by married couples in India as compared to vasectomy. The reversal of tubectomy requires expert microsurgery by opening the abdomen. Tubectomy can be done by the open method by a small incision on the abdomen below the naval or by a telescope - assisted device called a **laparoscope**.

In conclusion, the profound impact of family planning on socioeconomic and intellectual development has been recognized only in recent history, particularly after the world was divided into developed, developing, and underdeveloped countries.

There are concerns that changing global demography may lead to a predominance of elderly people over the age of 80, outnumbering the younger population.

Therefore, just as non - adherence to family planning can hinder human development, strict adherence to policies such as one child per couple or choosing to remain childless could potentially pose a threat to the survival of humankind.

Mother and Child Health (MCH) programs have been widely adopted by countries around the world, focusing on nutrition, birthing practices, and disease prevention. Improved living conditions, along with enhanced child and adolescent health, have contributed to increased overall survival rates.

Moreover, modern contraceptives have played a crucial role in liberating and empowering women, enabling them to live life on their own terms.

Chapter 23

Balanced Diet & Nutrition

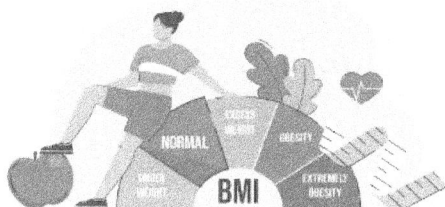

Learning Objectives:
• Process of digestion
• Significance of seven components of food - carbohydrate, protein, fat, water, vitamin, mineral, fiber
• Diseases caused by deficiency of nutrients
• Role of fiber or roughage in digesting food and strengthening gut flora
• Elements of 'Detoxification'

All living beings rely on food for survival, and their potential is largely influenced by their diet. A balanced diet is one that provides all the necessary nutrients in the right proportions to prevent diseases and maintain overall health. The choices we make about what to eat, what to avoid, and what to consume in moderation are crucial for our well - being. A balanced diet, sound sleep, and regular physical exercise are fundamental necessities of life.

When we eat, our tongue and teeth work together to grind and mix the food into a **bolus**, which is then swallowed and propelled through the esophagus, or food pipe, into the stomach. The enzyme **amylase**, secreted in saliva, begins the digestion process by acting on the starch in the food, converting it into maltose.

In the stomach, the acidic gastric juices further break down the food into a semi - liquid form called **chyme**. This chyme is then passed into the duodenum, the upper part of the small intestine, where it is further digested by enzymes from the **pancreas**. The nutrients are absorbed into the bloodstream in the small intestine, while the residual waste matter is passed into the large intestine and eventually excreted as **feces**.

The food we consume serves multiple purposes: it fuels basic metabolic functions, supports physical activity, and facilitates growth and tissue repair.

A healthy adult woman requires 1,800 to 2,400 calories per day, while a man requires 2,000 to 3,200 calories per day. However, individuals engaged in physical labor or intense physical activity may require 3,000 to 4,000 calories daily, as they burn most of the calories they consume. Conversely, people with sedentary lifestyles who do not engage in regular physical activity may struggle to burn off the calories they consume, leading to fat accumulation, particularly around the abdomen and neck.

The majority of people worldwide - over 7 billion of the 8 billion - consume a mixed diet that includes both plant - based and animal - derived foods. In India, a 'non - vegetarian' diet typically includes a significant number of plant - based foods (cereals, lentils, vegetables, fruits), along with some quantity of milk, milk products, eggs, and meat. A vegetarian diet, on the other hand, generally consists of plant - based foods along with milk and milk products but excludes eggs, meat, and fish. A **'vegan'** diet, which excludes all animal - derived products such as milk, milk products, meat, eggs, and fish, is relatively rare.

The daily diet must contain **seven components** known as nutrients. These are **carbohydrates, protein, fat, vitamins, minerals, water and fiber.** They are obtained from milk, cereals, vegetable - fruit - legumes - nuts, eggs, meat, fish, etc. Three of the above seven components provide energy to the body - carbohydrates, protein, and fat and are called **macronutrients.** Vitamins and minerals called **'micronutrients'** are required in small or minute quantities. Calories from carbohydrates are used mostly for energy production, calories from protein for body building and repair, while calories from fat are mostly stored in the body. Ultimately, all are interchangeable. The **balanced diet** or ideal diet must provide calories from all these three components of food.

Carbohydrates should be taken to provide 60% to 70% of the required energy. Proteins should be taken to provide 15% to 20% of the total calories, and fat should provide 18% to 25% of the body's energy requirement. Notably, carbohydrates give immediate kinetic energy to the body. Protein, being an important repairing agent, fabricates the tissues. Enzymes, many hormones, and body fluids are derived from proteins. Fat is responsible for building body contours and is the energy that is stored in the body in various forms.

Health reports elucidate that market food, unlike home kitchen food, is full of carbohydrates and fat. **Junk Food** or **fast food** is the lavish food of modern times, deep fried in oil. Add tobacco and alcohol, and a recipe for chronic diseases is ready.

More about the seven components of food:

1. **Carbohydrates** (**1 gm = 4 calories**): These are organic compounds present in foods in the form of starch, **sugars**, and cellulose. The ratio of hydrogen and oxygen in carbohydrates is the same as in water, i.e., 2:1.

   These typically break down quickly in the body to release energy. Wheat, millet, coarse grain, rice, lentils, potato, banana, sugarcane, beetroot, dates, **sugar**, raisins, fig, honey, etc., are the main sources of carbohydrates. Carbohydrates obtained from natural sweetening in fruit and vegetables are conducive to health. Carbohydrates can be classified into three groups viz;

   i) **polysaccharides** present in starch like rice, potato, wheat, and sago;

   ii) **Sugars** like sugarcane, fruit, and beetroot; and

   iii) **cellulose**.

Carbohydrate in cereals is digested by the enzyme amylase in saliva. Various types of **sugars** viz; **fructose** from fruits, **maltose**, **sucrose** from sugarcane, and lactose from milk are respectively digested by the enzymes maltase, sucrase, and lactase, etc. **Cellulose** carbohydrates (polysaccharides) derived from fibre are digested by **cellulase**. This enzyme is not produced in the digestive system of human beings but is found in animals like elephants, hippopotamuses, cattle, horses, deer, etc., and keeps them active and energetic. Extra carbohydrates are stored in the liver as **glycogen.** During starvation and critical situations, glycogen is a ready source of energy. Excessive intake of carbohydrates leads to **metabolic syndrome**, becoming the harbinger of **obesity, diabetes, cancer,** etc.

All types of carbohydrates are broken down into glucose and provide energy to the body. Carbohydrates with a high **glycemic index** lead to a quick and high rise in blood glucose after consumption. Such foods are avoided in diabetes.

2. **Protein (1 gm = 4 calories)** – Proteins are complex, large molecules containing nitrogen, oxygen, hydrogen, carbon, and sometimes sulfur. They help in building tissues. **Enzymes, antibodies**, and **hormones** are made of protein. Leguminous plants, meat, dairy products, fish, egg, wholegrain cereals, wheat, barley, millet, corn, lentils, ragi, *rajma*, white and brown beans, chickpeas (*chhole*), soybean, nuts like groundnut, almond, walnut – all these foods have high protein content. Proteins are made up of long chains of **amino acids**. There are about 20 amino acids, of which nine are essential, i.e., they cannot be synthesized in the body and must be provided in the diet. The arrangement and sequence of these 20 amino acids determines the protein formed. However, plant - derived proteins mostly have lower **bioavailability** than animal proteins. i.e., they are less efficiently absorbed and incorporated into the body. Whey protein and protein in cooked eggs are considered to have the highest bioavailability.

Protein supplements are advised to be taken by those who perform heavy physical exercises. Protein malnutrition causes swelling, fatty liver, skin fissures and breaches, infectious diseases, etc. The immune system of the body is strengthened by protein.

3. **Fat (1 gm = nine calories) – Clarified butter (desi ghee), plant oils, butter, and thick cream of milk (malai) are all sources** of fat. The calories in these products are twice the calories present in carbohydrates and protein. The fat intake ratio should be low in food, and the consumption of fat should be less than 20% of the total calories. Lipase enzyme breaks down fat into fatty acids, which are absorbed by the body. Fat gets stored in the adipose tissue, which is mainly found in **subcutaneous fat** under the skin and **visceral fat** inside the abdomen.

Fat provides energy during fasting; controls body temperature, provides contour to the physique, and is used for the synthesis of hormones.

Fat can be classified into three types –

(i) **saturated fat** found in milk, butter, cheese, and cream

(ii) mono - unsaturated fat, and

(iii) **poly - unsaturated fat.**

Vegetable oils such as olive oil, nuts, canola oil, avocado oil, sunflower oil, soyabean oil, walnuts, almonds, corn, soybeans, etc., are sources of unsaturated fat and are considered 'good fat.'

Consumption of these oils does not increase cholesterol deposits in the walls of the arteries. Saturated and 'trans' fats (partially hydrogenated fats) are considered 'bad.' Ghee is a saturated fat but has some advantages, such as high Omega - 3 fatty acid, vitamin A, and lower acrylamide – a toxic compound produced on heating. Two types of cholesterol are – low - density lipoprotein (**LDL)** and high - density lipoprotein (**HDL).** Raised LDL builds up plaques, which can block the arteries.

Thus, **LDL is called bad cholesterol,** while HDL is good cholesterol. Excessive consumption of fat may cause obesity, metabolic syndrome, high blood pressure, diabetes, heart disease, brain stroke, etc.

Deficiency of the above nutrients - carbohydrates, proteins, and fat - in the diet causes malnutrition and weight loss, while excess intake leads to obesity and being overweight. Minerals, vitamins, water, and fiber do not affect body weight but are important for body functions.

4. **Minerals** – Important minerals (inorganic substances) that are required in the diet are calcium, phosphorus, sodium, potassium, iodine, iron, chloride, zinc, chromium, magnesium, copper, sulfur, selenium, fluoride, etc. They provide necessary nourishment to the body, while their deficiency may cause specific symptoms and diseases. Cereals and lentils, leafy vegetables, seeds, nuts, groundnuts, cashews, walnuts, almonds, pistachio, shellfish, cabbage, broccoli, meat, egg, beans, avocado, berries, yogurt, cheese, milk, and milk products are the chief sources of minerals.

Calcium (Recommended dietary allowance (RDA) = **1000 mg/ day**). **Sources** – dairy products (milk, cheese), soybeans, leafy vegetables, figs, etc. Calcium is an essential mineral for bone strength, blood vessels, and cellular functions, especially blood coagulation, muscles, nerves, and the heart. Its deficiency may cause back and joint pains. Excessive calcium occurs in disorders of the parathyroid gland and causes abdominal pains, psychiatric symptoms, and stone formation in the kidney.

Phosphorus (RDA= **800 - 1000 mg/day**) – **Sources** – egg, *paneer*, curd, dark chocolate, cereals, meat, nuts, lentils, milk etc.

This mineral undergoes absorption in the small intestine. Its deficiency or **hypophosphatemia** may cause musculoskeletal weakness, fatigue, dizziness, etc.

Sodium, potassium, and calcium are important electrolytes. They are important for cellular functions, maintaining electrical neutrality in the cells and conducting impulses in the muscles of the heart and brain.

Sodium (RDA = **2000 mg/day**), **Source** – salt, value range in the blood is 135 - 145 milliequivalent/liter. Low level in the blood is known as **hyponatremia** and high level is called **hypernatremia**.

When sodium is low, as may occur in severe vomiting, diarrhea, and dehydration, there is nausea, lethargy, muscle cramps, confusion, loss of energy, weakness, seizures, and coma.

Hypernatremia occurs because of net water loss. The symptoms of excess sodium are extreme thirst, confusion, lethargy, irritability, muscle weakness, seizures, and unconsciousness.

Potassium (RDA = **3500 mg/day**) **Sources** – fruit and vegetables, value range in the blood 3.5 - 5.0 milliequivalent/liter. Low level in blood is known as **hypokalemia**, and high level is called **hyperkalemia**.

Potassium deficiency causes extreme tiredness, fatigue, muscle weakness, cramps and abnormal heart rhythms. Hyperkalemia generally occurs in kidney failure and presents as irregular pulse, numbness and sudden death.

Zinc – (RDA = **8 mg/day for women; 11 mg/day for men**)

Sources – egg, groundnut, garlic, fish, seed of watermelon, cashew, curd, nuts, chickpeas *(chhole)* etc. This mineral is neither produced nor stored in the body, but it is important because it helps build cells, heal injuries or wounds, and strengthen the immune system. Symptoms of zinc deficiency are diarrhea, poor wound healing, frequent infections, and hair loss.

Zinc is widely prescribed for **acute diarrhea in children**.

Iron (RDA = 8.7 mg/day, 14.8 mg/day for women aged 19 to 49 years) – this mineral is responsible for producing **hemoglobin** present in **red blood cells (RBC)** and certain enzymes.

Source – egg, nuts, green leafy vegetables, spinach, beetroot, lentils, jaggery, groundnuts, pomegranate, apple, gooseberry (amla), jamun, pistachio, walnut, raisin, etc. Its deficiency causes **anemia.** Iron deficiency anemia is the most common type of anemia in India.

Magnesium (RDA = 370 - 440 mg/ day) – **Source** – wholegrain cereal, vegetables, walnut, cashew, almond, fig, avocado, dark chocolate, etc. One cup of boiled spinach contains 100 - 157 mg of magnesium. This mineral is also important for the functioning of the nervous system. Its deficiency may cause fatigue, low appetite, nausea, vomiting, muscle spasms or tremors, abnormal heart rhythms, constipation, weight loss, dry skin, hair falling, etc.

Iodine – (RDA = 150 microgram/day) This element is not classified as a mineral but is an important constituent of food. **Sources** – radish, carrot, tomato, salt, spinach, potato, peas, seafood, meat, egg yolk, milk, cod liver oil, seaweed, etc. Deficiency of iodine causes certain thyroid problems, such as **goiter.** Deficiency of iodine in young children causes impaired physical and mental growth – **cretinism**. Salt in India is fortified with iodine, and this has drastically reduced the prevalence of goiter and cretinism.

5. **Vitamins** – These are complex organic compounds that do not provide energy to the body but are required in the diet and cannot be synthesized in the body. Insufficiency may cause **vitamin deficiency diseases.** Vitamins are frequently advised as a supplement which is often unnecessary.

Vitamins are classified into two groups viz: **fat - soluble (Vitamins A, D, E & K)** and **water - soluble vitamins (Vitamin B complex and vitamin C)**. Fat - soluble vitamins are stored in the body, and excess can cause toxicity, while water - soluble vitamins are not stored, and excess usually does not cause toxicity.

Vitamin A or Retinol – (RDA = 1000 mcg/ day), **Sources** – carrot, papaya, cod liver oil, egg, cereal, green - red - yellow vegetables, and fruit.

Its deficiency may cause dry and inflamed skin and mucosal surfaces, **night blindness**, infertility, and **corneal opacity**. Vitamin A deficiency is the most common cause of preventable blindness.

Vitamin B – This is a group of water - soluble vitamins B1, B2, B3, B5, B6, B7, B9, B12, folic acid etc.

Vitamin B1 or thiamine (RDA = 1.4 - 2.2 mg); **Sources** – cereals, fruits, vegetables, dairy products. It is an important vitamin required in carbohydrate metabolism and nerve impulse conduction.

Severe deficiency of thiamine may cause the disease **beriberi,** which may cause nerve and heart dysfunction.

Vitamin B2 or riboflavin (RDA = 2.0 - 3.2 mg/day), **Sources** – fish, rice, peas, lentils, yeast, egg yolk. This is important for the maintenance of healthy skin and the lining of the digestive system and various organs. Its deficiency may cause hyperemia, fissures of the corners of the mouth and lips, hair fall, and problems in the reproductive system.

B3 or niacin (RDA = male 14 - 23 mg/day, female 11 - 18 mg/day), **Sources** – groundnuts, sunflower - seed, mushroom, chicken, pea, almond, milk, egg, dates, tomato, carrot, leafy vegetables and nuts. Niacin preserves the health of the skin, nervous, and digestive systems. Its deficiency may cause **pellagra**, in which skin rash, dementia, and diarrhea occur simultaneously. This disease is caused by genetic disorders, malabsorption, and side effects of drugs.

Vitamin B5 or pantothenic acid (RDA = 5 - 6 mg/ day). Sources – tomato, husky bran, wheat flour, egg yolk, almond, walnut, plant seeds, orange - mandarin, grapes, milk, fresh beans, pea, lentil, liver, green leafy vegetable, potato, fruits, yeast, gram, coconut, pistachio, cabbage, curd, spinach, etc. B5 is an important vitamin in the building of blood cells and is beneficial to the skin, eyes, hair, liver, etc.

Vitamin B6 or pyridoxine (RDA = 1.2 - 1.5 mg/day). Sources – chicken, potato, corn, spinach, egg, chicken, carrot, sweet potato, banana, avocado, chickpeas (chole), fish, etc. Its deficiency causes fatigue, weakness, anemia, skin infections, lip fissures, **seizures, sleep disorders,** etc.

Vitamin B7 or biotin (RDA = 30 mcg/ day), Sources – egg - yolk, whole grain cereal, soybean, nuts, yeast, tomato, strawberry, etc. Its deficiency may cause decay of gut flora, hair loss, scratches around the eyes - nose - face and genital organs, depression, etc.

Vitamin B9 or Folic Acid (RDA = 220 - 300 mcg/ day), Source – spinach, *bathua*, fenugreek seeds, sprout cereals, mustard leaf, turnip, beetroot, soybean, salmon fish, whole grain, root vegetables, wheat, rajma, lentils, beans, avocado, orange - peel, milk, etc. Its deficiency may cause **anemia**.

It also has a role in the **prevention of neural tube defects** in the fetus if supplemented in the peri - conceptional period.

B12 Cyanocobalamin (RDA = 2.4 mcg/ day), Sources – milk, milk - product, egg, fish, chicken. It is to be noted that this vitamin is **only found in animal foods**, and vegan diets are deficient in this vitamin. Its deficiency may cause **tremors**, fatigue, muscle weakness, **anemia**, tingling and stiffness in hands and feet, pins and needles sensation, mouth ulcers, constipation, diarrhea, and symptoms of the nervous system, including weakness in lower limbs and dementia in severe cases.

Vitamin C or Ascorbic - acid (RDA = 75 - 80 mg/ day), Sources – citric juicy fruits (gooseberry, orange - mandarin, lemon, orange, grapes, tomato, guava, apple) banana, berry, jack fruit, turnip, mint, radish leaf, raisins, milk, beetroot, *chaurai* vegetable, cabbage, coriander, spinach, etc. Vitamin C plays an important role in collagen production – a protein important for the integrity of connective tissues like skin, bones, joints, and blood vessels. Its deficiency causes a condition called '**scurvy**' characterized by bleeding gums, easy bruising, and poor wound healing.

Two centuries ago, people who went on long cruises and sailed on high seas without a supply of fresh fruit suffered from scurvy. It was later realized that as soon the sailors came on land and were fed fresh foods, especially citrus fruits, their bleeding wounds healed. This is the story of the discovery of vitamin C. In 1937, the Nobel Prize was given for this discovery to a Hungarian doctor, Albert Szent–Gyorgyi who called it 'hexuronic acid.' Vitamin C is also an **antioxidant**.

Vitamin D (RDA = 600 IU/ day) – This vitamin, also considered a hormone, is produced in our skin from the sun's rays and is also obtained from our diet. Vitamin D plays an important role in the metabolism and utilization of calcium and phosphorus. Dietary **Sources** – fish, fish oils, egg yolk, mushroom, milk, cheese etc. Its deficiency may cause **muscle weakness, osteoporosis, osteomalacia** in adults, and **rickets** in children.

With severe and chronic vitamin D deficiency, calcium and phosphorus levels go down, and absorption of these from the intestine is also affected. This results in the activity of parathyroid glands to maintain blood calcium levels. The forms of vitamin D are **vitamin D_2** and **vitamin D_3**.

Calcitriol is the active form. Despite abundant sunlight, Vitamin D deficiency is extremely common in India. Vitamin D is now believed to play a **wider role in human health**, and there is some evidence linking vitamin D deficiency with cancer, cardiovascular disease, diabetes, autoimmune diseases, and depression.

Vitamin E or Tocopherols – **(RDA = 15 mg/day; 19 mg/day in lactating women) Sources** – sun - flower - seed, leafy vegetables (spinach, broccoli), vegetable oils, and nuts like groundnut, walnut, almond.

This compound acts as **an antioxidant.** This is an important vitamin for maintaining the health of skin and hair. The main symptoms of vitamin E deficiency are mild haemolytic anemia and nonspecific neurologic deficits.

Antioxidants are compounds that inhibit auto - oxidation and build up of harmful free radicals in the body (oxidative stress). Antioxidants are added to several food items and industrial products to preserve and increase their shelf life and stop the deterioration. Lipsticks and moisturizers are added with antioxidants.

Numerous dietary compounds vitamins A, E and C act as antioxidants in the body and prevent aging and disease.

Vitamin K or phylloquinone/menaquinones – (RDA = 120 mcg/kg/day for men; 90 mcg/kg/day for women).

One important source is bacteria present in the large intestine. This vitamin plays a role in coagulation of blood. Its deficiency may lead to bleeding.

Thus, though vitamins are not a source of energy, they play an important role in metabolism and are helpful in maintaining the good health of various organs of the body.

All the vitamins may be easily obtained from daily diet or from vitamin tablets.

The following table gives a quick review of Vitamins:

Vitamin Types	Symptoms /Diseases due to deficiency
Fat soluble Vitamins	**A, D, E and K**
Vitamin A or Retinol **Source:** Carrot, papaya, egg, green, red, yellow vegetable, avocado, green chilli, sweet potato, spinach, egg, meat, fish	Night blindness, corneal scar
Vitamin D or Cholecalciferol **Source:** Sunlight	Rickets in children, osteomalacia, osteoporosis, colon cancer
Vitamin E or Tocopherol **Source:** Sunflower seed, leafy vegetable, almond, avocado, groundnut, olive oil	Increase and decrease in cholesterol, mental disorders

Vitamin K or Phylloquinone **Source:** Dairy products, intestinal bacteria, soyabean	Coagulation disorder, sterility
Water soluble Vitamins **B Complex and C**	
Vitamin B1 or Thiamine **Source:** Cereal, fruit, vegetable, dairy product, pea, lentils	Beriberi, heart failure
Vitamin B2 or Riboflavin **Source:** Rice, lentil, fish, egg - yolk, milk banana	Inflammation of lips
Vitamin B3 or Niacin **Source:** Groundnut, Sunflower seed, milk, tomato, leafy vegetable, egg, lentils, brown rice	Pellagra (skin rash, dementia, diarrhea)
Vitamin B5 or Pantothenic acid **Source:** Groundnut, Sunflower seed, milk, tomato, leafy vegetable, egg, lentils, brown rice, flour with bran, tomato, fenugreek, chia seed, dry fruit, green vegetable, mushroom	Tiredness, sleep apnea, irritation, vomiting, stomach pain, lack of protein
Vitamin B6 or Pyridoxine **Source:** Corn, green vegetables, avocado, green chilli, milk, chickpeas, seed, chicken, egg, fish	Anemia, skin infection, epilepsy, brain tumor
Vitamin B7 or Biotin **Source:** Whole grain, soyabean, nuts, green vegetable, egg - yolk	Hair fall, stress

Vitamin B$_9$ or Folate **Source:** Dark leafy vegetables, fruits and fruit juices, nuts, beans, peas, seafood, eggs, dairy products, meat, poultry and grains	Weakness, fatigue, Irregular heartbeat, shortness of breath, difficulty concentrating, hair loss, pale skin, mouth sores
Vitamin B$_{12}$ or Cyanocobalamin **Source:** Milk product, egg, fish, chicken, sea food. Not present in plant foods.	Tiredness, mouth ulcer, nervous system weakness
Vitamin C or Ascorbic acid **Source:** Citric juicy fruit, guava, green chili, broccoli, tomato, mango, gooseberry, green coriander (parsley)	Scurvy, cataract, skin disease, bad digestion

Vitamins & mineral supplements – Vitamins and minerals need to be supplied in the diet and are not **synthesized** in the body. They have many health benefits. It is preferable to get the daily requirements through a varied diet. Controlled studies have shown little or no benefit of supplements, except in special groups like pregnant women, children etc.

Supplements of water - soluble vitamins usually do not cause harm and are easily excreted from the body. On the other hand, fat soluble vitamins are stored in the body and can build up to toxic levels if supplemented. It is rare to get toxic levels through diet. One of the important fat - soluble vitamins is Vitamin D which is often found to be deficient even in a sunny country like ours and often needs to be supplemented.

6. **Water** – Water is available in nature from rivers, waterfalls, springs, groundwater, lakes, oceans etc. Water from natural sources contains dissolved and suspended molecules and may be contaminated with dangerous microbes. **Potable water** is that which is fit for human consumption but is not so abundant.

To be potable, water should be free from contamination by microbes and harmful elements and compounds. Water makes up about **60% of the human adult body** and the proportion is higher in children.

The proportion is different in various organs – about 73% in brain and heart, 83% in lungs, muscles, 79% in kidneys and 31% in bones. Water is required by every cell of the body for **vital life processes**. It helps in regulating our internal **body temperature** and in **metabolism** of carbohydrates and proteins. Through circulation it helps in **transportation** of metabolites and cells. It assists in flushing waste from the body mainly through urination and acts as a **shock absorber** for brain, spinal cord, and fetus and also forms saliva and joint fluid. Water is a necessary element for the incessant flow of life.. Water gets excreted from our body in different ways viz; 500 ml from sweat, 1500 ml from urine and 200 ml from defecation and rest as **'insensible loss'** through skin.

Taking at least this amount of water from liquid or solid food is needed to maintain good health. Frequent water drinking during the day keeps the body detoxified. Adults should take 2 - 3 liters of water every day – more water drinking is not harmful if kidney function is normal.

Many diseases like amoebiasis, colitis, cholera, typhoid and hepatitis are caused by consumption of contaminated water. Low level water consumption causes dehydration. Drinking slightly excessive water keeps the body healthy and sturdy.

7. **Fibre (RDA = 25 - 30 gm/ day)**, Source – husk - bran, wheat flour, gram flour, lentils, semolina *(suji)*, porridge or gruel *(dalia)*, apple, papaya, grapes, cucumber with peel, tomato, green - leaf onion, spinach, *chaurai* vegetable, mustard leaf, dill - fenugreek *(soya - methi)*, *bathua*, bottle gourd *(lauki)*, zucchini *(taroi)*, coarse food – all contain good amount of **fiber, roughage** or **residual diet**. Though fiber or roughage does not provide energy, it keeps the digestive system healthy. Fiber in the diet is conducive to growth of **gut flora**. Roughage in whole grain cereals, fruits and vegetables contains cellulose along with fiber. Fiber has great significance for keeping the digestive system of human beings functional and effective.

Fiber preserves the gut flora, prevents diabetes, arthritis, cancer etc. and softens the stool. The deficiency of gut flora may cause metabolic disorder and weakened immune system. High fiber diet prevents constipation, increases digestive efficiency, impedes weight gain and obesity and also prevents various cancers. Low fiber diet - refined flour and carbohydrates as used in samosa, pizza, noodles and white bread.

Benefits of millets – Recently, a lot of importance is being given to millets in the diet. These include finger millet (*Ragi*), sorghum (*Jowar*), pearl millet (*Bajra*) etc. Millet are ancient grains often used for feeding livestock and birds. Millets are adaptable grains – **cheap** and **easy to store**.

They are **fast - growing**, **hardy** crops which are drought resistant, and require low input.

Millets are a **good source of protein, fiber, key vitamins, and minerals**.

They have **low glycemic index** which means consumption of millets is not associated with immediate and high rise of blood sugar as compared to wheat flour.

The potential health benefits of millet include protecting cardiovascular health, preventing the onset of diabetes, helping people achieve and maintain a healthy weight, and managing inflammation in the gut.

Dietary systems of the world – Local availability, environment and season, habit and value system determine the dietary patterns and cooking habits. When harmful effects of traditional diets were seen, health interventions changed the value system and the diets.

For example, use of *Khesari dal* (Grass Pea Dal) in central India caused paralysis in lower limbs, red meat consumption in Scandinavian countries causes stomach cancer, diet mainly consisting of meat, potato and rum in British Armed Forces caused cancer colon and lack of iodine caused goitre in the Sub - Himalayan belt. These were checked by appropriate dietary corrections.

Some notable types of diets are as follows:

1. **Vegan diet** – Vegetarian diet that excludes everything from animal sources like milk and milk products and egg and fish. This type of diet may cause deficiency of Vitamin B_{12}.

2. **Low carb diet** – Eating fat and protein diet viz; nuts and seeds and abstaining from carbohydrates.

3. **Low fat diet** – Eating low quantity or oil free foods.

4. **Vegetarianism** – has been popular for millions of years in the Indo - Gangetic plains and evidence has been found that rice was cultivated thousand years BC. As practiced in India, a vegetarian diet includes milk and milk products but no other animal product.

   Some research reveals that vegetarian diet enhances human health. Deficiency of certain vitamins and minerals may be prevented by supplementation. Condemning meat eating Bertrand Russell said, "My stomach is not a graveyard...", Dr Michael Greger, USA in his book "How not to die...", holds that vegetarian diet bestows long life to man.

5. **Intermittent fasting** – consists of generally low carbohydrate diet but strictly taken within 8 hours and then strict 12 - 16 hours fasting.

6. **Mediterranean diet** – This diet includes leafy vegetables, nuts - seeds - beans - lentils, whole grain cereals, potato, avocado fruit, spices, fish, sea foods, poultry items like eggs, chicken, yogurt and red meat eaten very seldom. Food is cooked in olive or avocado oil only.

7. *Ayurveda* **Diet** – Since ancient times, age old Indian medical systems prescribe certain tenets for living moral and virtuous life of which the diet of 3 types –*Rita Bhukha* (ऋत भुख) – Eating as per season, *Hita Bhukha* (हित भुख) – Eating conducive to health, *Mita Bhukha* (मित भुख) – Eating in low quantity.

Maintaining fast once or twice a week, drinking excess of pure water, abstaining from salt, sugar and fat, creating momentum in the body by exercises and *Pranayama*, discarding irritation, anxiety and depression, waking and sleeping timely, living an active life while discarding lethargy and laziness.

Indian food manifests the cultural values of this subcontinent. Impact of *shuchita* (शुचिता) and *parhase* (परहेज) as instructed in *Ayurveda* is visible in the divergent cuisines of Indian people.

The bread or *chapati* of any sole cereal viz; whole wheat, gram, barley, millet, corn or mixture of these or various other cereals, lentils and legumes, seasonal vegetables and fruits, green salad, curd, sauce of mint or coriander, pickle, wafer (*papad*) roasted over the flame, cow - milk - *deshi* - *ghee* for cooking food and jaggery *kheer* or sweet as a dessert are the delicacies of Indian food. Eating whole wheat flour makes it rich in fiber. Eating different cereals and different vegetables on different days according to the season or climate has been the popular custom of Indian lifestyle – these food varieties has been attracting people belonging to different cultures. *Idli, dosa, vada, sambhar* in the southern states, *rice and lentil* preparation along the fish or sea food in Bengal and other coastal areas, *mishti - doi* (mixing honey or jaggery in the curd) and *paneer* - sweet. Dates and jaggery extracted from dates have a long reaching effect in repairing health.

Lancet - the world - famous medical journal has described that 2000 calorie from Indian diet is the average necessity. Lentils and - rice soaked in water for ½ to 1 hour then washed and squeezed of toxic phytate and tannins and then cooked. Nutrients of boiled vegetables and lentils remain preserved. Boiled vegetables mixed with meagre fried cumin seed, ginger, black pepper, lemon, vinegar being fresh is easily digested. Frying asafoetida, cumin and coriander seed with meagre sprinkling in *Deshi Ghee* or healthy oil increases the taste of the food.

Turmeric is a very important item in spices with antibacterial, antioxidant and anti - inflammatory properties. *Rai, Methi* (fenugreek), *kalonji* (Nigella Sativa), dry coriander seed powder, carom seed, cinnamon, fennel and various other such spices are enriched with number of properties conducive to health.

Vegetarians and vegan diet followers do not eat meat. Inhabitants of **5 blue zones** eat meat but as determined in their custom. These populations follow healthy dietary practices and cook their food in olive or avocado oil etc. Vegetable oils prevent diseases like obesity, diabetes and arterial plaques. Boiling, frying, roasting and baking for long periods destroy vitamins. Foods viz. *sohal, gujhiya*, pizza and noodles which consist of refined flour (*maida*) are harmful for health.

Detoxification – in daily life means a good intake of water, and good urine output, and good digestion with complete sense of bowel clearance. Some daily exercise with sweating, good inhalation and exhalation also should ideally detoxify the body. External surfaces and orifices need to be cleaned and washed with bathing, hair wash and clipping of nails.

In *Ayurved, panch karma* forceful vomiting, complete purging and sauna steam bath is practiced as part of detoxification. The key to a healthy diet lies in knowing what to eat, what to avoid, and what to consume only occasionally. While everyone aims to eat healthily, many are not fully aware as to which foods are beneficial, and which are harmful.

A balanced diet should include proper proportions of the seven essential components: carbohydrates, proteins, fats, minerals, vitamins, fiber, and water. It is now widely accepted that refined sugar and carbohydrates should be minimized in our diets. Natural sugars found in fruits, sugarcane, vegetables, and jaggery are considered healthier alternatives. Similarly, refined flour, commonly used in white bread, noodles, cakes, biscuits, and pizza, should be restricted. Salt intake should be moderate, as excessive salt can lead to high blood pressure (hypertension).

Fats in the diet should be primarily unsaturated rather than saturated. Cooking with unsaturated fats is advisable, but it's important not to use excessive amounts of even healthy oils. About five teaspoons of unsaturated oil per day is sufficient.

Additionally, the diet should be rich in fiber or roughage. Such a diet can help protect against various illnesses, including obesity, diabetes, high blood pressure, constipation, and cancer.

What to eat:

Fruits and Vegetables – Seasonal fruits, fruit juice, mixed vegetable juice or soup, and salad are all beneficial for health. Whether cooked or raw, fruits and vegetables in any form, including their juices, soups, or smoothies, contribute positively to well - being. However, raw fruits and vegetables must be thoroughly washed before consumption to remove any potential infections or pesticides.

How to Cook – Cooking food is crucial because heat kills germs. Freshly cooked, hot food is safer than stored or uncooked food, as it reduces the risk of infection. Try to cook with a minimal amount of healthy oil, as **five teaspoons of healthy oil per day** is sufficient. Over - roasting or excessive frying can diminish the nutritional value of food. Cooking with balanced spices and salt can enhance digestion and nutrient absorption.

However, some cooking methods may reduce key nutrients, especially water - soluble vitamins like vitamin C and B vitamins, which are sensitive to heat. Water - based cooking can significantly reduce the content of these vitamins, so it's important to cook with a reasonable amount of water to retain up to 90% of vitamins and minerals while improving food quality.

Including a small bowl of curd daily, which is rich in probiotics, has been a staple in Indian diets for centuries. A healthy breakfast consisting of barley or wheat porridge (*dalia*), semolina (*suji*), puffed rice (*lai*), crushed and parched rice (*chura*), roasted gram, sprout gram, *moong dal*, and seasonal fruits is advantageous in the long run. A good breakfast is essential for optimal school performance. Avoid eating while watching television, mobile devices, or laptops. Minimize the intake of carbohydrate - rich foods like potatoes, rice, sugar, and sweets. Use salt sparingly and avoid adding it at the table. Limit the use of excessive red or green chili and spices.

Incorporate protein - rich foods such as lentils, egg whites, and fish into your diet. Consume meat in small quantities, not more than once a week, and limit it to two servings. Green leafy vegetables should be part of the daily diet. Avoid stale food.

When eating out, opt for hot, freshly prepared food, and avoid chopped salads. Try to eat whole grains and vary your grains and vegetables frequently.

Drinks and Beverages – Aim to drink 12 - 15 glasses of water daily. Drink lukewarm water after meals but avoid sipping or swallowing water while eating. It's advisable to drink water at least one hour after meals. Choose milk with the cream removed or opt for skimmed milk Avoid soda or fizzy drinks, as they are high in sugar. Acidic beverages should be consumed only occasionally, such as during ceremonies or parties.

Indian Beverages – Low quantities of lemon juice, raw boiled mango juice, fruit juice, squash, *kewra* - fragrance sherbet, rose - water sherbet, salty - spicy - thin - curd *lassi*, buttermilk, and coconut water are good for maintaining a healthy gut.

What to eat very seldom:

Deep - Fried Foods – Items like patties, samosas, pooris, kachoris, and deep - fried potato chops should be eaten only occasionally. Dry fruits and nuts can also be consumed occasionally. Food items preserved in cans or packets should be avoided. Consuming semolina, porridge, lentils, fruits, vegetables, and *Isabgol* is beneficial for preventing and treating constipation.

What not to eat:

Many societies and cultures have a tendency to consume substances that can lead to delusions, hallucinations, lethargy, and inertia.

Therefore, substances like tobacco (betel, *gutkha, khaini, bidi,* cigarettes, etc.), alcohol, and intoxicating drugs (cocaine, cannabis, LSD, etc.) should be avoided as they are addictive and harmful to health in the long run.

Chapter 24

Metabolic Syndrome, Susceptibility to Disease, Obesity & Bariatric Surgery

---

Learning Objectives:

- Signs, symptoms and criteria of metabolic syndrome
- Causes and effects of metabolic syndrome
- How to manage metabolic syndrome
- Significance of bariatric surgery for control of obesity

Metabolic syndrome is a condition that has gained significant attention in recent years, particularly in India, which is often referred to as the "*diabetes capital*" of the world.

A syndrome refers to a group of symptoms and/or signs that may have various causes. **Metabolic syndrome** involves multiple, interrelated risk factors of metabolic origin that are strongly associated with type 2 diabetes.

These risk factors include **disordered blood lipids, elevated blood pressure, high blood glucose levels, a predisposition to blood clotting, and inflammation**.

As we age, **atherosclerosis**, or the thickening and hardening of the arteries due to plaque buildup in the inner lining of the artery, becomes more common. **Plaque** consists of **deposits of fatty substances, cholesterol, cellular waste products, calcium, and other materials**. Metabolic syndrome appears to directly contribute to the development of atherosclerosis, increasing the risk of **arterial blockages** in the heart and brain. Such blockages can lead to serious adverse events like **myocardial infarction (heart attack) and stroke**.

Risk factors for metabolic syndrome include obesity, insulin resistance (as seen in type 2 diabetes), aging, genetic or ethnic predisposition, a sedentary lifestyle, smoking, and hormonal imbalances.

Polycystic ovary syndrome (PCOS), a condition that affects fertility, is also associated with metabolic syndrome. Epidemiologic studies have linked adverse early - life conditions with the risk of metabolic syndrome in later life.

This theory – **Fetal Onset of Adult Disease** (FOAD) was first propounded by Dr David Barker in 2009 – also called the **Barker hypothesis**. Maternal undernutrition during gestation and **intrauterine growth retardation** and **low birth weight** were found to be associated with features of metabolic syndrome later in adulthood.

The mechanism is believed to be through a kind of developmental **'re - programming of the biological clock'**.

Criteria have been formed to diagnose metabolic syndrome, which include:

- Abdominal obesity with high waist - hip ratio (>1).
  Fat deposits more around the waist.

- Body Mass Index above 25

- High triglycerides

- Low HDL cholesterol (good cholesterol)

- High blood pressure (> 120/80 mm Hg) or using medicine to lower blood pressure

- Insulin resistance and Type - II diabetes – fasting blood sugar>100 mg%, 90 minutes after meal blood sugar>180 mg%, HbA1C>6.5

- Increased blood clotting

Management – Metabolic syndrome is treated by addressing all the modifiable risk factors. These include lifestyle changes like regular exercise and consuming a balanced diet low in saturated fats and trans fats, cholesterol, salt, refined sugars, and flour, and high in vegetables, fruits, lean protein, beans, and whole grains. The Mediterranean diet, which is high in fruits, vegetables, nuts, whole grains, and olive oil, has an anti - metabolic syndrome effect. Diabetes should be controlled by oral drugs and/or insulin so as to maintain Hemoglobin A_1C levels below 7.

Obesity should be reversed - again by diet and exercise. **Body Mass Index (BMI)** is a simple calculation using a person's height and weight. The formula is **BMI = kg/m²** where kg is a person's weight in kilograms and m² is their height in meters squared. A BMI of 18.5 to 24.9 in adults is in the healthy weight range; 25 to 29.9 is in the overweight range; 30 to 39.9 is in the obese range and 40 or above is in the severely obese range. Hypertension must be properly controlled with drugs. Antiplatelet drugs such as aspirin and clopidogrel are used to prevent clotting. Cholesterol lowering agents are used to lower the 'bad cholesterol' or LDL in the blood.

Obesity – Objective criteria for this term have been laid down on the basis of **Body Mass Index (BMI)** as given above. Causes of obesity may be both genetic and environmental. Obesity is a feature of some genetic conditions, such as Prader–Villi syndrome and Bardot - Beidl syndrome.

In other cases, there is a familial predisposition. Hormonal problems – hypothyroidism and Cushing's syndrome are also associated with obesity. High - calorie intake coupled with low levels of physical exercise leading to **not enough calories burnt** is the most common extrinsic cause. Obesity also results from nutritionally 'deprived' fetal life, as postulated in the FOAD hypothesis. Obesity itself can result in **less inclination** for exercise, thus leading to a **vicious cycle** of sedentary life and obesity.

Obese people are often beset with **mental health problems** and **depression**. They are prone to **Type 2 diabetes, hypertension, heart disease, snoring, sleep apnea, and osteoarthritis**. Excess body weight is a major cause of early death. It is said that every kilogram of excess weight contributes to years of life lost.

Management - It is well known that extrinsic obesity can be reduced by striking a healthy balance between caloric intake and exercise. Fatty foods should be avoided, and salads should be eaten instead. This may not be so easy to follow.

Surgical Management of Obesity – Obesity in a few people is represented as a familial or hereditary symptom. Most of the people carry on with obesity and are unable to reduce their obesity. Obese people get afflicted with metabolic diseases like diabetes, high blood pressure, knee and joint pain, etc. Often, obese people appear jovial and happy on the surface but, in reality, are most often sad, lonely, alienated, and depressed. In some selected cases, surgery remains the only way to retrieve and rejuvenate the concerned despondent person. During the last decade, surgery has been undertaking the big task of removing the fat from belly - waist etc. The surgery undertaken for the removal of fat is known as **bariatric surgery.**

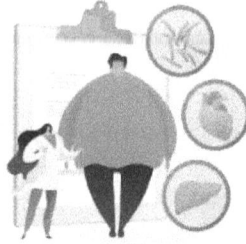

Bariatric surgery - This type of surgery is also known as **metabolic surgery or weight loss surgery.** The aim of this surgery is to reduce appetite by making a bypass in the digestive system. As a result, the number of calories taken by the patient is limited because hunger is completely satiated with a limited quantity of food.

Bariatric surgery not only controls obesity but at the same time, it proves helpful in controlling blood pressure, diabetes, cholesterol, etc. Bariatric surgery is therefore also called **'milieu restorative surgery.'**

Previously bariatric surgery entailed a number of risks like opening the whole abdomen and performing anastomoses in intestine. However, after the advent of the laparoscope, it has become easy and convenient. The **laparoscopic** minimal access surgery is performed by making small stomata (openings) in the abdomen.

Bariatric surgery is undertaken in overweight and obese patients with BMI in the range - 30 - 35 only. Types of procedures are:

1. **Sleeve Gastrectomy** – In this operation, approximately 80% of the stomach is removed using the laparoscope. The remaining stomach is the size and shape of banana. The new stomach holds less food and liquid helping reduce the amount of food and thereby less calories are consumed. By removing the large portion of the stomach "**hunger hormone**" production is also curtailed.

The few side effects of this surgery are onset of esophageal reflux and heart burning, which may be controlled and treated by medicines.

2. **Roux - en - Y Gastric Bypass (RYGB)** – This is performed by laparoscope stapler. A small pouch the size of an egg is constructed at the top of the stomach and a larger lower portion of the stomach is bypassed. Thus, it no longer processes and digests the food. This small pouch is connected with the jejunum of the small intestine. The feeling of satiety comes early, and food passes directly into the small intestine. Calorie consumption is reduced – as a result obesity is also reduced. Supplements of vitamins and minerals are given after surgery to prevent deficiencies.

3. **Laparoscopic Adjustable Gastric Band (LAGB/AGB)** - In this surgery, a silicon band is placed around the top portion of the stomach pouch, which is made to be pressed to reduce it to a very limited size. Thus, the appetite is reduced, and the patient feels satiated earlier. Obesity and weight are lost gradually but perpetually. Living non - abstemiously may need several adjustments of the silicon band. The risk of vitamin - mineral deficiency is low.

4. **Biliopancreatic Diversion with Duodenal Switch (BPD/DS)** – This is somewhat similar to sleeve surgery and gastric bypass surgery. In this procedure the duodenum of the small intestine is attached to the lower part of the small intestine. Gallbladder and pancreatic tube are attached to this bypass pathway which helps in digesting dietary fat and carbohydrate. This surgery is also known as biliopancreatic surgery. Thus, food in the last portion of the intestine is processed promptly. Deficiency of nutrition does not occur. Vitamins - minerals are taken as per medical advice.

5. **Single Anastomosis Duodeno - Ileal bypass with Sleeve gastrectomy (SADIB - SG)** – This is somewhat similar to bilio - pancreatic diversion with duodenal switch. In this surgery the sleeve of the stomach (sleeve as made in the sleeve gastrectomy) is attached to the dissected first portion of the small intestine and the remaining portion of the small intestine is attached to the duodenum.

Thus, the appetite and obesity get contained and controlled – as a result of less hunger and reduced fat intake, type - 2 diabetes and symptoms of metabolic syndromes remain well controlled. **Esophageal reflux** may occur due to acidic stomach contents that may return spontaneously in the mouth. Acidity and burning may be felt in the upper stomach and chest. All these disorders get controlled by healthy diet and medicines.

Bariatric surgery triggers multifarious mechanical and chemical alterations – the body makes efforts to accommodate the alterations. The fat around the waist and neck and fat over the abdomen recede, and obesity is abolished. However, if the patient leads a non - abstemious lifestyle after surgery, he is likely to regain weight and become obese within 5 years.

Liposuction and body contouring – Liposuction is a surgical procedure primarily performed by plastic and cosmetic surgeons to remove excess adipose tissue (fat) from various parts of the body, such as under the chin, neck, abdomen, navel, upper arms, and thighs. The procedure is designed to improve body contours and enhance aesthetic appearance.

During liposuction, negative pressure (suction) is applied to remove fat deposits, which are first liquefied by the administration of specific chemicals. This technique allows for the targeted removal of fat while minimizing damage to surrounding tissues.

It is important to note that liposuction is distinct from bariatric surgery, which is performed to treat obesity and related metabolic disorders such as diabetes. Unlike bariatric surgery, liposuction does not affect the digestive system or alter metabolic functions, nor does it address or control diabetes or related health conditions. Instead, it is a cosmetic procedure aimed at reshaping specific areas of the body to achieve a more desirable appearance.

Chapter 25

Gut Flora – Gut Microbiome

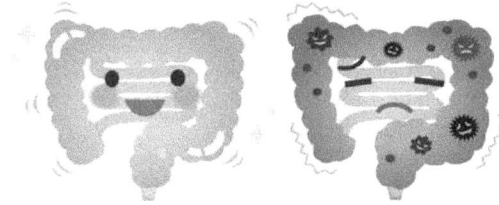

Learning Objectives:

- Gut microbiome - an ecosystem of micro-organisms in the gastrointestinal tract

- Excessive medication, sedentary lifestyle, substance abuse, poor nutrition in pregnancy or infancy disturbs gut microbiome

- Conditions which may result in **gut dysbiosis** or overgrowth of pathogenic bacteria - poor digestion, hectic lifestyle, travelling

- Role of prebiotics and probiotics

- Gut Brain axis

The gut microbiome has recently gained significant attention in medical science, with its importance being increasingly recognized over the last 3 - 4 decades as central to human health.

The term "**gut**" refers to the intestines or gastrointestinal tract, which is also known as the digestive system. "**Microbiome**" refers to an ecosystem of a large number of microorganisms. The gut microbiome or flora consists of trillions of bacteria, as well as viruses, fungi, and parasites present in our gastrointestinal tract . Collectively, these organisms coexist in a **symbiotic** relationship with the human body, deriving shelter and nutrition from it while providing various beneficial functions in return.

The microbiota dwelling in our intestines can be broadly categorized into **friendly bacteria** and **harmful bacteria**. The functions of gut microbiota and their significance in human health are currently subjects of intense interest and research.

Location of the Gut Microbiome

The "gut," or gastrointestinal tract, includes the stomach, small intestine, and large intestine (colon). Gut microbiotas exist in various parts of this tract, including the mouth, esophagus, stomach, small intestine, duodenum, colon, and rectum. However, **the majority of these microorganisms reside in the colon,** where they float in the lumen or attach to the mucous lining of the colonic wall.

Types of Bacteria in the Gut Microbiome

The bacteria that inhabit our colon are distinct from those found elsewhere in the body. Colonic microbes are mostly **anaerobic**, meaning they thrive in low - oxygen environments. The upper gastrointestinal tract has higher oxygen levels, a greater quantity of digestive juices, and faster gut movement, all of which inhibit microbial colonization. The **composition of the gut microbiome is dynamic**, changing in response to dietary alterations and other factors.

This dynamic ecosystem plays a crucial role in maintaining our overall health, influencing everything from digestion and metabolism to immune function and even mental health.

How gut microbiome develops – The gut of infants is nearly sterile at birth, but it becomes a community of trillions of microbiomes within weeks and reaches adult levels over a period of 2 - 3 years after birth. Breastfeeding provides nutrients and good bacteria to the infant and enables it to fight off pathogens. Scientists have proven that the relationship between co - existence and symbiosis of gut microbiota plays an important role in making us healthy and building the capacity to fight pathogens.

Functions of the gut microbiome – The anaerobic microbes in the gut perform important functions. Firstly, they **help break down indigestible fibers**, and secondly, they **produce essential nutrients** that we cannot otherwise get.

They also help to **keep the harmful (pathogenic) bacteria in check.** However, these microbes are only helpful to us if they remain within their natural habitat. If they settle in the small intestine in greater numbers, they interfere with digestive functions, and in case they invade the wall of the colon, they can cause infection of the bloodstream.

Factors affecting the composition of the gut microbiome – Our diet, chemical exposures, disease - causing organisms, and bowel movement regularity are the factors that affect the composition of the gut microbiome. A **high - fiber plant - based diet helps the microbiome to thrive,** producing short - chain fatty acids that nourish our gut and lower the pH inside, favoring the more beneficial organisms (or 'good' bacteria). On the other hand, a diet high in sugar and saturated fats favors the less helpful types or 'bad' microorganisms.

Chemicals like alcohol, tobacco, pesticides, and antibiotics can reduce both good bacteria and bad bacteria. **Medications,** like acid blockers, can also affect our microbiome by changing the pH inside. Acute and temporary exposure to these can be overcome, but chronic exposure can change the composition of the gut microbiome.

Gut motility also determines the composition of the microbiome. This is how the "crop" of microorganisms turns over. The movement of food and waste through the colon distributes the microbes along the way. Here, they help break down undigested compounds into nutrients, and many also come out with stools.

While excessive sugar, protein, and fat can damage the gut flora, certain oils found in plant - based foods like mustard, groundnuts, cashews, walnuts, sesame seeds, coconuts, flaxseeds (rich in omega - 3), avocados, olives, and neem are beneficial for gut health. These oils, particularly from flaxseeds, *neem*, and nigella (*kalonji*), are also known to help manage cholesterol levels and arthritis, further supporting overall health and well - being.

Division of gut flora – It is important to understand how the diversified gut flora are distributed in the upper and lower GI tract. Microorganisms found in the stomach and small intestines are very few in number and species as compared to the microorganisms found in the colon.

Harmful bacteria, along with friendly bacteria, always remain present in the colon, rectum, and anus. Sugar, salt, and fat taken in excessive quantities breed harmful bacteria in the colon, rectum, etc. The microbiota of the colon obtains nourishment only from fibrous food.

Friendly & inimical microbiota – Various species of microorganisms are found in our stomach and intestine, for example, firmicutes, Bacteroides, actinobacteria, proteobacteria, fecal bacterium, streptococcus, peptostreptococcus, Escherichia, lactobacillus, etc., various fungus viz; candida, saccharomyces, aspergillus, penicillium, etc. Archaea, like rhodotorula, may cause inflammatory bowel disease. However, the process of fermentation goes on in the gastrointestinal tract (GI tract), which is facilitated by gut microorganisms.

Some of the bacteria and microbiota dwelling in our gut play friendly and inimical (harmful) roles side by side. Friendly bacteria keep digestion efficient and healthy and make the body, mind, and immune system strong, dynamic, and capacitated. Gut bacteria are believed to play an important role in conditioning $CD8^+$ T (immune) cells.

How the inimical bacteria cause injury and impairment to the physical system is an enigma. These bacteria cause ulcers in the small intestine, may damage the digestive acidic elements in the intestine and are even linked to nervous system diseases like **Parkinson's disease**. Research in medical science has also described some good effects of inimical bacteria like **helicobacter** which control **T - cells** of our stomach and intestine.

Gut dysbiosis – Gut dysbiosis occurs due to the profusion of pathogenic (harmful) bacteria. The delicate balance of good and harmful bacteria can get disturbed. It may be a lack of 'good' bacteria, overgrowth of 'bad' ones, or lack of overall bacterial diversity in the microbiome colony. Thus, our gut becomes prone to various conditions and diseases.

- **Infections** – If pathogenic food or water infect our gut, its lining is damaged and dysentery, diarrhea, and inflammation (colitis) occur frequently. When these bad bacteria infiltrate into the bloodstream, **systemic infection** may also occur. Systemic infection may be prevented in case we are cautious to rebuild our gut health.

- **Motility disorders** – When gut motility slows down, bacteria from the large intestine may migrate, settle, and overgrow in the small intestine.

- **Inflammatory Bowel Disease** (IBD) – This is a group of autoimmune conditions including ulcerative colitis, Crohn's disease and microscopic colitis. The exact reason for these serious diseases is not understood. They are regarded to be due to gut microbiome dysbiosis.

- **Atherosclerosis** – Certain 'bad' gut bacteria produce a substance called **trimethylamine N - oxide (TMAO),** which increases atherosclerosis (hardening of your arteries).

- **Other conditions** – that may be indirectly related to gut dysbiosis include allergies, asthma, autism, chronic fatigue syndrome, diabetes, anxiety, depression, fatty liver, irritable bowel syndrome, cancer of the liver, colon, and pancreas, multiple sclerosis, obesity, rheumatoid arthritis, and neurodegenerative diseases.

Common signs or symptoms of gut dysbiosis – Typical symptoms of gut dysbiosis include excessive gas, bloated stomach, poor digestion, diarrhea, constipation, lower abdominal pain, leg pains, and muscular cramps.

Care of gut microbiome – The following steps improve the health of the gut microbiome

- **Diet & lifestyle** – A diverse and plant - rich diet with a variety of whole grains, vegetables and fruits is conducive to gut health as they offer plenty of dietary fiber and micronutrients. On the other hand, processed and refined foods do the opposite.

- **Fiber** is an important constituent of food. The microbiome manufactures small chains of fatty acids, acetic acid, and butanoic acid – which in turn provide sustenance to the microbiome dwelling in the intestine. The microbiota absorbing vitamins B and K maintains the balance of the bile in the body, due to which hormones are produced.

Eating food in varying dietary styles in our daily routines goes a long way in maintaining and safeguarding our health. Some people traveling from place to place complain of constipation, diarrhea, etc. Such bowel problems occur due to changes in water, which also change gut microbiota. Thus, foods lacking in fiber, food soaked with sugar, salt, and oil, and cooked and deep - fried food augment harmful bacteria, causing disorders and diseases of the gut.

- **Prebiotics and Probiotics** – Probiotics and prebiotics can be taken in supplement form or from foods. **Prebiotics** are the fibers present in diet. **Probiotics** are helpful microbes that you can ingest through fermented foods (such as yogurt, cheese, sourdough bread, pickle) or supplements. They are available in the market. The food enriched with probiotics promotes friendly bacteria.

- **Antibiotics** – Overuse of antibiotics can kill your good bacteria and create imbalance between the good and bad bacteria.

Some people are deprived of gut microorganisms, i.e., they are deficient in microbial colonies in their digestive system. Due to this deprivation, they severely suffer from relapsing, sometimes fatal infection with **Clostridium difficile**. Such people are administered with **fecal (stool or poop) microbiota transplantation** (FMT) into their gastrointestinal tract – that is, the administration of fecal matter from a donor into the intestinal tract of a recipient in order to rebuild microbial composition and confer good health benefits to them.

Gut - Brain Axis – Anticipating and assessing the sensitivity of the gut, the doctors of many medical systems draw the inference that there exists a very close relationship between the gut and the brain – this **relationship between the two is that of an axis.**

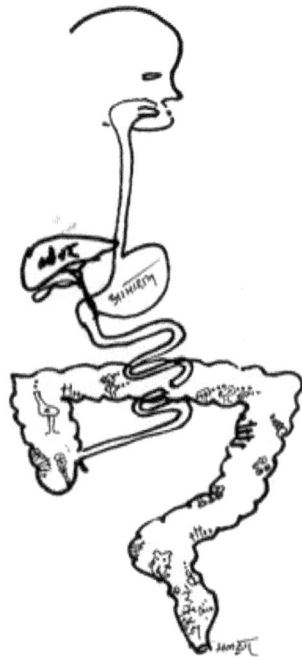

Dr Giulia Enders elucidates and expounds that the **gut - brain axis** is physically established through the **vagus nerve**. This nerve on the right and left sides passes through the diaphragm, lungs, heart, and esophagus and reaches the brain. Dr. Enders calls the intestine nervous plexus the 'brain of the gut.'

Healthy and Effortless Defecation in the morning hours eliminating toxins from the body keeps the body detoxified and disease free with strong immunity.

Further, Dr Enders, in her exploration of the differences between Eastern and Western lavatory systems, emphasizes that the traditional Asian method of squatting during defecation is superior to the Western practice of sitting on a commode. She argues that squatting strengthens the muscles of the abdomen, stomach, and waist, whereas sitting weakens the excretory system and enfeebles the nerves of the colon, rectum, abdomen, and waist.

Squatting, therefore, is believed to facilitate a more complete emptying of the colon. In contrast, the Western habit of eating fiberless, non - vegetarian food and not washing the rectum with water after defecation can lead to constipation, piles, and fissures. Recently, Western countries have started installing bidets to address these concerns.

In conclusion, we all aspire to maintain good health and stay disease - free, and this can be achieved by consuming a balanced diet and engaging in regular physical exercise. These practices support the beneficial gut flora that coexist with us, promoting overall health. Detoxifying the body, particularly the gut, and ensuring proper gut motility are key strategies for achieving and maintaining health, well - being, and vitality. Gut health revolves around the balance and function of bacteria in gastrointestinal tract. The findings of research revalidate the age - old Indian conviction that good health revolves around the gut.

Chapter 26

Addictive Substance Abuse (ASA)

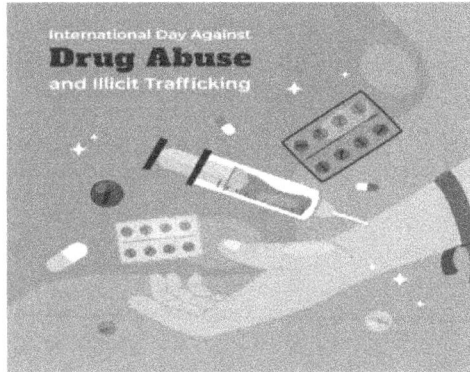

International Day Against
Drug Abuse
and Illicit Trafficking

Learning Objectives:

- Addiction to tobacco, alcohol and drugs like cannabis, opium, cocaine, etc. are common forms of substance abuse
- Addictive Substance Abuse harms physical and mental health
- Criteria for labelling addiction-dependence on substances
- Effects of different addictive substances

There are many substances – usually devoid of nutritive value which cause **addiction**. Some addictions have been known since ancient times.

Typically, they include tobacco, alcohol, and drugs. Such substances have addictive potential, i.e., propensity to cause addiction. 'Addiction' is a mental health condition in which a person's dependence on a substance causes distress, impairs their lifestyle, and ultimately decays their mental state and life years. Such addicts often refrain from social life or are not accepted by society. Tobacco, alcohol, and substances like cannabis, opium, and cocaine do not contain nutritional value and are therefore not considered food.

The habitual use of these addictive items, especially when consumed daily or multiple times a day, is known as **substance abuse. Craving** is the intense, uncontrollable desire to use a substance. Over time, **tolerance** develops, meaning that increasingly larger amounts of the substance are needed to achieve the same effect. This can lead to **dependence - ** a compulsive behavior that may drive a person to extreme measures, such as selling personal belongings or even committing crimes to obtain the addictive substance. This state of physical and mental dependency is a serious health condition. When the substance is no longer available, **withdrawal symptoms** can occur, further entrenching the addiction. A person may abuse more than one substance at a time, such as alcohol and cocaine, leading to multiple substance use disorders simultaneously. Substance abuse can severely impact an individual's health, relationships, and overall quality of life and may even be life - threatening.

Substance abuse affects people of all races, ages, genders, and socioeconomic classes, and it can sometimes affect children as well. Social and scientific research indicates that drug addiction is more prevalent among males aged 18 to 25 years. The reasons for addiction can vary widely depending on age, life circumstances, and personal challenges. Many substances provide an immediate or near - immediate sense of euphoria or a "kick," which contributes to their widespread use. Substance abuse is a global issue, with over 20 million people in the United States alone affected by at least one substance use disorder. Among these, tobacco use is the most common form of addiction worldwide.

Nature unveils herself in innumerable ways, and we humans interpret and decipher various facets of Nature according to our innate inclination. It is noteworthy that most of the addictive constituents originated from natural substances. Tea, coffee, coco, fermented fruits, *mahua*, Cannabis indica (source of cannabinoids), and Papaver somniferum (source of opioids) are rich sources of **psychoactive substances**.

These are stimulant, seductive, depressive, sleep - inducing, hallucinating, diuretic, attention enhancing, altering judgment, falsely relieving tension, habit forming, addictive, upgrading criminal instincts, debilitating, tormenting, and threatening life. Nature also provided **receptors** for cannabinoids such as CB1 and CB2 and receptors for opioids – endorphins and enkephalins in the human nervous system and tissues – these are the receptors (chemical moiety that binds with the drug or agent) that bind cannabinoids and opioids in the body.

Addiction to certain substances like tea, coffee, or caffeine products causes harm mainly to gut health. But substances like tobacco, alcohol, psychoactive, hallucinogenic, narcotics, or sedatives are hazardous to our personal and social health. Let us now discuss briefly some of the substances that cause addiction.

1. Caffeine is commonly consumed in the form of drinks such as tea and coffee, which are popular in homes, offices, restaurants, and roadside stalls. Its widespread use dates back about 100 years, with tea drinking becoming prevalent among the English in the 19th century, who then introduced it to India. Roadside vending and the culture of tea - making have created an impression that tea is essential for invigorating life. Today, many food items like chocolate, cake, ice cream, and colas also contain caffeine, which is regulated under statutory guidelines. Tea and coffee are often consumed to alleviate fatigue and refresh the mood. In small quantities, caffeine can reduce weight, relieve tiredness, and seemingly boost productivity. Tea and coffee contain xanthine, which increases the tendency to urinate. However, excessive consumption of tea and coffee, especially when mixed with sugar, can cause restlessness, nervousness, sleeplessness, increased urination, dysbiosis, muscle twitching, and elevated blood sugar levels.

2. Nicotine, the primary active ingredient in **tobacco**, is consumed in various forms, including:

    a. Smoking: Cigarettes, *beedis, hookahs*, cigars, *churutas, chilams*, and pipes.

    b. Chewing: Betel with tobacco, *khaini, gutkha*.

    c. Snuffing: Refined powdered tobacco inhaled deeply into the nostrils.

    d. Rubbing: Tooth powder mixed with tobacco (such as *lal - dant - manjan, gulmanjan*) and toothpaste containing tobacco.

    e. Drinking: *Tuibur and hidakphu*, which are tobacco - water products prepared by passing tobacco smoke through water, are common in Manipur and Nagaland.

Tobacco, which was cultivated in South America, was introduced to India in 1605 AD by the Portuguese. Today, India is the third - largest producer of tobacco, following the United States and China. Gujarat is the largest producer of tobacco among the Indian states. The global tobacco market has a turnover of about USD 900 billion, making it a significant source of excise duty revenue for governments. Approximately 20 - 30% of adults worldwide use tobacco. Workers in the tobacco industry often become addicted to tobacco products and gradually fall victim to various diseases. Tobacco stimulates the central nervous system, creating a false sense of relief from fatigue and apathy. However, excessive tobacco use can lead to lethargy and a decline in daily activities.

Chewing and smoking tobacco are behaviors that breed illness. While tobacco addiction is harmful to health, it does not typically lead to social crimes. Excessive tobacco use is linked to several diseases, particularly respiratory and cardiovascular diseases, and various cancers, including **lung, oral, esophageal, and stomach cancer.** These effects may take years to develop, and the risk of cancer increases with the amount of tobacco consumed over time. Besides lung cancer, smoking leads to respiratory problems and chronic conditions like **chronic obstructive pulmonary disease** (COPD). Heart disease and stroke are also related to tobacco use. These harmful effects are often depicted on tobacco and cigarette packaging. According to the World Health Organization, tobacco kills more than 8 million people worldwide each year, including an estimated 1.3 million non - smokers exposed to second - hand smoke. Around 80% of the world's 1.3 billion tobacco users live in low and middle - income countries. In 2020, 22.3% of the world's population used tobacco: 36.7% of men and 7.8% of women.

3. Alcohol has been widely consumed as a beverage for ages. It is produced from fruit pulps and juices through fermentation, malting, mashing, and distillation processes. Common alcoholic beverages include fermented drinks like beer, wine, whisky, and distilled spirits like vodka, rum, gin, and country liquor (made from sugarcane, fruits, herbs, and spices). Whisky, made from fermented grain mash such as barley, corn, rice, and wheat, contains the highest proportion of alcohol. Wine production often coincides with grape or fruit harvesting, involving steps like crushing, fermentation, clarification, aging, and bottling.

Enjoying alcohol has been a social practice in various cultures for a long time. People typically consume alcohol to foster familiarity, demonstrate etiquette, and formally welcome guests. It induces a temporary sense of emotional uplift and pleasure. Alcohol is consumed socially by all groups, including the rich, poor, academics, and intellectuals.

When consumed in moderation (2 - 3 pegs), alcohol acts as a stimulant, relieving tension and providing a pleasant effect. However, excessive consumption can lead to hyperactivity, which is harmful. The acute effects of alcohol appear almost immediately, impairing decision - making abilities. Long - term use can result in **liver cirrhosis**, potentially leading to **hematemesis** (vomiting of blood) and, ultimately, liver failure. Additionally, alcohol can adversely affect the esophagus, stomach, intestines, nerves, and balance.

a. *Mahua* (**Madhuca longifolia**) is a tropical tree native to India. The Mahua tree is a botanical treasure of India, offering a range of valuable properties. Its edible flowers, which contain a high sugar content (about 70%), are a rich source of alcohol. The seeds of the Mahua tree are also a good source of oil. Mahua juice is traditionally fermented by mixing it with water, jaggery, and *'navshar'* (ammonium chloride). Tribal communities in Odisha prepare a country liquor known as *'mahuli'* from this fermented juice. Although Mahua may have some apparent benefits, such as alleviating headaches and gastrointestinal disorders, it is similar to other addictive substances and is particularly known to cause infertility and hypoglycemia in diabetics.

b. **Taadi or Toddy** is extracted from the sap of palm trees. It is a sweet drink that is typically consumed fresh in the early morning for its soothing effect. Toddy contains a variety of nutrients, including protein, carbohydrates (sugar), vitamin C, yeast, potassium, zinc, magnesium, iron, and B group vitamins. Toddy is an integral part of the cultural fabric of the Bhil community in Madhya Pradesh and certain parts of Kerala. It is considered a natural alcohol and a healthy drink. Toddy has an alcohol content of about 8.1%. People may consume toddy both for its health benefits and for its intoxicating effects.

Additionally, toddy is used as vinegar in many southern Indian dishes to enhance their flavor. While the sale of date palm juice is not illegal, many toddy sellers adulterate it with liquor, sleeping pills, urea, and other sedatives. Common side effects of consuming toddy include nausea, vomiting, dry mouth, dizziness, sleepiness, headaches, and other similar symptoms.

4. Psychoactive Drugs are another category of substances that cause addiction and can lead to rapid physical and mental decay. Drug intoxication gradually diminishes physical strength in multiple ways - slowing down various bodily systems such as the digestive, circulatory, respiratory, excretory, reproductive, and nervous systems. It also impairs sensitivity and cognitive abilities. Drug addicts often become alienated from society, retreating into their own imaginary worlds. They frequently participate in rave parties - events where young people dance under the influence of illicit drugs. Psychoactive drugs can be consumed in various forms, including orally, through inhalation, snuffing, or injections. Below are some examples of these drugs:

a. **Sedatives, Hypnotics, and Depressants** – This category includes drugs such as amphetamines, lysergic acid diethylamide (LSD), and barbiturates. **Amphetamine** was discovered in 1887 by Romanian chemist Lazăr Edeleanu. It gained popularity in the form of Benzedrine inhalers and was initially prescribed for conditions like coryza, rhinitis (runny nose), itching, sneezing, asthma, narcolepsy, Parkinsonism, and **attention deficit hyperactivity disorder (ADHD).** However, it was later found to be highly intoxicating and addictive. Amphetamine use affects the central nervous system (CNS) by disrupting neurotransmitters, leading to various adverse effects, including cardiac issues, hyperpyrexia (extremely high fever), ataxia (loss of coordination), euphoria, ADHD symptoms (paradoxically), acne, blurred vision, tactile hallucinations, and psychosis.

b. **Barbiturates** – are central nervous system depressants or sedative drugs that became popular around 1903. These drugs, which include brands like secobarbital, pentobarbital, and amobarbital, produce effects ranging from mild sedation to general anesthesia. Barbiturates were initially used for their tranquilizing properties, relieving pain and distress by inducing alterations in consciousness and slowing down bodily activity. However, they are highly addictive and can be abused, leading to serious health risks.

c. **Benzodiazepines** – Drugs such as diazepam and alprazolam (commonly known as Xanax) became popular for treating anxiety, insomnia, and symptoms of alcohol withdrawal. However, these hypnotic drugs themselves became subjects of abuse, leading to addiction and intoxication. Benzodiazepines work by enhancing the effect of gamma - aminobutyric acid (GABA), a neurotransmitter that inhibits activity in the brain, but this effect can be harmful when abused, leading to impaired cognitive and motor functions, dependence, and other severe consequences.

d. **Narcotics** – These are substances primarily used to treat pain but are also known for their high potential for addiction and inducing drowsiness. Common narcotics include cannabis, opium, heroin, smack, brown sugar (opioids), and cocaine.

Cannabis (Cannabis sativa) – This herbaceous plant, also known as *Sativa indica* in India - Pakistan and parts of Central and South America, is widely known for its psychoactive properties. Cannabis, extracted from hemp seeds or marijuana, contains the psychoactive compound **tetrahydrocannabinol** (THC). While hemp seed proteins are used in some medicinal products, cannabis contains over 400 chemical constituents, including 50 that are intoxicating and harmful, such as *Ganja, Bhang,* and *Charas*. The effects of cannabis intoxication can range from increased appetite to severe hunger suppression, trembling, irritation, anxiety, shuddering, insomnia, red eyes, dry mouth, and eventually, dependence syndrome. Prolonged use can lead to depersonalization and detachment from reality. Cannabis use can be detected in urine tests.

Opium – Extracted from the seeds of the *Papaver somniferum* plant, also known as the Opium poppy or Breadseed poppy, opium has been cultivated in the Mediterranean region since 5000 BC. In Northeast India, it is known as '*Kani*,' and its cultivation is legally permitted in selected regions like Madhya Pradesh, Uttar Pradesh, and Rajasthan. However, illicit trafficking and smuggling of opium and its derivatives are rampant in regions bordering India, such as Pakistan, Afghanistan, Burma, Thailand, and Laos.

The plant is rich in alkaloids, many of which are used medicinally for their analgesic, anti - cough, and anti - spasmodic properties. Poppy seeds are also a rich source of iron and are known to increase hemoglobin levels. Opium is the primary source of several narcotic drugs, including morphine, codeine, heroin, smack, and brown sugar. Morphine, a potent painkiller, is used for analgesia during major surgeries. Some users consumed opium and its derivatives by smoking, while others, particularly during the British period, used heroin injections, which are twice as intoxicating. Morphine is sometimes administered through intramuscular or intravenous injections. The effects of opioid intoxication can include a slow pulse, low blood pressure, shortness of breath, bronchial crises, subnormal body temperature, and delayed reflexes. Treatment for opioid intoxication typically involves three approaches: overdose management, antidote - naloxone, and maintenance therapy.

Cocaine *(Erythroxylum coca)* – This tropane alkaloid, extracted from the coca plant or shrubs like the blackthorn bush, is a powerful central nervous system stimulant with a high potential for addiction. Cocaine has been used for thousands of years, particularly in Bolivia and Peru, where natives chew and ingest coca leaves. The drug was discovered by Albert Niemann in 1860, and its anesthetic properties were later described by renowned psychologists Sigmund Freud and Karl Koller. Cocaine, also known as "crack" among addicts, rapidly affects neurotransmitters, leading to feelings of euphoria, pleasure, and heightened arousal.

Cocaine can be consumed by swallowing, snorting, smoking, or injection, with the latter method providing the most intense effects. Chronic use can lead to gum problems, pupil dilatation, tachycardia (rapid heart rate), hypertension, nausea, and vomiting.

Cocaine intoxication impairs judgment and can lead to hypomanic episodes. Treatment for cocaine intoxication may involve oxygen therapy and medications such as thiopentone and diazepam to relax the muscles and alleviate symptoms.

Hallucinogens – Drugs like Lysergic acid diethylamide (LSD) and Phencyclidine (PCP) alter consciousness, perception, and mood, causing psychedelic effects. LSD, discovered in 1938 from morning glory seeds, initially treated conditions like ADHD.

Users of these drugs aren't typically physically dependent but may experience tachycardia, tremors, loss of coordination, dilated pupils, and hyperactivity. PCP, available as a white powder, has similar effects to LSD.

Inhalants & Volatile Solvents – These substances, such as toluene, benzene, acetone, and gasoline, vaporize quickly and are harmful to health. Frequent exposure can lead to burning sensations, hyperactivity, respiratory issues, vision disorders, neuropathy, coordination loss, cardiac or brain diseases, amnesia, liver and kidney damage, and cancer.

Cough Syrups containing codeine and tramadol were once sold widely but were found to be addictive. Now, dextromethorphan is used in new cough syrup brands, but overdosing can cause intoxication similar to ketamine. Children using these syrups can become addicted.

Prevalence of ASA in India – Addictive substances like tobacco, alcohol, cannabis, opioids, cocaine, sedatives, inhalants, stimulants, and hallucinogens are prevalent in India.

Risk Factors for Addictive Substance Abuse (ASA) several factors contribute to ASA, such as:

Home and Family: Substance addiction in the family, broken family ties, and unhappy childhoods can predispose children to substance abuse.

Peers and School: Peer pressure in school and college can lead to experimentation, which may escalate to addiction. Poor academic performance and social skills increase this risk.

Exposure to Addictive Substances and Symptoms of ASA:

According to the American Psychiatric Association (APA):

1. Frequent abuse of prescribed psychiatric drugs

2. Withdrawal symptoms create resistance to treatment

3. Delusions of fulfilling obligations due to substance abuse

4. Continued use despite distorted relationships

5. Depersonalization from society

6. Increasing substance use due to tolerance and withdrawal symptoms

7. Substance abuse often starts experimentally and progresses to addiction

8. Genetic predispositions, mental health conditions, and adverse childhood experiences contribute to the development of substance abuse.

Behavioral Transformation in Substance Abuse (ASA) - The progression of ASA is a complex process driven by access to and exposure to addictive substances, leading to significant changes in brain chemistry. This often results in surges in dopamine, which alters the brain's reward system and influences behavior. Over time, individuals may exhibit changes in personality, such as confusion, neglect of personal appearance, and cognitive deterioration. The affected person may also become secretive or hostile when confronted with their addiction.

Diagnosis of ASA - Diagnosing ASA is not straightforward, as it involves not just physical symptoms but also behavioral changes that can carry a stigma. There is no single test that can diagnose substance use disorder.

Instead, healthcare providers conduct a thorough evaluation of the individual's medical history, focusing on behaviors and thought processes related to substance use. Drug tests may be ordered, and prescription drug monitoring program reports might be reviewed.

Additionally, assessing the individual's mental health history is crucial, as ASA often coexists with mental health conditions. According to the APA, a diagnosis of ASA requires the presence of at least two symptoms or signs over a 12 - month period. The severity of ASA is categorized based on the number of signs present: 2 to 3 signs indicate a mild form, 4 to 5 signs suggest a moderate form, and six or more signs reveal a severe form of ASA.

Treatment for Substance Abuse Disorder (ASA)

Treatment for ASA is highly individualized, with various approaches required at different stages.

Given the high propensity for relapse, long - term care is crucial. It's essential for care providers to recognize and address any concurrent mental health conditions. Treatment can occur in intensive care units, outpatient or inpatient settings, and within families, communities, or self - help groups.

The main forms of treatment include:

1. **Detoxification**: This involves stopping the use of the substance, either abruptly or gradually.

2. **Cognitive and Behavioral Therapies**: These therapies, including psychotherapy, help modify harmful behaviors and thought patterns.

3. **Medication**: Certain medications can assist in altering brain chemistry to treat specific ASAs, relieve cravings, and manage withdrawal symptoms. For example, nicotine patches, sprays, gums, or lozenges are used for tobacco de - addiction. Bupropion or varenicline may also be prescribed for tobacco cessation. For alcohol withdrawal, the FDA - approved drugs include naltrexone, acamprosate, and disulfiram. Opioid addiction can be treated with methadone, buprenorphine, and naloxone.

How to Prevent ASA

Preventing substance abuse starts with instilling strong family values that children learn at home from parents, grandparents, relatives, and family friends. Schools play a critical role in reinforcing these values. Education in schools, communities, and families helps prevent the initial use of substances or the misuse of prescription medications. It is essential to follow prescriptions strictly and dispose of leftover medications according to regulations. The risk of ASA is heightened during times of stress, such as during a divorce, job loss, or the death of a loved one. Teenagers may find moving house, parents' divorce, or changing schools particularly stressful. During these times, it's important to cultivate healthy coping mechanisms like exercising, meditating, or learning a new hobby.

Being surrounded by supportive people is vital, and consulting a mental health professional may be beneficial in these circumstances.

Prognosis for Addictive Substance Abuse

The outcome of ASA depends on several factors, including:

1. The specific substance used

2. The severity of ASA, degree of dependence, and withdrawal

3. The individual's motivation for abstinence

4. The duration of treatment

5. Genetic predisposition

6. Coping mechanisms

7. Family and community support

While ASA can be a lifelong condition, recovery is possible, and individuals can lead full lives.

The key to recovery lies in treating the individual with empathy during cravings. Different strategies work for different people, but ongoing therapy and self - help groups (such as Narcotics Anonymous) are effective for many.

Disorders and Diseases in ASA syndrome

- **Relapse** – ASA is a relapsing disease. Recurrence can happen years after treatment. Ongoing and restart of treatment is required

- Memory loss, overall cognitive issues, personality changes, mood dysregulation, loss of nerve function, stroke, seizures, heart failure, nasal septal perforation, respiratory depression, etc.

- Certain cancers - for example, tobacco habit is associated with cancers of the mouth, tongue, tonsils, esophagus, stomach, throat or larynx, bronchus, lungs, and urinary bladder

- Alcohol addiction is well known to cause fatty liver, cirrhosis of the liver, and psychosis

- Blood - borne virus infections are the most dangerous diseases contracted, especially in drug addicts. These are due to the sharing of needles and syringes used for drugs. Diseases like hepatitis B (HBV), hepatitis C (HCV), and the human immunodeficiency virus (HIV - AIDS) do not occur so uncommonly in drug addicts

In conclusion, substance abuse is an **'illness breeding behavior'** that severely damages family and social relationships. The pursuit of sensual pleasure or the need to satisfy cravings through substance abuse erodes spontaneity and closeness within society. Addictive Substance Abuse syndrome undermines social ethics and values, leading to unnatural behavior, greed for unethical gains, and participation in illicit activities.

Many addicts sacrifice their lifetime belongings to satisfy their cravings. Despite stringent rules and laws, mafia networks and syndicates continue to thrive, fueling smuggling and drug trafficking. This not only deteriorates the youth but also plays a catastrophic role in fostering terrorism.

Chapter 27

Abdominal Problems –
Gas, Indigestion, Constipation,
Gastro - Intestinal Manifestations
of Stress

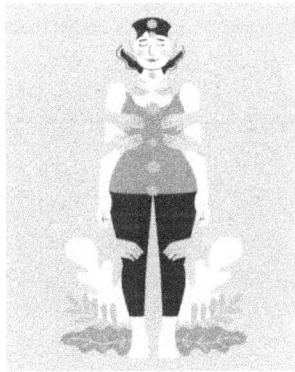

Learning Objectives:
• Understanding abdominal cavity
• Abdominal symptoms of nausea, vomiting, burping or belching, gas, heartburn, stomach bloating, diarrhea, constipation, acute, chronic and recurrent abdominal pain
• Liver diseases - Common symptoms and causes
• Gall bladder disease

Our abdomen, or the peritoneal cavity, houses the gastrointestinal tract, or hollow viscera - lower esophagus, stomach, small intestine with the duodenum, jejunum, ileum, and large intestine with ascending, transverse, and descending colon, sigmoid colon, and rectum. Other organs include the liver, gall bladder, spleen, pancreas, and the genito - urinary system (kidneys, ureters, and urinary bladder). The loops of the small intestine are held together by layers of the peritoneum or mesentery.

Gastrointestinal symptoms like bloating, nausea, vomiting, constipation, diarrhea and abdominal pain are common.

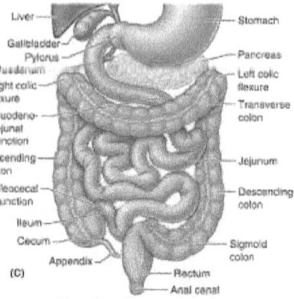

Often, these symptoms are caused by mental states - "stomach is the mirror of feelings; it blushes in anguish, turns pale with rage, gets fueled in anger, shrinks and shrivels with fear." It is now well recognized that there is a strong gut - brain interaction, and many acute and chronic symptoms of the gut are manifestations of unrevealed psychological states.

Several symptoms of gastrointestinal dysfunction are described here:

Nausea and Vomiting – Many times, a gruesome sight or a bad stink may bring on nausea and vomiting. Travel, heights, and riding on a 'merry - go - round' result in motion sickness or nausea and vomiting in some. Whenever the **chemo - receptor - trigger zone** (CTZ) of the brain is stimulated, emesis or vomiting occurs. Hormonal changes in pregnancy cause **'morning sickness,'** which actually occurs at any time of the day.

Migraine headaches, epilepsy, and raised pressure in the brain are causes of vomiting. Many medicines, especially cancer chemotherapy, gastritis, some antibiotics, and infections of the gastrointestinal tract cause nausea and vomiting – this shows that the gut - brain axis plays a certain role.

Diarrhea – Frequent passage of loose or watery stools is diarrhea. Most commonly, diarrhea is caused by an infection of the intestine – viral, bacterial, protozoal, or other. In India, as in many other countries, amebic infection is very common. Diarrhea may be watery, or it may be loose and associated with mucus and abdominal tenesmus with or without blood. Diarrhea with blood and mucus is **dysentery** – it is usually a bacterial or amebic infection. Often, dysentery is an infection of the large intestine (colon).

Colitis may be associated with cramps in the lower abdomen just before and during the passage of stool. Other causes of diarrhea are increased gut motility due to mental stress, use of antibiotics, food allergies, intolerance, and hyperthyroidism (excess thyroid hormone).

Intolerance to lactose in milk or milk products due to lactase enzyme deficiency also leads to diarrhea, cramps, and bloating. Continued watery diarrhea, especially in children, can cause dehydration.

If severe, this can result in low urine output, renal failure, and shock. **Diarrheal dehydration** in children was, and still is, an important cause of child mortality. It is treated with **oral rehydration solution** (ORS) and zinc salts. These two interventions have drastically reduced child mortality due to diarrhea.

Constipation – Infrequent and often difficult passage of hard stools is called constipation. This is an extremely common complaint – not really an illness but a part of life for many. Constipation may simply be a reflection of the type of diet one consumes – **a low - fiber Western diet** is constipating. **A sedentary lifestyle, lack of exercise and irregular schedule, traveling, lack of access to a comfortable toilet, etc.,** may contribute. Rarely, constipation may be a symptom of a systemic disorder like **hypothyroidism** (low level of thyroid hormones) **Hirschsprung disease** (congenital deficiency of nerves in the colon) in a baby causes severe constipation with distension of the abdomen) and is generally treated by surgery. **Cancer of the colon** causes painful and difficult motion with a feeling of incomplete evacuation.

Constipation may result in a feeling of discomfort, incomplete defecation, and being bloated. Frequent and prolonged constipation may result in piles, rectal prolapse, fissure, perianal abscess fistula, etc. Defecation four times a week or up to four times a day may be normal. As to how many times a person will defecate in a day depends on food habits, healthy gut flora, and the current mental state. The Indian system of squatting for defecation straightens the angle between the rectum and anal canal, raises the intra - abdominal pressure, and facilitates evacuation, which the Western commode may not.

The best way to avoid constipation is to drink a lot of water, consume habitually a **high fiber diet** found in vegetables, salad, seasonal whole fruits, whole grain flour *roti*, brown rather than white bread, *suji* (semolina), whole wheat porridge, millet - based foods, lentils with husks, liquid substances, etc.

Constipation can be redressed by adopting a disciplined lifestyle. Exercise and *yog* are also helpful in keeping constipation at bay. Home remedies are frequently used to relieve constipation.

Normally, *isabgol* - husk mixed with water, milk, curd, etc., controls constipation to a great extent. Other domestic remedies are *amla* or gooseberry, *hada, baheda* (*terminalia bellirica*), dates, *munakka, chhuhara, triphala churna,* flax seed, and various other ayurvedic *aushadhi.* These domestic remedies generally do not harm or damage the digestive system. Castor oil or chemical laxatives, which are strong cathartic agents, may affect the myenteric plexus in the colon, disturbing spontaneous mobility of the bowel. Diarrhea and **electrolyte imbalance** may result. Medicines like bisacodyl, *sena,* docusate sodium, lactulose, milk of magnesia, paraffin liquid, sodium picosulfate, prucalopride, etc., are advised with caution by practitioners of modern medicine.

Acute pain in the abdomen – also called '**acute abdomen.'** This is often an emergency. Pain frequently occurs due to some infection, inflammation, or obstruction in abdominal organs, especially the gall bladder (cholecystitis), appendix (appendicitis), pancreas (pancreatitis), etc. Hepatitis, colitis, gastritis, and cystitis (inflammation of the urinary bladder) usually do not cause such acute pain. Another cause is **intestinal obstruction** – **with symptoms of acute colicky pain, vomiting, abdominal distension,** and **complete constipation**. The latter may be caused by a hernia, tuberculosis, adhesion, kinking of the bowel, tumor, etc.

Intestinal cramps are often **colicky** in nature – which means that acute pain comes intermittently for short intervals, disappearing in between.

Appendicitis - the appendix is a **vestigial** organ (i.e., non - functional and incompletely developed) at the junction of the ileum and large bowel cecum. It may become inflamed, causing acute severe pain in the right iliac fossa.

Cholecystitis – Inflammation of the gall bladder presents as acute pain in the right upper abdomen, often radiating to the back.

Pancreatitis – The pancreas is a solid organ towards the back. Inflammation causes the release of digestive enzymes.

Pain radiates to the back. Pancreatitis may be a severe, life - threatening condition. Another cause of acute abdominal pain is **renal colic** due to renal or ureteric stones. **Chronic or recurrent abdominal pain** is a very common symptom. Pain in lower abdomen accompanying dysentery is called **tenesmus**.

Chronic ulcer in the stomach (**peptic ulcer)** may occur. Pain occurs at a fixed point especially when the stomach is empty and is relieved after meals. **Diverticulosis** is a condition of out - pouching or **diverticulum in the colon which** can lead to chronic, recurrent abdominal pain or acute abdomen if inflamed **(diverticulitis)**. Another common cause of recurrent abdominal pain, especially in children, is **worm infestation.** Chronic abdominal pain or sometimes low - grade boring pain in the abdomen, continuing for months, may be a recurring problem. Such recurring pain may be **functional** in nature. **No objective sign** is found, and tests are also normal. Many **psychological issues** may be related to such chronic pain. Gastrointestinal disorders include **functional dyspepsia** (FD) and **irritable bowel syndrome** (IBS).

These may also cause some abdominal pain and discomfort. Chronic lower abdominal pain in women is frequently due to chronic urinary tract infections, pelvic inflammatory conditions, and ovulatory problems.

Pain in the Right Iliac Fossa – Some young women may feel pain in the right iliac fossa. This pain is not related to digestive or functional defecation disorder. It is felt in the right pelvic region due to **menstrual cycle disorder**.

On examination, the pelvic region may feel stiff and tender. Laboratory examinations show everything normal, but tests are done to exclude diseases like **appendicitis, ovary cysts, or Crohn's disease**. Mild to severe mid - menstrual cycle pain in women may be due to a condition called endometriosis, which is sequestration (spillage) of the endometrium (lining of the uterus) outside the uterine cavity into the pelvis. Chronic infection in the pelvic cavity can be a cause of lower abdominal or right iliac fossa pain.

A structured history is prepared by modern physicians in patients with abdominal pain consisting of the type of pain, site of pain – finger pointing, radiation of pain to back, shoulder, and other areas of the abdomen, aggravating and relieving factors, relation to meals, association with nausea, vomiting, fever, loose motion, etc. Clinical history is followed by abdominal examination with inspection, superficial and deep palpation, percussion, auscultation, and finally, digital examination of oral/rectal/vaginal cavities.

Next investigations may be conducted viz; **abdomen X - ray, ultrasound, CT scan, MRI** – these are analyzed by an experienced physician and surgeon to make a final diagnosis – surprising causes may spring up from the abdomen - 'a magic box'.

Dyspepsia and Bloating – Discomfort in the upper abdomen is called dyspepsia or indigestion. Often, it is a feeling of fullness or bloating. Occasional indigestion is common and not serious. If it happens after a large meal, it can be relieved by sitting upright or walking, using a digestive enzyme, or an antacid. Indigestion that lasts longer than one meal or that occurs frequently is less simple. Sometimes, there is an organic cause, like peptic ulcer or acid reflux disease. In some people, no obvious cause is found. This is called **functional dyspepsia (FD)**. 'Bloating' is a feeling of tightness, pressure, or fullness in the abdomen, which may or may not be associated with a visibly distended (swollen) abdomen. It can result from eating heavily, swallowing air with food (aerophagy), gulping without chewing much, eating too fast, taking liquids and fizzy drinks, etc.

Usually, bloating is relieved by antacids, anti - flatulent, fruit salts, digestive enzymes, etc. Many patients suffer from troublesome **repetitive belching** called **eructation**. Intestinal motility can be maintained by medicines like **domperidone, levosulpiride, peppermint oil,** etc. Stomach bloating may also be caused by amebiasis, spastic colon, mucous colitis, irritable bowel syndrome (IBS), etc.

Common diseases of the bowel

Gastroesophageal Reflux is a common condition. Recently ingested food with gastric juices and acid regurgitating or flowing back into the esophagus (food pipe) and mouth (water brash) with burning in the chest area is called gastroesophageal reflux. This occurs more commonly after certain foods and drinks – such as alcohol, coffee, and fatty or spicy foods.

Reflux is more commonly seen in those overweight, smokers, and pregnant women. If frequent and persistent, it is **gastroesophageal reflux disease (GERD)**. Symptoms of severe GERD are upper abdominal pain, heartburn, sudden waking up from sleep with acid stomach contents in the throat or mouth, and a bout of incessant cough. This occurs when the **lower esophageal sphincter** (the circular muscle between the esophagus and stomach) becomes loose and incompetent.

Chronic regurgitation of stomach acid can lead to inflammation and eventually **narrowing (stenosis)** of the lower esophagus. Treatment includes avoiding tobacco and alcohol and also large meals just before sleeping. Medicines like antacids and **proton pump inhibitors** (omeprezol, pantoprazol, esomeprazole, etc.). Sleeping with the head end elevated and staying upright for a few hours after meals prevents gastroesophageal reflux. Severe cases may require surgery.

Irritable Bowel Syndrome (IBS) – This is a common chronic condition with an obscure cause, most often stress. Some medical scientists designate IBS as a **neuro - gastrointestinal disorder**. IBS is also known by various other names, viz, spastic colon, mucous colitis, unstable colon, adaptive colon, etc. This condition occurs in the large intestine. How the brain and gut coordinate mutually with each other in maintaining the overall functionality of the gut is an enigma. Whenever the coordination between the two is disrupted, IBS may present as diarrhea or constipation. Symptoms may occur with the onset of the menstrual cycle, certain foods, and stress, which may act as triggers of IBS. Other symptoms are abdominal discomfort, cramps, pain, the excessive passage of wind (farting), constipation, inflammation, loose motion, gas, and bloating, which may occur singly or collectively. Although it is a chronic condition, IBS usually does not damage the digestive tract or increase the risk of colon cancer.

In IBS, a cramp or tenesmus in the gut is felt below the navel towards the left or right side of the pelvis region. This feeling is relieved after defecation. In this disorder, loose motion and constipation may alternate one after another. Endoscopic examination and biopsy of the colon (large intestine) only show mucosal hyperemia. Diverticulosis and diverticulitis may cause symptoms mimicking IBS. Recurring amebic or bacillary dysentery may also simulate IBS.

Management of IBS: IBS can generally be managed by medications, diet, and lifestyle changes. There are no laboratory tests for making this diagnosis, but tests are done to exclude other diseases.

Treatment includes:

(i)   anti - depressant medications like imipramine, laxatives, probiotics, antispasmodics, and diazepam

(ii)   dietary changes – increasing fiber in the diet while limiting dairy products, fatty foods, and gluten - containing foods and drinking plenty of water,

(iii)   lifestyle changes viz; regular exercises, *yog - pranayam,* and sound sleep.

Splenic Flexure Syndrome – The highest segment of the colon, attached to the undersurface of the diaphragm, known as the transverse colon.

This continues to the descending colon on the left side of the abdomen. The curvature is called **splenic flexure**. Splenic flexure syndrome has similar symptoms to IBS. In this syndrome, gas builds up in the splenic flexure of the colon. This gas not getting released causes bloating and a feeling of fullness in the upper left abdomen, along with pain in the left iliac fossa. A large, loaded sigmoid colon can kink on its axis.

This is called the **volvulus of the colon**. Colon volvulus leads to complete intestinal obstruction and is generally treated by surgery.

Ulcerative Colitis (UC) – This is a chronic **autoimmune** condition associated with inflammation and small ulcers on the inner lining or mucosa of the large intestine – the colon and rectum in most cases. This condition may be mild to severe. It mostly affects lean and thin people from 15 - 30 years of age, but it can occur after the age of 60. Race or ethnicity also plays a role, as people of Jewish descent are at higher risk. UC tends to run in families, with a risk of up to 30% of people in close relations.

Symptoms include recurrent pain all over the abdomen, tenesmus, abdominal cramps, and copious amounts of mucous and fresh blood in stools. There is a painful desire to defecate many times a day.

Health never builds up. Endoscopic examination of the rectum and colon shows leathery inner lining mucosa with punctate ulcers.

Patients of UC have an increased risk of severe bleeding, anemia, dehydration, perforation of the colon, blood clots in veins and arteries, joint inflammation, problems in skin, eyes, and bone (osteoporosis), and developing colon cancer at a later age. Total removal of the colon may be advised in severe cases.

Treatment includes dietary modification, nutritional supplementation, and immunosuppressive agents. The last recourse may be surgery. The foremost measure should be to avoid milk and dairy products like curd and cheese, red meat, processed meat, alcohol, carbonated drinks, refined sugar, and its preparations like chewing gum, mints, candies, sweets, etc.

High - sulfate foods like nuts and high - fat - containing foods should also be avoided. This condition responds to **5 - ASA or acetylsalicylic acid compounds, mesalazine,** and **corticosteroids**. All these can be used orally or as an enema.

The aim of medical treatment is to keep patients free of troubling symptoms of bleeding, tenesmus, and frequent mucus in stools without the use of corticosteroids. In severe conditions, drugs like cyclosporine, tacrolimus, azathioprine, 6 - mercaptopurine, and TNF alpha antibody – infliximab are used. Many more immunomodulatory agents are being tested to treat UC. Surgery is performed in extremely severe conditions of the toxic megacolon, perforation, and to avoid the future probability of cancer.

The total colon and rectum are removed, and this is called **panprocto - colectomy**. After surgery of total colon and rectum removal, stool frequency is high but gradually settles with time.

Munchausen Syndrome – This is a fictitious disorder associated with severe emotional difficulties. The patient who is not really sick repeatedly and deliberately acts as if suffering from some physical illness and often feigns acute and piercing pain in the abdomen. The 'patient' intentionally assumes a 'sick role' or 'victim card' by pretending to be sick so that they are the center of attention. They also try to delude the doctors.

During the 1950s - 60s, surgeons, bewildered by the pretensions of the patients, would even open up the abdomen and fail to find any convincing pathology inside. Nowadays, surgeons equipped with readily available radiological diagnostic tools do not fall into this trap. Patients with this syndrome are referred to psychologists for counseling.

Globus Hystericus – This is a specific form of conversion disorder – in which psychological problems lead to the physical sensation of a lump in the throat which causes discomfort in swallowing.

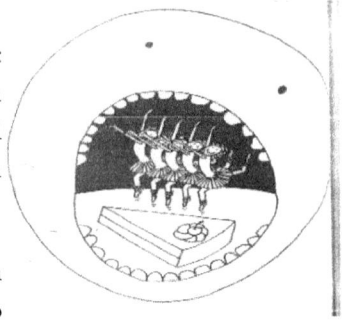

The sensation may also be of choking in the esophagus. The patients pretending to have such symptoms are referred to psychotherapists.

Liver Diseases: The liver is one of the organs in the abdominal cavity. It is located on the right upper part just below the **diaphragm -** the arched muscular sheet that separates the chest and abdominal cavities.

Normally, the liver lies behind the rib cage and is not felt during abdominal palpation. The liver performs many functions – the metabolism of carbohydrates, fats, and proteins; synthesis of plasma proteins such as albumen and clotting factors; storage of glycogen; enzyme activation; production of bile; and excretion of bilirubin, cholesterol, and drugs.

Symptoms of liver disease are **jaundice, enlargement of the liver, firm consistency (as occurs with cirrhosis), excessive bleeding due to deficiency of clotting factors, and finally,** coma in liver failure (hepatic coma).

The degree of jaundice is measured by the level of bilirubin in the blood. Jaundice occurs in 60 - 70% of normal newborns in the first week of life due to immaturity of enzymes and regress spontaneously. This is called the **'physiological jaundice of the newborn.'** However, if the bilirubin level rises to a very high level, it is pathological jaundice and can cause brain damage in newborns.

Hepatitis or inflammation of the liver usually occurs due to **viral** infection. There are a group of viruses which can infect the liver **Hepatitis A, B, C, D and E.** Hepatitis A and E are acute and self - limiting infections, while B, C and D cause acute or chronic infection. Symptoms are fever, loss of appetite, nausea, vomiting, jaundice and liver enlargement with pain. Vaccines are available against Hepatitis A and B.

Cirrhosis refers to permanent scarring and shrinking that changes the consistency of the liver from soft to firm. It usually occurs over months or years. Causes are chronic hepatitis due to virus infections, alcohol, drugs, and metabolic disorders.Hematemesis (blood in vomit), ascites, and swelling in the feet and body may occur due to low plasma proteins. Cirrhosis damages the liver and can lead to liver failure.

Non - alcoholic fatty liver disease (NAFLD) is a liver problem that affects people who drink little to no alcohol. It is mostly seen in overweight or obese people. NAFLD is due to too much fat building up in the liver. It is becoming more common as the number of obese people rises and has become the most common form of liver disease worldwide.

Liver failure - With severe liver damage, liver failure may set in with drowsiness, disorientation, coma, jaundice, bleeding tendency, fluid in the abdomen (ascites), and swelling in the feet and body.

Tremors and a peculiar musty odor may be present. The patient is treated in an intensive care setting. Occasionally, a **liver transplant** may be required.

Apart from the above, the liver is affected by various space - occupying lesions like hydatid cysts, abscesses, and **tumors** (metastatic cancer and primary hepatoma). Investigations done for liver disease are **liver function tests** – serum bilirubin level, liver enzymes, serum proteins, **blood clotting tests**, **antigen and antibody** levels for hepatitis viruses, biopsy and **imaging** by ultrasound, CT scan and MRI. The **gall bladder** is a small sac just below the liver. It stores and concentrates the bile excreted by the liver.

The bile then passes into the **common bile duct** and is released into the **duodenum** (the first part of the small intestine). The gall bladder may get inflamed (**cholecystitis**) or develop stones. Treatment is surgical by removal of the gall bladder – **cholecystectomy**.

Removal of diseased gall bladder does not cause any deficiency in the human body. The **spleen** is another organ in the abdomen located within the rib cage on the left side. It is part of the **reticulo - endothelial system**.

It is enlarged in many blood disorders, malaria, kala azar and infections and also in cirrhosis of liver. The spleen must be enlarged to at least twice its size to be palpable below the rib cage.

Kidneys, ureters and urinary bladder are also housed in the abdominal cavity behind the peritoneum. They are discussed under the chapter on Urinary and excretory system.

To conclude, gastrointestinal disorders are common to all humans, from childhood to adulthood and into old age. Some gut problems are inherited, while others arise due to lifestyle choices and certain behaviors. Long - standing gut issues can even lead to substance abuse. Consuming excessive sugar, salt, oily products, and processed foods exacerbates these problems. Gut health should be nurtured gently.

Maintain a healthy and well - functioning gut by following a balanced diet and regular exercise. Live a life full of vigor, surrounded by wise friends and elders.

Chapter 28

Hypertension

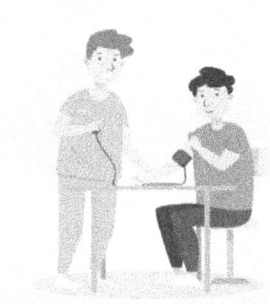

Learning Objectives:

- Relation between atherosclerosis (arterial stiffness) and hypertension
- Systolic and diastolic blood pressure
- Normal variations in blood pressure
- Measuring blood pressure
- Difference between stage I & II hypertension
- Difference between primary and secondary hypertension
- Treatment and drugs for controlling hypertension

Hypertension, often abbreviated as HTN by doctors, refers to persistently **elevated blood pressure**. The heart, located on the left side of the chest, beats at a rate of 60 - 80 times per minute, which is the heart rate or pulse rate. With each beat, the heart pumps blood into the aorta from the left ventricle. The pressure exerted on the artery walls when the heart contracts is called **systolic blood pressure.** When the heart muscle relaxes, the pressure on the arteries is called **diastolic blood pressure**.

The difference between these two measurements is known as **pulse pressure**. As people age, systolic blood pressure tends to increase, while diastolic pressure remains relatively stable, leading to systolic hypertension. This condition results from the gradual loss of arterial elasticity due to **atherosclerosis**, which is the buildup of **plaque** made up of fatty substances, cholesterol, calcium, and other materials inside the arteries. Atherosclerosis is a slow process that often begins in youth and is exacerbated by factors like high cholesterol, high triglycerides, smoking, diabetes, obesity, stress, and lack of physical activity. Hypertension and atherosclerosis create a vicious cycle, as one contributes to the worsening of the other.

While high blood pressure is more common in adults, it can occasionally affect infants, children, and adolescents due to other underlying causes. Blood pressure varies by age, sex, and height, and it is not a fixed number. It fluctuates based on rest, exercise, stress, and emotional state. To diagnose hypertension, blood pressure should be measured multiple times over different occasions.

Traditionally, doctors used a mercury **sphygmomanometer** to measure blood pressure, later replaced by the aneroid manometer. Nowadays, sensor - based devices like self - recording BP machines, available for home use, are common. Another tool, the ambulatory BP monitor, can record blood pressure over a 24 - hour period, providing a detailed analysis of blood pressure variation throughout the day, including during activities like running, sleeping, eating, and driving.

Blood pressure tends to follow a diurnal rhythm, rising in the morning, peaking around midday, and dropping in the evening, typically being lowest at night during sleep. A normal adult blood pressure is around 120/80 mmHg, but prolonged elevated blood pressure increases the risk of further atherosclerosis and other cardiovascular issues.

Some people have lower blood pressure – like 90/60 mmHg, which is healthy for them. **Low blood pressure is not a chronic disease**.

Acutely low blood pressure is an acute condition that may represent **shock** due to inadequacy of water, salt, or sodium or acute loss of blood in the body.

Types of Hypertension – Two main types of hypertension are **primary** and **secondary**. Primary hypertension is also known as **Essential Hypertension,** which has no definitive or identifiable background cause like any acute or chronic biological disorder in the body. Primary Hypertension is what we see commonly. **Primary hypertension has no symptoms** of its own. It develops very slowly and tends to run in families. Putatively, hurry and worry, hasty lifestyle, mental tension, intemperate and even sedentary life, disturbed sleep and sleep disorder cause low - grade slow inflammation and atherosclerosis in the arteries. High salt (sodium) intake is also related to hypertension.

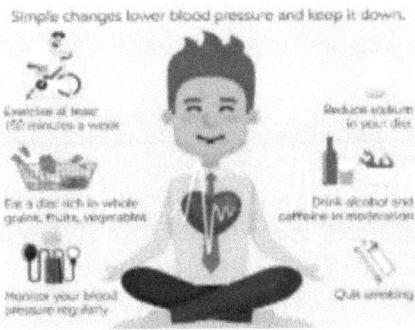

Simple changes lower blood pressure and keep it down.

Secondary hypertension occurs as a manifestation of certain medical conditions in the body. Chronic kidney disease, adrenal disease, endocrine disorders, coarctation (constriction) of aorta, sleep apnoea etc. leads to persistent increase in blood pressure – secondary hypertension.

Symptoms of hypertension – It has to be emphasized that increased or escalated blood pressure **does not generally cause any symptoms** on its own. However, prolonged and persistent raised blood pressure damages the blood vessels and other organs **silently**. The heart has to pump against a higher pressure in the arteries, and over a period of years, this places a strain on the heart muscle, causing it to become thicker (**hypertrophic**).

Eventually, uncontrolled hypertension causes decreased efficiency of the pump or **heart failure**. Hypertension accelerates atherosclerosis and is an important risk factor for **coronary artery disease, brain stroke, and kidney failure**. Therefore, it is important to check your blood pressure now and then, especially after the age of forty.

Stages of Hypertension – The Joint National Committee – JNC8 on Prevention, Detection, Evaluation, and Treatment of High Blood Pressure has laid down the following criteria -

Pre-Hypertension	BP in mm of Mercury or Hg
Systolic	120–139
Diastolic	80 – 89
Stage–I	
Systolic	140–159
Diastolic	90 – 99
Stage–II	
Systolic	≥ 160
Diastolic	≥ 100

Prehypertension and **stage - I hypertension** can often be managed effectively through lifestyle changes without the need for medication. Key modifications include reducing salt intake, managing body weight, maintaining a balanced diet, and incorporating practices like *yog - pranayam*, physical exercise, and sports into daily routines. Many households have successfully decreased their salt consumption or switched to low - sodium salt (LoNA). Additionally, substituting regular table and cooking salt (sodium chloride - NaCl) with potassium salt (potassium chloride - KCl) is another strategy to lower sodium intake and control blood pressure. These changes can help prevent further progression of hypertension and promote overall cardiovascular health.

Stage - II hypertension – if the BP reading remains above the limits and continues for 3 - 4 days, drug treatment is necessary. The aim of treatment is to regulate and maintain the systolic and diastolic BP as per the standards of JNC8. The BP range according to age group is as follows –

- **Below 60 years** – BP range < 140/90 mm Hg

- **Above 60 years** – BP range < 150/90 mm Hg

The medicines are to be regulated as per the advice of the physician. BP has to be monitored carefully. Medicines for controlling BP can be classified into 4 groups viz.

1. **Diuretics** – such medicines are given to increase the excretion of sodium and water from the kidney and control BP.

2. **Renin - Angiotensin function control** – such medicines control the Renin - Angiotensin system and control BP.

3. **Calcium channel blockers** – such medicines reduce the resistance of the arteries and control BP.

4. **Vasodilators** – such medicines act as sympathetic inhibitors for Alpha and Beta receptors. They improve elasticity and dilate the arteries, reducing peripheral artery resistance.

Medicines used for control of BP

Diuretics	*Rennin - Angiotensin function control (RAAS)*	*Calcium channel blockers*	*Vasodilators Alpha/Beta sympathetic inhibitors*
Hydrochlorothiazide	Captopril	Verapamil	**Direct Vasodilators** Diazoxide Hydralazine
Chlorthalidone	Enalapril	Diltiazem	Nitroprusside Sodium
Frusemide	Lisinopril	Nifedipine	
Torsemide	Ramipril	Felodipine	**β - Blocker** Propranolol
Spironolactone	Losartan	Amlodipine	Metoprolol Atenolol
	Telmisartan	Nicardipine	

Hypertension

	Olmesartan	Cilnidipine	α & β - Blocker Labetalol Carvedilol
	Azilsartan		
	Valsartan		α Blocker Prazosin Terazosin Doxazosin Phentolamine

Drugs safe in pregnancy	
Methyldopa	Clonidine
Nifedipine	Hydralazine
	Labetalol

Emergency hypertension – The emergency stage of hypertension is when it escalates to the range – 220/110 mmHg. In such situations, medicines like Nicardipine, labetalol, and Sodium Nitroprusside are given intravenously.

In conclusion, elevated blood pressure or hypertension often presents without noticeable symptoms, leading many individuals to neglect their condition despite consistently high readings. Some people, due to obstinacy or fear of side effects, may resist modern medication, opting for *AYUSH* or alternative treatments instead. Unfortunately, this disregard can result in sudden and severe outcomes like brain strokes or heart attacks. Strokes may cause paralysis, loss of speech, or even coma.

Wisdom lies in regular blood pressure monitoring, consulting experts, adopting necessary lifestyle changes, and consistently taking prescribed antihypertensive medications to maintain healthy blood pressure levels.

Chapter 29

Diabetes

SYMPTOMS OF DIABETES

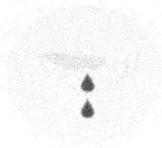

WOUNDS HEAL SLOWLY   EXTREME FATIGUE   HIGH BLOOD SUGAR

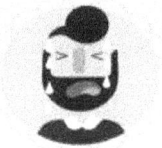

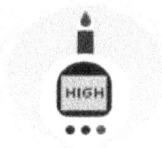

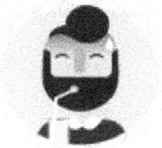

ALWAYS THIRSTY   PRESSURE

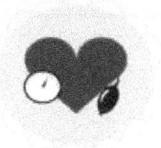

Learning Objectives:

- Three types of diabetes – Diabetes mellitus (types 1 & 2), and gestational diabetes
- Genesis of type 2 diabetes (T2D) – sedentary lifestyle, neglecting physical exercises in routine life, stress, anxiety and not taking balanced diet or eating intemperate food
- Symptoms and complications of T2D
- Diabetes diagnosis and monitoring - measurement at home by glucometer, or 24 hours measurement by sensor equipment with chip fixed to the body (**continuous glucose monitoring**)
- Treatment of T2D by lifestyle changes, medicines and insulin
- Concept of glycemic index in the food we eat
- Types of drugs and insulin used
- Condition of hypoglycemia in diabetics – cause and treatment

Diabetes is a chronic metabolic disorder affecting the body's ability to process carbohydrates, fats, and proteins due to either **insufficient insulin production** or **insulin resistance**. Insulin, a hormone secreted by the pancreas' beta cells, is crucial for directing glucose into cells to generate energy. In insulin resistance, although insulin is present, glucose cannot effectively enter cells, leading to elevated blood sugar levels.

Previously, two types of diabetes were recognized: **diabetes insipidus** and **diabetes mellitus**. Diabetes insipidus, now referred to as Arginine Vasopressin Deficiency (AVP - D), is distinct from diabetes mellitus. This chapter focuses primarily on **type 2 diabetes (T2D)**, which is the most common form of diabetes mellitus.

Glucose, the primary sugar used for energy, is derived from the digestion of carbohydrates, proteins, and fats in the diet, with carbohydrates being the main source. After digestion, carbohydrates are broken down into glucose, proteins into amino acids, and fats into fatty acids. Glucose then travels through the bloodstream to energy - demanding tissues like muscles. There, it enters cells (a process facilitated by insulin) and is converted into energy in the form of **adenosine triphosphate (ATP),** which is the body's ultimate energy currency. Glucose can also be stored in the liver and muscles as **glycogen,** which can be used during physical activity.

If insulin is absent or ineffective, glucose cannot enter the cells and remains in the blood, causing elevated blood sugar levels. When blood glucose levels exceed 180 - 200 mg/dl, glucose spills into the urine, a condition known as **glycosuria**. Normally, glucose is absent in the urine of healthy individuals.

Food digestion is processed in two stages. Primary digestion takes place in the intestine, where food is digested with many intestinal juices and their enzymes, after which it is converted into glucose, amino acids, and fatty acids.

Digested forms of food are absorbed into the blood and pass through the portal venous system, reaching the liver, where they are metabolized. Some elements of assimilated food in the liver are consumed like 'current account' by the tissues and organs of the body, and the rest is stored as glycogen and fat like 'term deposit.'

Secondary digestion – The secondary digestion of the food takes place in cells and tissues. Here, glucose is consumed with the help of insulin, as a result of which energy and carbon dioxide are produced. Thus, diabetes is a disorder of secondary - level digestion. Extra glucose in the blood, which is unable to enter cells, causes diabetes – the body feels weak and feeble; it is the condition of **starvation amidst plenty**. Despite excess glucose in the blood, the body is deprived of energy.

We usually consume sugar in 3 - 4 forms: glucose, galactose, fructose, and sucrose. Glucose is burnt in the body by exercise, activities, and sports. The risk of diabetes is increased by sedentary habits and other illness - breeding behaviors, i.e., lack of exercise. Consumption of excess carbohydrates (starches and sugars), along with low insulin levels, increases susceptibility to diabetes. Persons engaged only in intellectual activity and not doing any physical activity also become prone to diabetes.

Diabetes mellitus may occur in **two types viz: type - 1 and type - 2.**

Type 1 diabetes presents at a young age and occurs due to autoimmunity, i.e., the body's own immune system destroys the β cells in the pancreas that produce insulin. **Type 1 diabetes patients do not produce insulin**. It is far **less common** than type 2. People with type 1 diabetes **must take exogenous insulin** so as to regulate their blood sugar levels; therefore, it is also referred to as **insulin - dependent diabetes** or **juvenile diabetes**, as it usually affects children and young adults but may occasionally present in late adulthood.

Type 2 diabetes (T2D) is more intricately related to lifestyle, but both genetics and environmental factors play a role. It usually occurs after the age of 45 years, but more and more younger people are also getting affected. Environmental risk factors known to impact the development of T2D include mental stress, obesity, a sedentary lifestyle, excess food containing carbohydrates, low birth weight, etc. It is a chronic condition that develops when the body is unable to use insulin properly **(insulin resistance)** or is unable to produce enough insulin for its needs. In both situations, glucose builds up in the blood but cannot be used for energy. An increase in blood glucose levels leads to various health complications. This type of diabetes is treated by lifestyle changes, especially the type of food and habits, medicines, and insulin.

Gestational diabetes mellitus (GDM) – A third type of diabetes may occur during pregnancy. Recently, GDM has been seen commonly. Gestational diabetes or GDM is associated with excess weight gain during pregnancy, heavy baby in the womb, heavy birth weight > 3.5 kg, **polycystic ovary syndrome (PCOS)** earlier in life, sugar in urine test, family history of diabetes mellitus, hypertension, low range HDL and sedentary lifestyle. Blood and urine glucose should always be tested during pregnancy, especially during the second trimester (24th - 28th weeks' gestation). GDM generally abates after the birth of the baby.

However, these ladies are at higher risk of developing diabetes later in the fourth decade of their lives. They should keep on testing blood and urine sugar as a routine screening and consume a diet with fewer carbohydrates and low glycemic index. An active lifestyle is always beneficial. For reasons not yet identified coherently, type 2 diabetes is extremely common in Asia. In India, approximately 10.1 crore adults are affected.

In fact, our country is 2nd only to China in diabetes load. One of the reasons for the high prevalence is attributed to poor nutrition in the intrauterine period. Poor maternal nutrition results in adverse health of neonate – **intrauterine growth retardation**. According to the **Barker hypothesis**, in such babies, there is a resetting of the biological clock, due to which there is a predisposition to develop **'metabolic syndrome'** later in life. This syndrome has the components of high blood pressure, obesity, high blood triglycerides, low levels of HDL cholesterol, insulin resistance, and obesity.

Genesis of Type 2 diabetes (T2D)

Risk factors for T2D include – age of more than 45 years, ethnicity, overweight or obesity, sedentary lifestyle, mental stress, high lipid levels, high intake of sugars in the diet, low birth weight, history of type 2 diabetes in the family, history of gestational diabetes and certain medical conditions (hypertension, stroke, polycystic ovary syndrome, etc.). Although habitual high intake of sweets in the diet is a known risk factor, the relationship between sugar intake and T2D is not clearly explained – the relationship between the two is neither proportionate nor ruled out. It is believed that the pancreatic β cells fail to keep pace with the demand for insulin.

Ultimately, **excessive consumption of sugar over time induces insulin resistance**. Sugar also causes weight gain, which is a risk factor for developing diabetes. Risk factors like weight gain, insulin resistance, and inflammatory responses can lead to prediabetes, which is a condition with higher - than - normal glucose levels not enough to be labeled as T2D. If prediabetes is not addressed, it can develop into type 2 diabetes in about five to 10 years.

Symptoms of T2D – Some of the most prominent symptoms are – **polyuria** (urination in increased frequency and volume), **polydipsia** (feeling excessively thirsty and drinking excess water), **polyphagia** (feeling excessively hungry and eating excessively), and, ironically, losing weight. Diabetes is like a hidden mite in the body, damaging many organ systems and their functions. It plays a vicious role in the decadence of the body. Diabetes or increased blood sugar is not manifested by normal symptoms. Diabetes is often a dormant disease – certain peculiar symptoms may manifest at times but may not draw our notice. Diabetes may be identified only after falling prey to various acute and chronic complications and diseases - such as skin boils, non - healing leg or foot wounds, urinary infections, kidney failure, eye trouble, etc. In such situations, testing of blood sugar may yield a high value. Many a time, diabetes is detected, and it is the first time it is diagnosed during general medical checkups – this is the outcome of modern - day routine blood screening tests.

Complications – Diabetes opens the threshold to many diseases. This disease silently accelerates atherosclerosis. **Vasculopathy** of various organs occurs, which ultimately develops into vascular aging. Diabetes is the precursor of fatal diseases of various organs **viz; nephropathy** (kidney function deteriorates), **retinopathy** (retina of the eyes are affected), **neuropathy** (weakness, tingling, and numbness), coronary artery disease – (CAD) and brain stroke. In addition, **diabetes predisposes to infections of the skin and urinary tract.** An acute life - threatening complication that is much more common in Type 1 diabetes is **diabetic ketoacidosis.**

Tests for diabetes – A **fasting blood glucose** (after more than 8 hours fast) less than 100 mg/dL (5.6 mmol/L) is normal, 100 to 125 mg/dL (5.6 to 6.9 mmol/L) is suggestive of prediabetes, while 126 mg/dL (7.0 mmol/L) or higher on two separate tests is diagnosed as diabetes.

A **random blood glucose** measurement at any time of the day exceeding 200 mg/dl or a hemoglobin A1c (HbA1c) of more than 6.5% is also suggestive. The latter is a reflection of the degree of control over the previous 2 to 3 months and is useful for monitoring purposes.

HbA1c is the percentage of red blood cells that have glucose - coated hemoglobin – a relatively new and very useful **biomarker of diabetes**. Apart from the above tests, sometimes doctors suggest glucose tolerance tests, which are represented in a graph. First, a fasting blood glucose level is done, and then a meal or about 75 gm of glucose is given to the patient, following which blood glucose is measured at intervals. If glucose in the blood increases beyond 180 mg/dl, it passes out in the urine. The presence of glucose in the urine is always abnormal. Thus, after necessary laboratory tests and clinical examination, doctors may suggest other tests of organ function in the evaluation of T2D.

Preventing T2D – The importance of preventing diabetes is apparent by the distressful conditions described above. T2D can be prevented by lifestyle changes and health - seeking behavior.

Measures to prevent diabetes are:

(1) A Balanced diet, regular meals, and a disciplined lifestyle;

(2) Taking exercises, walking 2 - 4 km per day, sports, and *yoga - asana*

(3) Eating food containing a low glycemic index; i.e., less sugar, sweets, wheat bread, rice, and potato would help reduce body weight also and reduce chances of other diseases like coronary artery disease and stroke.

Monitoring – Chronic diabetic patients must understand the consequences of diabetes, and they should purchase a domestic glucometer (approximate price Rs 800 – 1500), which helps the patient to keep the disease well controlled. **HbA1C** measurements should be done regularly. **A continuous glucose monitoring sensor device is a software technology in which a blood sample by venous puncture or by needle is not required,** and the blood sugar is measured and continuously informed on your mobile phone App and warning communicated at once that blood glucose is high – be aware of intemperance. It automatically teaches which foodstuff is causing a rise in blood sugar.

After diagnosis, regular evaluation and monitoring of T2D under the expert guidance of your physician is necessary to prevent hypoglycemia with antidiabetic medicines. Sugar and protein should be checked periodically in urine samples. Patients should also take care of their eyes and consult an ophthalmologist from time to time. Taking appropriate and timely treatment for foot injuries or infections will enhance wellness in the long run. Injuries and wounds may adversely affect diabetic patients and should be attended to early.

Glycemic index – It is important, especially for diabetics, to understand the concept of glycemic index. This reflects the speed by which blood glucose peaks after the intake of a particular food item. The quantity of food ingested multiplied by the value of **the glycemic index gives the value of the glycemic load**. Certain food items increase blood glucose instantaneously and are known to have a **high glycemic index**. The ratio between the two phenomena is called the indexing of glycemic level in a particular food. If diabetes is to be controlled with or without medicines, food having a high glycemic index, such as carbohydrates, should be avoided. It needs to be reiterated here that though high amounts of fat - containing food items are not included in glycemic indexing, fat should be avoided because it can convert into carbohydrates, which again inflates the level of sugar in the blood.

Glycemic Index (GI)	Glycemic Load (GL)
Carbohydrate food increases glucose in the blood	Carbohydrate food increases the amount of glucose in the blood
Measurement of the quality of carbohydrate	Both the quality and quantity of carbohydrate food determine the glycemic load.
High GI food > 70 Sugar, jaggery, fried/boiled potato, rice, wheat flour, refined flour etc. **Medium GI 56 – 69** Multigrain flour (*missi ka atta*), besan, *jowar flour, semolina (suji), gram, corn, honey, roots – beetroot, mango,* etc. **Low GI < 55** Almost all vegetables, berries, popcorn, tomato, guava, kiwi, etc.,	High GL > 20 Medium GL 11 – 19 Low GL < 11 **How to calculate glycemic load:** Glycemic Index x Weight of the carbohydrate in grams per 100 grams of the food.

Food Groups	Low glycemic index (0–55)	Medium glycemic index (55 – 69)	High glycemic index (> 70)
Cereal	Barley, oats, quinoa, porridge, *Dalia*	Wheat flour, mustard seed, brown rice, *basmati* rice	White rice, bread, puffed rice, poha, refined flour, instant oats, cornflakes, cake, biscuit, Maggie, bakery products
Pulses & legumes	Green gram, split pigeon peas, lentils, beans, soybean, chickpeas (*chole*), kidney bean	Almost	Almost
Vegetables	Green leafy vegetables like – spinach, fenugreek leaf, amaranth (*chaulayi*), brinjal, green beans, cauliflower, cucumber, snake cucumber, green, papaya, tomato, broccoli	Peas, potato, sweet potato	Pumpkin, potato
Fruits	Apricot, apple, sweet lime, orange, kiwi, potato plum, pear, berries, mango, banana	Papaya, banana, muskmelon, mango, fig, pineapple, raisins	Watermelon, muskmelon, dates

Milk and milk product	Milk and milk products like curd and buttermilk	Ice cream	Rabri, cream scraper
Others	Vegetable soup, peanut, flax seed, almonds, walnut, cashew nut, pumpkin and sunflower seed, egg, meat, spices	Soft drinks, honey	Energy drinks, pizza, fast food, sugar, jaggery, chocolate

Note:

People in India consume almost 5 to 20 grams of white sugar and 100 - 200 grams of potato per day. Both these have a high glycemic index, leading to a higher glycemic load. Some items have huge quantities of water, and therefore, despite their high glycemic index, they do not build up high blood sugar levels. For example, watermelon and pumpkin do not increase blood sugar despite consuming 200 grams.

Low glycemic index food items increase the sensitivity for insulin secretion in natural processes, which is why blood sugar is also controlled. Low glycemic index foods item, besides controlling hunger, preventing T2D and heart disease help to lower cholesterol. Instead of using lentils without peel, taking **whole lentils** is beneficial. Cereals full of fiber and brown/multigrain bread keep the gut healthy and prevent an increase in blood glucose.

White rice, white bread made of refined flour, and cereals without fiber should be avoided. Vegetables enriched with fiber and leaf, such as green beans, brinjal, carrot, cauliflower, tomato, cucumber, broccoli, spinach, salad, and salad leaves, should be necessary constituents of routine food. Vegetables full of starch, like potatoes, should be avoided.

Walnuts, almonds, peanuts, nuts, flax seeds, sunflower seeds, seafood, lean meat (low - fat content), and white eggs have a low glycemic index and do not increase blood sugar as much.

Treatment of diabetes – Diabetes is commonly treated by family physicians or specialists who very well understand its symptoms and keep diabetes treated and controlled. That the reversal of T2D is possible is being claimed and advertised by many protagonists in the open commercial market – most of their strategy is to replace a high glycemic index diet with a low glycemic diet, monitor blood glucose, weight reduction, etc.

However, severe advanced diabetes, often in a thin - built person, may not be reversed. Obese diabetics practicing good restraint on diet and exercising with a regulated lifestyle may reverse diabetes.

Evidence shows that diabetes reversal is best achieved under the surveillance of dieticians, but as soon as this supervision is withdrawn, diabetes returns. It is to be reiterated once again that incomplete examination and treatment of T2D by the quacks may be injurious to health in the long run. So - called diabetes experts are in plenty on social media.

Curing diabetes without medicine – As already stated, maintaining good health and wellness through long walks, sports, jogging, *yog*, physical workouts, etc., must be a daily routine. Attempts should be made to reduce carbohydrates in the diet as they tend to quickly increase blood glucose. These lifestyle changes help to prevent T2D in normal and prediabetics and are advised to all diabetics as well. Early T2D and prediabetes can be cured by these changes in lifestyle alone.

Treating diabetes with medicines – If blood sugar is not controlled by the lifestyle changes described above, medicines, such as anti - diabetic drugs or insulin, should be taken as per medical advice. It is important to understand that **the timing** of food should be such that episodes of hyperglycemia and hypoglycemia may not occur.

Food intake and medicines/ insulin should be **synchronized** properly to avoid these episodes. It is also emphasized that anti - diabetic drugs or insulin do their proper function when the concerned person also remains vigilant and is devoted to lifestyle changes and taking the drugs in adherence to the timing as advised in the prescription. T2D may be treated by two types of medicine, indicated in Tables 1 and 2.

Table 1 Types of Oral Anti - Diabetic Drugs

S. No	Group	Effect	Side Effect
1.	**Biguanides** Metformin	Lower blood glucose levels by decreasing the amount of glucose the liver produces and releases in the bloodstream. It also helps lower sugar levels by making skeletal muscle tissue more sensitive to insulin so it can absorb glucose for energy. Transfers glucose from the blood into the cells	Muscular pains and wasting Pain in arms & legs. Stomach discomfort & gas Constipation loose - motion Anxiety
2.	**Sulfonylureas** Glibenclamide, Glimepiride, Tolbutamide, Gliclazide	Release insulin secretion from *beta - cells of the* pancreas. Sulfonylureas close ATP - sensitive K+ channels in the *beta - cell* to initiate a chain of events that release insulin in the blood	It can drop blood sugar quite dramatically Increased insulin secretioncan cause rebound hypoglycemia
3.	**Meglitinides** Repaglinide, Nateglinide	Directly stimulate the release of insulin from pancreatic beta cells and thereby lower blood glucose.	Weight gain hypoglycemia
4.	**Thiazolidinedi ones** Pioglitazone, Rosiglitazone	Improve insulin sensitivity via activation of the nuclear receptor peroxisome proliferator - activated receptor gamma (PPARγ)	Swelling in feet & fluid retention, ankle swelling

5.	*Dipeptidyl Peptidase (DPP - 4)Inhibitors* Incretin enhancers, Teneligliptin, Sitagliptin, Saxagliptin, Vildagliptin, Linagliptin, Alogliptin,	DPP - 4 inhibitors inhibit the degradation of incretins, glucagon - like peptide - 1 (GLP - 1), and glucose - dependent insulinotropic peptide (GIP). Thus, GLP1 remains in blood circulation for a longer time. This increases incretin, leading to an increase in insulin secretion. When sugar levels are high, it signals the liver not to make more glucose.	
6.	*Alpha Glucosidase inhibitors* Acarbose, Miglitol, Voglibose	Inhibit the absorption of carbohydrates from the small intestine. Inhibit enzymes that convert complex non - absorbable carbohydrates into simple absorbable carbohydrates. These enzymes include glucoamylase, sucrase, maltase, and isomaltase.	Gas in stomach
7.	*SGLT2 inhibitors Sodium - glucose Co - transporter use* (suffix used is gliflozin) Dapagliflozin Canagliflozin Empagliflozin	Lower plasma glucose levels by blocking the reabsorption of filtered glucose in urine, causing glycosuria. It reduces the renal threshold for glucose excretion. Thus, they do not usually cause hypoglycemia.	SGLT2 inhibitors modestly decrease blood pressure and weight

8.	**_Incretin Mimetics – GLP1 receptor agonist_** Exenatide, Liraglutide, Dulaglutide, Lixisenatide, Semaglutide	These incretin drugs work by mimicking the incretin hormones that the body usually produces naturally to stimulate the release of insulin in response to a meal. They are used along with diet and exercise to lower blood sugar in adults with T2D.	Nausea and vomiting, weight loss
9	**_Combination Drugs_** – (combination drugs) Several medicines are combinations of medicines, as mentioned above. **These medicines should be taken strictly as per doctor's advice.** This information is given in brief. Sometimes more than one medicine, apart from insulin and other oral medicines are given in acute diabetes. In the treatment of diabetes, **monitoring** should be done continuously or at some intervals.		

Side effects of diabetes medications are common and may include dizziness, vomiting, gut disturbances, skin rashes or eruptions, allergies, fast heart rate, and loss of appetite. Diabetic patients need to be cautious about using certain medications, such as pain killers, as some are contraindicated.

Other medications, such as blood thinners (like warfarin), beta - blockers (like metoprolol), diuretics, corticosteroids, and lipid - lowering drugs, should be discussed with the doctor to avoid harmful interactions with diabetic treatments.

Diabetic medicines should be taken either half an hour to one hour before meals or after meals, depending on the doctor's instructions, to prevent sudden drops in blood sugar levels. Insulin therapy is recommended for type 2 diabetes patients with an initial HbA1C level greater than 9% or when blood glucose remains uncontrolled despite optimal oral hypoglycemic treatment.

Table 2 Types of Insulin

1	**Immediate acting** Works in 5 - 15 minutes; effect lasts for 2 - 4 hours	Insulin Lispro, Insulin Aspart, Insulin Glulisine
2	**Short - acting** Works in 30 minutes – one hour; effect lasts for 3 - 6 hours	Isophane Insulin, (Lente) Insulin, Regular Insulin
3	**Delayed acting** Works in 1 - 2 hours; effect lasts for 14 - 24 hours	Insulin Glargine Detemir & Degludec
4	**Mixed insulin pen** It works for 5 hours, and the effect lasts for 10 - 24 hours.	Insulin Lispro Protamine & Insulin Lispro, Insulin Aspart Protamine & Insulin Aspart, NPH Insulin & Regular Insulin
5	Insulin is also available in the form of powder, which is administered intranasally.	

Hypoglycemia is a condition where blood glucose levels drop abnormally low, even though diabetes is typically associated with high blood sugar.

This can happen as a result of anti - diabetic drugs, eating very little, or other factors that create an imbalance between insulin/drug intake and food consumption, such as skipping a meal. Low blood sugar can severely impact the body's energy supply, leading to symptoms like confusion, incoherent speech, sweating, loss of consciousness, heart palpitations, weakness, shakiness, anxiety, and depression. In severe cases, hypoglycemia can lead to sudden death.

Family caregivers should be aware of these symptoms, as hypoglycemia is usually easily treated by checking blood glucose with a glucometer and giving sugary foods or drinks like glucose water, jaggery, chocolates, sweet biscuits, or fruit juices.

If the patient becomes unconscious, immediate medical intervention with intravenous glucose is needed. In such emergencies, it's important to carry the patient's medical records and prescriptions to the nearest hospital or clinic for prompt treatment. Other methods of treating diabetes include surgical options such as implanting a **sensor insulin pump**, similar to a pacemaker, which automatically releases insulin based on blood glucose levels, thereby regulating blood sugar. Another approach involves **transplanting pancreatic β cells**, the source of insulin production, although this procedure is still experimental and complex. Bariatric surgery, often used in obese patients, not only addresses obesity but has also been found to reverse metabolic syndrome, including obesity, diabetes, hypertension, and dyslipidemia.

In conclusion, those who adopt a balanced lifestyle while allowing occasional indulgence can manage their health and prevent diabetes or other lifestyle - related diseases, leading to a long and healthy life.

Low - carbohydrate diets are often prescribed to reverse diabetes, but they are difficult to follow and sustain. Although some individuals manage to adhere to such diets, they usually find it challenging to maintain them over time. As a result, despite temporary reductions in diabetes medication, they often need to resume treatment to keep their blood sugar levels in check.

Chapter 30

Cardiac and Vascular Diseases

Learning Objectives:

- Structure and functions of the heart and Circulatory System

- Diseases of heart – hypertensive heart, congestive heart failure, pulmonary heart disease, arrhythmias, valvular heart disease, rheumatic heart disease, congenital heart disease, etc.

- Diseases of the vascular system – arteries and veins

- Investigation of cardiovascular disease

The Cardiovascular system, also called **the circulatory system, consists of three main components viz: heart, blood vessels, and blood**. Blood vessels or vascular systems consist of three types of vessels – arteries, veins, and capillaries. In medical science, the study of heart diseases is called **cardiology**. Some important functions performed by the cardiovascular system are as follows:

1. This system while maintaining blood circulation incessantly in the body supplies **oxygen (O2)** to the tissues and removes **carbon dioxide (CO2)** back to the lungs.
2. Besides providing oxygen which is important for every cell and tissue of the body, the blood and circulatory system also carry **nutrition**.
3. Carrying **waste** material from the cells for excretion through the lungs (for removal of carbon dioxide), liquid waste through kidneys and sweat, and other waste from different organ systems through metabolic activity
4. Preventing infection through its white blood cells and antibodies
5. Stopping the blood oozing out from injuries and wounds
6. Maintaining the **body temperature**
7. Producing **hormones** and **transporting** them to various organs of the body.

Components of the cardiovascular system – The heart, blood vessels, and blood make up the circulatory system. Of these, blood is discussed in a separate chapter.

Heart – This is a unique hollow organ made of strong muscles that function tirelessly and **ceaselessly, contracting and relaxing from fetal life till death** of the individual. The heart beats more than one hundred thousand times (1,00,000) in a day. Due to the incessant pumping by the heart, the blood in the vessels travels around 60,000 miles in a day. The right side of the heart, after receiving oxygen - depleted blood, pumps it into the lungs to get oxygenated. The veins from the lungs carrying oxygenated blood empty into the left side of the heart, which pumps it into all the tissues of the whole body. There are three layers in the heart: the endocardium (inner layer), epicardium (outer layer), and **myocardium** (middle layer – thick layer). The heart is covered by a membrane called **pericardium.** This is a protective fluid - filled sac that covers the roots of major blood vessels and encloses the heart and the great vessels. There are four chambers in the heart, viz. **i. right ventricle ii. left ventricle iii. right atrium** and **iv. left atrium.** The ventricles are located at the lower side of the heart, while the atria are located on the upper side. The left and right atria receive blood, and the left and right ventricles pump blood out of the heart. Oxygen - depleted blood from the whole body is received in the right atrium and then passes into the right ventricle. The latter pumps de - oxygenated blood through the pulmonary arteries into the lungs (**pulmonary circulation**) to get oxygenated. From the lungs, the pulmonary veins carry oxygenated blood to the left atrium.

From the left atrium, this oxygenated blood passes into the left ventricle, which pumps it to all the tissues of the body (**systemic circulation**). The two circulations are arranged in series. Thus, the pulmonary arteries are the only arteries in the whole body carrying de - oxygenated blood, and the pulmonary veins are the only veins in the body that carry oxygenated blood. Contraction of the heart is called **systole,** and relaxation is called **diastole.** There is **a sinoatrial node (SA node) or natural pacemaker** in the heart. This node generates electrical impulses regularly, i.e., a wave of conduction through the heart muscle, and keeps it contracting and relaxing 60 - 90 times a minute (in adults) throughout life. These impulses are responsible for the normal **rhythm and rate** of the heart.

Each of the four chambers of the heart has valves that allow only the forward flow of blood. These four valves are

(i) **the tricuspid valve,**

(ii) **the pulmonary valve,**

(iii) **the mitral valve, and**

(iv) **the aortic valve.**

When the blood moves from one chamber to another chamber, it has to flow through these valves. The contraction and relaxation rhythms of heart muscles induce the valves to open and close simultaneously. These valves are unidirectional flaps. Blood flowing through the valves cannot return back in the reverse direction. Both the ventricles and atria are separated by a thick muscular wall called **interventricular septum and interatrial septum,** respectively. Structural and functional defects of the heart are tested by color Doppler – echocardiography, ECG (echocardiogram), etc.

Diseases of the Heart

Heart Failure – This is a general term and end result of many diseases affecting the heart. When the heart is unable to pump blood according to the needs of the body, the condition is known as **congestive heart failure (CHF)** or just heart failure. The strength of contraction and relaxation of the left ventricle is affected. Heart failure can be acute or chronic.

Many diseases like hypertension, ischemic heart disease, myocardial infarction, valvular heart disease, cardiomyopathy, and some metabolic disorders may cause heart failure. As forward flow is reduced, there is a build - up of blood in the lungs and liver. Cardinal symptoms and signs of CHF are shortness of breath, especially on lying flat (orthopnea), fast pulse rate, fatigue, tender enlargement of the liver, swelling of feet, and raised pressure in the neck veins.

Enlargement of the heart or **cardiomegaly** occurs because of dilatation. Investigations to confirm CHF include an **X - ray** (radiography) of the chest, **an echocardiogram to measure ejection fraction,** and **pro - brain natriuretic peptide (Pro BNP).**

CHF is treated with oxygen, raising the head end, diuretics to increase urine output, drugs like digoxin to increase the strength of cardiac contractions, and drugs to decrease systemic resistance (to decrease the workload of the heart). Treatment also includes pacemakers, cardioverter defibrillators, ventricular assist devices, and heart transplantation. The goal of treatment is the gradual rehabilitation of the patient.

Cardiomegaly – This term simply means **enlargement of the heart.** It can be detected clinically and also by imaging, like an X - ray chest. Enlargement of the heart is a feature of congestive heart failure due to any cause – like coronary artery disease, rheumatic heart disease, or hypertensive heart disease. It may be due to many conditions like hemochromatosis, cardiomyopathy, pericardial effusion, anemia, valvular heart disease, heart attack, heart failure, etc. Features of CHF may be present.

Coronary Artery Disease (CAD) or Ischemic Heart Disease – Heart muscle requires nutrition and oxygen throughout for its lifelong, never - ceasing beating. When the blood flow in the arteries supplying the heart itself is obstructed due to atherosclerosis, the heart muscle suffers from a relative lack of oxygen and nutrients. Due to the atherosclerotic **plaque** build - up in the walls of the arteries, they are narrowed, and blood flow in the arteries is blocked or limited. Arteries are thickened, and their elasticity is altered. If physical activity exceeds the blood reaching the heart muscle, a severe pain in the chest called **'angina'** results. This manifests as chest pain, pain in the shoulder and left arm, and sometimes even back pain.

Angina usually subsides if the patient stops physical activity or takes medicines (nitroglycerine or sorbitrate) to dilate coronary arteries. However, if the reduced blood supply is prolonged or severe, it may **permanently** damage the heart muscle and cause a 'heart attack,' also known as **myocardial infarction**, due to the death of some part of the cardiac muscle. A symptom of myocardial infarction is severe chest pain with a feeling of impending doom. Sometimes, this is mistaken for 'indigestion,' etc. Infarction may also affect the heart's conductive system. A large area of infarction may lead to congestive heart failure or sudden death. Blockage in the coronary artery is tested by **coronary angiography, and blockage is removed by angioplasty, stent,** or **bypass graft surgery**.

The heart disease resulting from CAD is called **ischemic heart disease**. Medicines like aspirin, clopidogrel, and nitroglycerine prevent blood clotting and narrowing of cardiac arteries.

Hypertensive heart disease – Chronically raised blood pressure (for a long period of time) results in increased load on the heart causing **hypertrophy** or thickening of the heart muscle of left ventricle.

However, if the high load on the heart continues unabated, the heart muscle finally becomes weak and fails, leading to congestive heart failure. All the features of heart failure set in.

Congenital heart disease (**CHD**) – There are many congenital malformations of the heart that can cause symptoms from early childhood. Many results in CHF. They can be classified as **acyanotic** and **cyanotic** (bluish tinge of tongue and lips due to low oxygen level). Acyanotic defects include **ventricular septal defect, atrial septal defect, and patent ductus arteriosus,** which are due to the shunting of blood from **the** left to right side of the heart (**left to right shunt**). Another acyanotic congenital condition is **co - arctation of the aorta,** which causes hypertension. Examples of cyanotic congenital heart diseases with **right to left shunt** are **Tetralogy of Fallot, Transposition of great arteries,** etc.

Rheumatic Heart Disease – This used to be the most common heart disease in young people in India till a few decades ago. It is primarily due to a bacterial infection of the throat by **Group A beta - hemolytic streptococci**. This leads to an **autoimmune** disorder affecting the heart, joints, and brain. In the heart, all three layers – endocardium, myocardium, and pericardium are involved, but the greatest damage occurs to the **heart valves**, leading eventually to **heart failure** (CHF). The heart valve which is most commonly involved is the **mitral valve,** followed by the **aortic valve**.

Symptoms include severe pain and swelling of joints (fleeting arthritis), cough, shortness of breath, and all features of heart failure. Treatment includes prophylaxis against recurrent streptococcal throat infection with penicillin, valvuloplasty, or valve replacement surgery. This disease is much less common now due to better living conditions. Treatment includes long - term antibiotics, balloon valvuloplasty and biological or mechanical valve transplantation.

Valvular heart disease – Four valves in the human heart function as flaps during blood circulation. The blood may pass through these valves but cannot return in the reverse direction. In valvular heart disease, the function of one or more of the four valves may be disrupted due to various reasons viz; aging, congenital abnormalities, but the most common cause of valvular dysfunction is **rheumatic heart disease** discussed above.

Other causes are mostly congenital – like congenital mitral stenosis and congenital diseases of collagen.

The **valvular dysfunction** may be of two types –

    (i)   **valvular stenosis** or narrowing and

    (ii)   **Valvular regurgitation** (reflux or insufficiency).

Dysfunction of heart valves can cause '**murmurs**' heard on auscultation and lead to **congestive heart failure**. The treatment of valves is done through surgery, viz valve replacement or percutaneous balloon mitral commissurotomy (PMBC).

Cardiac arrhythmias - Abnormalities in the rate and rhythm of the heartbeats result due to disorders of impulse formation and conduction through its conducting system. Cardiac arrhythmia is easily diagnosed by electrocardiogram or EKG. The impulse causing contraction of cardiac muscle originates in the **sinus node** in the upper right part of the heart.

With dysfunction of the sinus node or conducting system, the heart rate may become very fast, known as tachycardia (tachyarrhythmias), or very slow, known as bradycardia (Brady - arrhythmias or **heart blocks**). The rhythm may remain regular or become irregular. **Palpitations, which are unpleasant awareness of one's own heartbeats,** may occur. Cardiac arrhythmia may be caused by ischemic heart disease, certain infections, autoimmune diseases, genetic defects, etc. Treatment is by medicines, **pacemakers, defibrillation,** etc.

Cor Pulmonale – Cor Pulmonale is a heart disease that occurs due to acute or chronic pulmonary (lung) disease. Lung disease may cause high blood pressure in the arteries of the lungs. High pressure in pulmonary circulation may lead to increased load on the right ventricle.

Ultimately, right ventricular failure occurs. **The clinical manifestations of right - sided heart failure are increased pressure in neck veins, enlarged and tender liver, and feet swelling.**

_ **Inflammatory Heart Disease** – Various infections with viruses, bacteria, fungi, parasites, and toxic materials cause inflammation of the heart:

- **Endocarditis** – This is inflammation of the inner lining of the heart or **endocardium**. Valves are also part of the endocardium, and valvulitis may occur in **rheumatic heart disease**. Alternatively, infections by bacteria reach the heart through the bloodstream. These usually infect heart valves, which are already damaged due to rheumatic heart or other causes.

- The resulting illness is called **subacute bacterial endocarditis**. Lesions in the heart valves occur wherein platelets, fibrin, and micro - organisms develop small colonies called **vegetations.**

- Symptoms and signs are fever, pallor, enlargement of the spleen, chest pain, palpitations, and change in pre - existing murmur. Rheumatic heart disease used to be an important type of endocarditis and valvulitis. The treatment may include medicines like intravenous antibiotics, anticoagulants, diuretics, and surgery of heart valve, etc

- **Pericarditis** – This means inflammation of the outer lining of the heart **(pericardium)** – usually due to **viral or bacterial infection**, metabolic causes such as renal failure **(uremia)** and autoimmune disorders such as Still's disease or systemic lupus erythematosus. Pericardial fluid can be tapped, examined and drained. Treatment is given according to cause.

- **Myocarditis** – Here the myocardium or middle layer of the heart muscle is inflamed. Usually, this is caused by various infections viz; echovirus, Epstein - barr virus, rubella, streptococcus, diphtheria, Trypanosoma cruzi, toxoplasma etc. It may also be caused by cancer chemotherapy and autoimmune diseases like rheumatic heart disease, lupus etc. All features of CHF are set in.

- **Cardiomyopathy** – These are intrinsic diseases of the heart, often of unknown cause.

This disease of the heart muscle is of 3 types.

i) **Hypertrophic cardiomyopathy** – in which heart muscle becomes abnormally thick and makes the heart stiff to take in and pump the blood.

ii) **Dilated cardiomyopathy** – when the heart muscle becomes weak, leading to usually massive enlargement, decreased forward flow, and congestion of the lungs. Viral infections, genetic and metabolic disorders, heart attacks with damaged heart muscle, toxic effects of mercury, lead, bismuth, and drug abuse (alcohol, cannabis, cocaine), etc,may cause this condition.

iii) **Restrictive cardiomyopathy** - the ventricles of the heart get stiff and weak. Though the heart is able to squeeze the blood well, it is not normally able to relax between the beats, which is why blood cannot fill the heart well. Causes are amyloidosis, sarcoidosis, and some types of chemotherapy.

Blood Vessels – Blood vessels are channels that carry the blood throughout the body. They are spread through the body in loop - like circuits that begin and end at the heart.

There are two main types of blood vessels, viz.

i) **Artery** – which carries blood from the heart to the periphery of various organs;

ii) **Vein** – which carries blood back from the periphery to the heart.

There are two types of circulation:

(i) **systemic circulation** - in which blood is circulated to the whole body except the lungs and

(ii) **pulmonary circulation** - in which blood is circulated from the heart to the lungs and back to the heart.

In systemic circulation, blood flowing through arteries is oxygenated blood.

This **oxygenated blood** reaches throughout the body from the left ventricle of the heart through the aorta and maintains vitality throughout various cells, tissues, and every organ of the body.

The aorta is the largest artery of the body and is a cane - shaped vessel. The aorta, carrying blood from the heart, transports the same to the whole body through various arteries.

Arteries, being hollow tubes full of elasticity, branch into smaller and smaller **arterioles,** which carry blood in the **capillary network** in tissues where they bathe the cells, allowing the **exchange of gases, nutrients, waste, etc**. Capillaries provide nutrients and oxygen to all the tissues of the body.

The capillaries then join and widen to become the radicles of venules, which in turn widen and converge to become veins. The blood flowing into the veins is **deoxygenated** blood. Veins take the deoxygenated blood from the tissues and carry it back to the heart.

All the blood from the body ultimately drains into two large veins of the venous system –

i)   **Superior vena cava** and

ii)   **Inferior vena cava**.

These two large veins carry **oxygen - depleted blood** from the upper and lower part of the body, respectively, back to the heart.

Both these large veins (Superior and Inferior vena cava) drain into the right atrium of the heart. Veins below the skin are visible discretely, and these veins are punctured to collect the blood samples and administer intravenous medicines and fluids. There are valves in the veins of lower limbs that open towards the heart, and the blood in these veins flows towards the heart.

If these valves are damaged, blood tends to collect here, and these veins become prominent and tortuous. This disorder is known as **varicose veins, venous insufficiency, or venous hypertension causing swelling, pain, black patches,** and itching occurring in the lower limbs.

Diseases of blood vessels

Atherosclerosis – The main disease of arteries is atherosclerosis, which advances with age. **Plaques** made up of blood clots, fat, cholesterol (mostly LDL), cellular waste products, calcium, fibrin, etc., are deposited in the inner lining of arteries (endothelium). Plaques may be stable for a long time and may become unstable and rupture and obstruct the blood flow in the arteries of various organs – thus, the supply of nutrition and oxygen to the tissues is depleted, and illnesses of various organs may be caused.

The process of atherosclerosis is accelerated by smoking, high blood cholesterol, chronic diabetes, hypertension, sedentary lifestyle, stress, etc. all of which must be kept in check to prevent its dangerous complications.

Peripheral Arterial Disease (PAD) – PAD is primarily related to the buildup of atherosclerotic or fatty plaque in arteries of the upper portion of the lower extremities or legs. The supply of oxygen and nutrition to the legs is hindered.

Pain in the legs may occur on exercise causing **intermittent claudication**. **Rest pain** may also occur. Such diseases occur due to frequent smoking, drug abuse, chronic diabetes, hypertension, kidney disease, atherosclerosis, high blood cholesterol, etc.

Cerebrovascular Disease (CVD) is discussed in the Chapter on Neurological Disorders.

Renal Artery Stenosis (RAS) – The narrowing of the artery supplying the kidney is called renal artery stenosis. It can occur due to atherosclerosis (plaque build - up) or **fibromuscular dysplasia** in the artery. RAS may lead to serious health problems, including high blood pressure and ultimately to coronary artery disease, stroke, chronic kidney disease, or kidney failure. This is known as **renovascular hypertension,** and it is classified as **secondary hypertension**. It is treated with medications for high blood pressure, lifestyle changes, and surgical procedures to restore blood flow to the kidneys.

Aortic Aneurysm – The aorta is the main artery (large cane - shaped vessel) carrying oxygen - rich blood from the heart through the chest to the abdomen to the pelvic region, that is, the torso/whole body.

In fact, this large artery supplies oxygen - rich blood to all the tissues. Certain genetic conditions and defects in collagen, like Marfan's syndrome or trauma, may damage or weaken the walls of the aorta. Weakness in the wall of the aorta causes a bulge (aneurysm). Blood may leak from it, or the force of blood pumping may split the layers of the artery wall, allowing blood to leak between them (dissection). Tearing or rupture of the aorta may damage various functions.

The rupture of an aortic aneurysm causes acute sudden pain in the chest or abdomen along with features of shock like faint pulse, cold, clammy skin, dizziness or faintness, fast heartbeat, numbness, tingling in limbs, etc.

Varicose veins – Varicose veins are tortuous enlarged veins, most commonly appearing in the lower legs and feet. Any vein close to the skin's surface may become varicose. The cause of this condition is not known. Weak walls or valves in the feet impede blood flow from the feet to the heart – which is an underlying circulatory problem; thus, aching and discomfort remain persistent. Treatment involves compression stockings, exercise, or surgical procedures to close or remove the leaking, incompetent, and varicose veins.

This condition is also discussed in the Chapter on Aching Legs.

Cerebral venous sinus thrombosis present with symptoms of stroke. Many local and systemic diseases can result in thrombosis of venous sinuses in the brain. These are meningitis, infections/ injuries in head and neck region, dehydration, nephrotic syndrome etc. In addition, there are a group of **hereditary** conditions associated with tendency to thrombosis, called **prothrombotic** disorders which should be looked for and excluded.

Investigation of cardiovascular diseases

For CAD or ischemic heart disease, baseline **electrocardiography (EKG),** stress EKG (with treadmill exercise), myocardial biomarkers – troponin – T and Pro BNP and CT angiogram of the heart are non - invasive tests.

An echocardiogram is done to evaluate **ejection fraction. X - ray chest** is done to assess cardiac size. Ultrasound and contrast CT imaging of blood vessels are done to assess renal arteries and kidney size, etc.

Serum cholesterol, triglycerides, and lipids are assessed to get an idea of the metabolic status of the subject. **Coronary angiography** is an **invasive** procedure in which a catheter is passed through the radial artery (at the wrist) or femoral artery (in the groin) to study the exact anatomy of the coronary arteries and their branches supplying the heart, with the percentage of the block. At the same sitting, intervention by stent or balloon may be done. Intravascular ultrasound and MRI may be performed.

For peripheral arterial disease or **PAD** ankle - brachial index (ABI – ratio of the systolic BP of ankle and arm), doppler ultrasound (non - invasive test), angiography, etc., are done.

Investigation of renal artery stenosis includes urine protein level, renal arteriogram, abdominal ultrasound for renal size and scarring, nuclear scan, etc. In arrhythmias stress - non - stress EKG, BP in various postures is examined using a tilt table test, and an electrophysiological test is performed by electrical impulses. For inflammatory heart disease, anemia, EKG, trans - esophageal echocardiogram, chest x - ray, biopsy, and CT scan are performed. For cardiac valvular disease, EKG, X - rays, MRIs, radionuclide scans, and contrast dye angiogram tests are performed. For rheumatic heart disease, throat swab culture and ASO titer in blood are specifically done for evidence of streptococcal infection.

In conclusion, the heart and brain are the two vital organs that must function continuously for life to continue. Poetically, emotions like love, loyalty, and passion have been attributed to the heart, but it is, in fact, the brain that governs all our thoughts, actions, and internal processes, including heart rate and digestion. The heart, however, maintains its own independent rhythm through its pacemaker, the sino - atrial node, ensuring constant circulation of blood throughout life.

This chapter has highlighted the heart's critical role in circulation and how both the heart and the vascular system, comprising arteries, veins, and capillaries, are susceptible to various diseases.

Chapter 31

Blood & Blood Disorders

Learning Objectives:

- Elements of Blood – (i) **Plasma** or liquid part of blood, (ii) Blood Cells – **RBC, WBC** and **Platelets**
- Basics of Blood Groups
- Disorders of Blood – Anemia, Polycythemia, Bleeding disorders – platelet defects and coagulation defects, Leukemia, Lymphomas
- Blood tests – blood group, blood culture for infection, complete blood cell counts or CBC – Hemoglobin, total and differential WBC, RBC and Platelet counts, hematocrit and other blood cell parameter, tests of antigen, antibodies, tumor markers, genes in the blood

---

Blood is the fluid that circulates within the cardiovascular system and is pumped by the heart to deliver oxygen, nutrients, and other essential substances to every tissue in the body. The study of blood and its disorders is known as "**hematology.**" The lymphatic system runs parallel to the venous system and consists of lymph vessels, lymph nodes, and the fluid called **lymph.** Its primary function is to return excess fluid from tissues back to the heart.

Blood consists of **plasma**, which is the fluid part, and three types of cellular elements: red cells, white cells, and platelets. These cells are produced in **bone marrow**.

Red cells carry oxygen from the lungs to tissues, white cells defends the body against infections, and platelets play a crucial role in blood clotting to prevent excessive bleeding and maintain the integrity of blood vessels. The average total blood volume in an adult is approximately **5 liters**.

Plasma – Plasma forms roughly 55 - 60% of the blood volume, while cellular elements make up the remaining 40 - 45%. Plasma consists of water (92%), dissolved gases, proteins (albumin, globulin, antibodies, coagulation factors, etc.), minerals, salts, sugar, fat, hormones, vitamins, and waste products. Normally, the composition of plasma is maintained within a range of 'normal limits' through various life processes called **homeostasis.**

This is a state of **balance** whereby vital parameters, such as blood pH, oxygen, electrolytes, etc., are maintained within a narrow range so that bodily functions can occur normally. The pH value of blood in a human being ranges between 7.35 and 7.45.

Red Blood Cells (RBC) – The normal RBC count in adults is roughly 5 million in males and 4 million in females per microliter (µl). RBCs are small, round, biconcave cells without a nucleus. They contain an iron - rich protein called hemoglobin, which has the function of carrying oxygen in the blood. The normal adult level of hemoglobin is 14 - 18 grams per 100 ml of blood in men and 12 - 16 grams per 100 ml in women. RBCs have a life span of roughly 120 days, after which they are destroyed in the spleen.

White Blood Cells (WBC) are also called **leucocytes**. The main function is to protect against infection. They are of **5 types** – polymorphonuclear leucocytes or neutrophils, lymphocytes, eosinophils, basophils, and monocytes. Normal total leucocyte count (TLC) is 4000 - 11,000/ µl while the differential count is neutrophils 40% to 60%, lymphocytes: 20% to 40%, monocytes: 2% to 8%, eosinophils: 1% to 4% and basophils: 0.5% to 1%. Neutrophil count increases in bacterial infections. Lymphocytes produce antibodies. The life span of WBCs is 12 - 20 days.

Platelets are tiny cell fragments without nuclei in our blood that form clots and help to stop or prevent bleeding. Normal platelet count is 1.5 to 4 lacs/ µl. The life span of platelets is 7 - 10 days.

Blood groups – there are four main blood groups defined by the ABO system. This blood group system was discovered by **Karl Landsteiner** in 1900 after extensive scientific research on serology, which paved the way for compatibility testing and subsequent transfusion practices. Every blood group is identified by antigens and antibodies in the blood. **Antigens** are protein molecules found on the surface of RBC.

Antibodies are proteins found in plasma. The ABO system is categorized as follows –

1. **Group A** – has A antigens on RBC with anti - B antibodies in the plasma

2. **Group B** – has B antigens on RBC with anti - A antibodies in the plasma

3. **Group O** – has no antigens, but both anti - A and anti - B antibodies are present in plasma

4. **Group AB** – has both A and B antigens on RBC but no antibodies

Receiving blood from the wrong ABO group may be life - threatening. For example, if someone with group B blood is given group A blood, their anti - A antibodies will attack the transfused group A cells – so group A blood cannot be given to group B blood. Red blood cells also have another antigen, a protein known as the Rh D antigen (Rhesus factor D). If this is present in the blood, the group is Rh positive, and if it is absent in the blood, the group is Rh negative. Thus, on the basis of the Rh factor, blood grouping is categorized into eight groups as follows –

(ix)   A RhD positive (A+),

(x)   A RhD negative (A -),

(xi)   B RhD positive (B+),

(xii)   B RhD negative (B),

(xiii) O RhD positive (O+),

(xiv)   O RhD negative (O -),

(xv)   RhD positive (AB+),

(xvi)   (AB RhD negative (AB -)

For a blood transfusion, the ABO blood group system is used to match the blood type of the donor and the person receiving the transfusion.

People with blood type O can donate blood to anyone and are called **universal donors**. People with type AB+ blood are **universal recipients** because they have no antibodies to A, B, or Rh in their blood and can receive red blood cells from a donor of any blood type. In an emergency, a transfusion of O - negative red blood cells can be given to anybody, and AB group individuals can receive any group of blood.

However, in practice, the transfusion is performed after properly matching the blood group and cross matching the blood samples of the donor and recipient. Blood is also tested for common blood - borne diseases like hepatitis and HIV. Pregnant women are always given a blood group test.

This is because if the mother is Rh - negative, but the baby has inherited Rh - positive blood from the father, it could cause complications in the form of severe jaundice in the newborn baby. This is because during pregnancy and childbirth some of the babies blood cells enter the mother's circulation and cause antibody production. These antibodies later cross into the baby's blood and cause lysis of baby's red cells. RhD - negative women of childbearing age should always only receive Rh - negative blood.

Anemia is the most common disorder of blood. The hemoglobin content of blood is below normal. In India, the prevalence of anemia is very high, at 52%. It is especially common in women of childbearing age and children. Symptoms are tiredness, lethargy and breathlessness. Signs are a pale appearance (**pallor**) of skin, brittle nails, lethargy and soreness of tongue. Anemia is not a diagnosis by itself, as the cause must be investigated and treated.

1. **Nutritional anemia** refers to cases of anemia in which one nutritional ingredient is deficient in the body. Most commonly, **iron deficiency anemia, deficiency of Vitamin B$_{12}$, and folic acid** are seen.

2. Anemia due to blood loss – acute or chronic

3. Anemia due to chronic illness or inflammation

4. Hemolytic anemia – anemia due to premature destruction of RBC

5. Aplastic anemia – anemia due to inadequate production in bone marrow

6. Anemia due to infiltration of bone marrow by malignant cells

Iron Deficiency Anemia is the most common type of anemia, caused by **low intake** of iron in the diet. It can also be caused by **blood loss** – acute or chronic, such as occult loss of blood from the gut. The RBCs are small in size (**microcytic**) and have low hemoglobin (**hypochromic**), which can be appreciated on peripheral blood smear examination.

The serum iron level is low, and iron binding capacity is increased. Iron deficiency is prevented by a diet rich in green leafy vegetables and is treated by giving iron - containing tablets or syrup, usually for up to 3 months, in order to also build up iron stores in the body. If the response to oral iron is poor, one must investigate blood loss or other causes of anemia.

Vitamin B_{12}/Folic acid deficiency anemia – Vitamin B_{12} and Folic acid are B complex groups of vitamins. Vitamin B_{12} (Cobalamin) is only found in animal foods, and deficiency may be seen in people with poor intake of animal milk and meat, as seen in a purely vegan diet. Deficient absorption of Vitamin B_{12} occurs in **pernicious anemia -** an autoimmune disease.

Folic acid deficiency may be found with the deficient intake of green leafy vegetables, fresh fruits, yeast, fortified cereals and meat, in alcoholics and those with malabsorption. Anemia is **macrocytic** in type, i.e., the RBCs are larger than normal.

Diagnosis is made by complete blood counts – high **mean corpuscular volume (MCV)**, peripheral smear for macrocytes, and large neutrophils with hyper segmented nuclei. Blood levels of vitamin B_{12} and/or folic acid are low. This type of anemia is treated with large oral or parenteral doses of these vitamins.

Anemia of chronic disease – Any chronic disease, infection or inflammation in the body can result in anemia, which is usually of **normocytic** (having normal size of RBC), **normochromic** (normal amount of hemoglobin in RBCs) type.

Hemolytic anemia – Here, the RBCs have a shortened life span. When RBCs are broken down, hemoglobin is released, and its iron is conserved, while the 'heme' is converted to bilirubin. Due to excess breakdown, the bone marrow tries to compensate by producing more RBCs rapidly.

Therefore, increased **reticulocyte (young RBC) count** and enlargement of the **liver and spleen** are seen almost universally in hemolysis due to any cause. **Jaundice** and **pigmentary gall stones** may also be seen. Hemolytic anemia may result from causes that are **extrinsic** to the RBCs (such as toxins, auto - antibodies, or certain drugs) and **intrinsic** to the RBCs.

The latter is mostly genetic and of the following types –

(i)   Defects in the RBC membrane as occur in **hereditary spherocytosis** or elliptocytosis.

(ii)   **Deficiency of enzymes** such as glucose - 6 - phosphate dehydrogenase (G6PD), which help the RBCs to function properly.

(iii)   Abnormal hemoglobin, as happens in '**sickle cell anemia,**' causing the RBCs to become deformed and clump together;

(iv)   Abnormal proportion of heme and globin chains of hemoglobin – the **thalassemias.** Of the above, thalassemia, sickle cell anemia, and G6PD deficiency anemia are especially prevalent in India.

Aplastic anemia – In this serious disease, the bone marrow fails and all the 3 types of cells in the blood are decreased (**pancytopenia**). Features of pancytopenia include anemia due to low RBCs, infections due to low WBCs and bleeding due to low platelets. Liver and spleen are not enlarged. Cause is often **autoimmune or** induced by toxins and drugs.

Anemia due to infiltration of bone marrow – This happens most often in leukemias, where normal marrow is replaced by **blast cells**. Other types of tumors can also invade bone marrow. The peripheral blood picture and symptoms may be those of pancytopenia.

Polycythemia – This is a much rarer condition in which, as opposed to anemia, the hemoglobin level is higher than normal i.e. increase in RBC counts. It may occur in response to chronic low oxygen as happens in **cyanotic heart disease**. The increase in RBC mass makes the blood thicker leading to strokes or tissue and organ damage.

Bleeding and coagulation disorders – Sometimes, the patient presents with abnormal bleeding. Of course, if the bleeding is from a specific site such as the rectum, nose, etc., the particular site must be carefully examined for a local cause. If bleeding is more generalized – as into the skin causing generalized rash (purpura), or from various mucus membranes, or there are repeated bleeding episodes from various sites, investigation for a blood disorder becomes necessary. Two types of abnormal bleeding are:

(i)   Platelet disorder and

(ii)   Disorder of coagulation factors.

As already explained, platelets help the blood to clot. A deficiency of platelets (especially if the platelet count falls below 20,000/μl) or defect in platelet function causes purpura – i.e., pinpoint reddish spots on the skin or bleeding from mucus membranes. Low platelets may occur in various infections, autoimmune disorders, drugs, infiltration of bone marrow, etc.

Besides platelets, our blood also has 13 coagulation factors or proteins that help in the coagulation of blood. When a vessel wall is disrupted, these factors get activated one after the other by a process called the **coagulation cascade**. Deficiencies of any of these factors are mostly inherited – the most common being deficiency of Factor VIII, which causes the disease **hemophilia**. Deficiency of coagulation factors generally results in large deep - seated collections of blood (**hematomas**), delayed bleeding, and bleeding into joints. Treatment is by replacement of the deficient factor or giving plasma or blood.

Leukemias – These are a group of cancers characterized by the rapid growth of abnormal blood cells in the bone marrow. The bone marrow becomes filled with immature white blood cells (blast cells). The cause of leukemia may be genetic changes in WBCs, which are acquired during life but not inherited. Certain inherited genetic syndromes (such as Down's syndrome) can increase the risk for acute leukemia, however.

Unlike other malignancies, leukemia does not result in solid tumors but causes abnormalities in cell counts. As the bone marrow gets filled with abnormal immature (**blast**) cells, **anemia,** infection **causing fever** and **abnormal bleeding** (all features of pancytopenia) occur.

317

Swelling of lymph nodes or **lymphadenopathy** and **enlargement of liver and spleen** are seen due to infiltration. Fatigue, lethargy and bone pains occur. Leukaemia is classified according to whether they are acute or chronic and secondly according to the type of cell of origin.

There are 4 main types:

1. **acute myeloid**

2. **acute lymphoblastic**

3. **chronic myeloid** and

4. **chronic lymphatic**.

Acute myeloid leukemia is the most common aggressive leukemia in adults, but it also occurs in children. Acute lymphocytic leukemia is the most common cancer in children, but it also occurs in adults. Chronic myeloid leukemia (CML) has a characteristic abnormal gene called *BCR - ABL*, which turns the cell into a cancer cell. CML often has very high WBC counts with all stages of premature white cells seen in peripheral blood and very large spleen size.

It is a fairly slow - growing leukemia but can undergo 'blast transformation' and turn into acute leukemia, which is hard to treat. Chronic lymphocytic leukemia, is very slow - growing and occurs at a mean age of 70 years. Treatment of leukemia is by chemotherapy and supportive measures.

Lymphomas – These are malignancies of the lymph nodes.

There are two main types:

1. **Hodgkins** and

2. **Non - Hodgkins**.

While Hodgkins lymphoma starts in a lymph node of the upper part of the body, and spreads in an orderly way to neighboring group of nodes, non - Hodgkins may start in lymph nodes anywhere in the body and spread is unpredictable. Diagnosis is by lymph node biopsy. Prognosis also depends on morphologic type.

Investigation of blood disorders

The most preliminary test is **peripheral blood smear** microscopy, which gives an impression of the morphology of RBC and WBC. **Automated complete blood count, i.e., CBCs, is the actual count of all blood cells and mean values of RBC volume, hemoglobin content,** and **concentration**. It also gives the distribution width of RBC and platelets, which are estimates of variation in their volumes. **Serum iron, ferritin, and iron binding capacity** measure iron deficiency anemia. Tests of **vitamin B$_{12}$** and **folic acid levels** are carried out when their deficiency is suspected.

Fever charting and cause is investigated in anemia of chronic illness. Investigation for hemolysis includes reticulocyte counts, serum bilirubin, and **hemoglobin electrophoresis** (for thalassemia and sickle cell disease).

G6PD levels are measured. An osmotic **fragility test** is done for hereditary spherocytosis. A **bone biopsy** is undertaken to diagnose aplastic anemia. For leukemias, **bone marrow aspirate** is examined for immature cells and type. Genetic tests for **the ABR - BCL gene and its level are** monitored for treatment response in CML. Lymph node biopsy is needed for histologic diagnosis of lymphoma. **Flow cytometry** analyzer, which measures cell size, cell count, cell morphology, cell cycle phase, etc., is gaining importance in the diagnosis and management of leukemia.

In conclusion, metaphorically speaking, blood relations symbolize consanguine bonds or 'kinship.' Our message to nurture these bonds reflects the purpose of our existence in the universe. The foundation of human rights was built to honor the existence of all races and communities that share human blood. Scientifically, blood plays a vital role in regulating our body's functions. It is essential to understand the critical roles of its various components, as well as the diseases that can affect the blood, in order to appreciate its significance in sustaining life.

Chapter 32

Respiratory Diseases

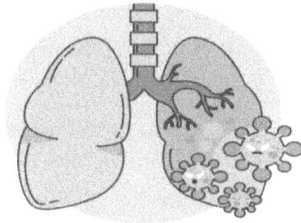

Learning Objectives:

- Structure of the lung

- Functions of the lung – respiration i.e. inhaling oxygen and exhaling carbon dioxide

- Effects of pollution on respiratory functions

- Infections of upper respiratory tract – pharyngitis, laryngitis, tonsillitis, sinusitis

- Infections of lower respiratory tract – pneumonia, pleural effusion, pneumothorax, TB, Covid-19

- Various other respiratory diseases viz; chronic obstructive pulmonary disease (COPD), interstitial lung disease, embolism of lungs, bronchiectasis etc.

- Lung cancer

- Examination and tests of respiratory diseases

Respiration involves the process of inhaling oxygen - rich air and exhaling carbon dioxide. In medical science, the study of the respiratory system is called pulmonology or pneumology, and specialists in this field are known as pulmonologists. Pulmonology is a sub - specialty of internal medicine and is closely associated with intensive care medicine, focusing on diseases and conditions affecting the lungs and respiratory tract.

The upper respiratory tract of the respiratory system includes the nose, mouth, pharynx, larynx, trachea, etc. The **lower respiratory tract** includes bronchi, bronchioles, and lung tissue. The **trachea** is divided into two main bronchi – left and right - which supply each lung.

The **bronchi** undergo several divisions into smaller and smaller bronchi and, ultimately, the **bronchioles**. The bronchioles open into air sacs or **alveoli**, which are the tiny balloon - like spaces around which the web of vessels (capillaries) is spread. Lungs are a pair of pinkish - grey, spongy cone - shaped organs. They are, therefore, like upside - down trees – the trachea being the trunk, bronchi being the branches, and alveoli being the leaves. The lungs are enveloped in a membrane called **pleura**. The lungs take up most of the space in the chest or thorax.

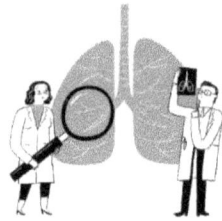

The diaphragm is the transverse muscle dividing the chest and abdomen. **The mediastinum** is the space within the chest that contains the heart, large vessels, aorta, esophagus, thymus, trachea, lymph nodes, etc.

It separates the chest into two compartments, viz, left and right pleural cavities, containing the left and right lungs. The structures and organs in the chest are protected by the sternum or breastbone in front, vertebral column behind, and rib care all around. The right lung consists of three lobes, and the left lung consists of two lobes.

The respiratory tract is lined by a **mucus membrane,** which keeps it moist. In day - to - day life, dirt, mud, smoke, sludge, bacteria, and viruses enter the respiratory system – which may cause dysfunction of the respiratory system. The mucus membrane has fine hairlike structures or **cilia** and long, thread - like structures called **flagella** found at one end of a cell. They sweep out the dirt, dust, toxins, etc., from the respiratory tract and keep it open and protected. During respiration, the diaphragm and muscles between the ribs (**intercostal muscles**) contract to enlarge the pleural cavities and lungs.

Due to the negative pressure generated, the air is inhaled through the nose or mouth, reaches the throat, from there through the larynx and trachea to the two main bronchi – right and left, and finally reaches the lung alveoli where gas exchange, i.e., mutual exchange of oxygen and carbon dioxide occurs – thus carbon dioxide comes out through the nose and oxygen enter the bloodstream. The normal rate of breathing in adults is 16 - 18 breaths per minute but is faster in young children, being about 40 breaths/minute in newborns.

Respiratory Diseases

Respiratory diseases due to air pollution - Ambient air pollution is becoming an important problem in recent times. This is an environmental health issue worldwide that is more specifically affecting developing countries. It is resulting from increasing industrialization.

Of all pollutants, it is the fine **particulate matter** that has the greatest ill effect on human health. Most of these come from burning fuel – either from vehicle engines, industry, power plants, households, or biomass combustion. The most important health effects of air pollution are acute and chronic obstructive lung disease, coronary artery disease, stroke, and lung cancer.

According to the World Health Organization, ambient air pollution is responsible for 43% of deaths due to chronic obstructive pulmonary disease (COPD), 25 % of ischemic heart disease deaths, 24% of deaths due to stroke, and 29% of lung cancer deaths worldwide.

The level of particulate air pollution is expressed as the **Air Quality Index** – varying from 0 to 500.

Respiratory tract infections – These infections are caused by bacteria and a group of respiratory viruses – rhinoviruses, influenza, parainfluenza, respiratory syncytial virus etc. Covid - 19 is also a respiratory virus.

Upper Respiratory Tract Infections (URTI): Rhinitis or common cold – This means inflammation of the mucus membrane of the nose. Usually, it is due to viral infection or **allergy**. The common viruses are rhinoviruses and other respiratory viruses like coronavirus, adenovirus, and respiratory syncytial virus. Symptoms include runny nose, nasal congestion, sneezing, itching, mild fever, and body aches. Later, secondary bacterial superinfection may cause thick nasal discharge and blockage of the nose.

Sinusitis – The sinuses are air - filled spaces in the skull surrounding and connected to the nose. They are located behind the forehead, nasal bones, cheeks, and eyes.

They are lined by mucus membranes, which may be infected with viruses or bacteria, causing **sinusitis**. Effective and regular drainage of the sinuses into the nose occurs naturally and keeps them healthy. Conditions like cold, climatic change, allergy, air pollution, and common structural defects predispose to sinusitis. Symptoms of sinusitis may include fever with light pain around the face, headache, mucus or pus discharge from the nose, or mucus trickling down the nasopharynx into the throat. Sinusitis may be acute but can also become a chronic and troubling condition.

An X - ray or CT scan may be done to diagnose the extent of the problem. Treatment is by gargling, Niti, steam inhalation, antibiotics, pain relief, and sometimes minimally invasive surgery is performed by balloon sinuplasty (enlarging the ostia or opening of the sinus) and lavage of the sinus for chronic or recurrent sinusitis.

Tonsillitis, Pharyngitis, and Adenoiditis – Tonsils are two masses of rich lymphatic tissues, like lymph nodes on both sides behind mucosal folds between the palate and tongue in the throat. Being a part of the lymphatic system, these helps filter the air entering the airway and trap the microorganisms like bodyguards. Infection and inflammation of the tonsils itself is a common painful condition called tonsillitis, which is due to viral or bacterial infections viz.Streptococcus pyogenes, respiratory viruses, etc. The pharynx is the passage at the back of the throat that connects the nose and mouth to the larynx and esophagus. Infection in the pharynx is known as **pharyngitis**.

Symptoms of tonsillitis/ pharyngitis are sore or scratchy throat, fever, dry cough, difficult and painful swallowing, muscle aches etc. Examination of the throat reveals enlarged and red (congested) tonsils and mucus membranes. Bacterial tonsillitis may show **exudates** or pus points on the tonsils and enlarged **tender** lymph nodes in the neck. Exudate is a fluid or pus made of dead cells, proteins, and solid materials. Bacterial tonsillitis/pharyngitis caused by **group - A beta - hemolytic streptococci** may be complicated by **rheumatic fever** and later **rheumatic heart disease**.

Treatment of acute tonsillitis/ pharyngitis is by gargles, steam inhalations, and paracetamol. If bacterial infection is suspected, an adequate course of antibiotics must be given.

Chronic pharyngitis also occurs due to smoking, smoky atmosphere, allergy, acidity, etc., and may enhance sinusitis and otitis media. Adenoids are also lymphatic tissue located in the back of the nose, which fights infections entering the body. Infection in adenoids is **adenoiditis**.Chronic adenoiditis causes nasal obstruction and discomfort. Treatment is similar to that of tonsillitis.

Laryngitis – This refers to inflammation of the voice box (larynx) in the throat. Laryngitis may occur due to infection or overuse of voice. Acute laryngitis is mostly caused by viruses. Smoking, smoky atmosphere, allergy, etc., may trigger acute infection. Chronic laryngitis is often caused by acid reflux from the stomach to the throat. Rarer types of laryngitis may be caused by diphtheria, fungal infections, etc. Common or acute laryngitis resolves on its own very shortly. Symptoms are fever, coughing, **hoarseness of voice**, pain, and swallowing difficulty. Treatment is by voice rest, steam inhalation, gargles, antibiotics, etc.

Otitis Media – This usually results from an infection of the middle ear, which reaches it from the nasopharynx through the **Eustachian tube**. Symptoms are pain in the ear, fever, and pus discharge from the ear. Sometimes, sterile fluid fills the middle ear without signs of acute infection, causing **otitis media with effusion** (**OME**). **Chronic suppurative otitis media** (**CSOM**) is a chronic bacterial infection of the middle ear with chronic/intermittent pus discharge. Complications include cerebral sinus thrombosis and brain abscess. Tests done are – a CT scan of the head, MRI, culture from pus, etc. Treatment is by antibiotics and sometimes surgery.

Lower Respiratory tract infections (LRTI)

Bronchitis – The lining of the bronchial tubes in the lungs are infected and inflamed. Two types of bronchitis may occur viz; acute bronchitis due to viral or bacterial infection, or chronic bronchitis due to smoking and air pollution. Symptoms are fever and cough. Cultures of sputum and X - ray of the chest are done.

Treatment is by antibiotics. **Bronchiolitis** is a serious disease affecting young babies. Viral infection (especially **respiratory syncytial virus**) of the bronchioles often occurs in the cold season. Symptoms are breathlessness, mild fever and cough. The chest may appear hyperinflated or barrel shaped. Liver and spleen may be palpable. Treatment is by oxygen inhalation, intravenous fluids and antiviral **Ribavirin** inhalation.

Pneumonia – Inflammation of the lung tissue is called pneumonia. Usually, it is due to bacterial, viral, or even fungal infection, which can affect part or whole lung, or it may be patchy, affecting both lungs (bronchopneumonia). The most important bacterial causes are **Streptococcus pneumoniae** and **Hemophilus influenzae,** and viral causes are respiratory viruses, especially respiratory syncytial viruses.

Such viruses circulate the world over. In young children or the elderly, pneumonia can be a killer disease, resulting in death. The elderly are advised to take the pneumonia vaccine. Inflammation of lung tissue causes the alveoli to fill up with fluid and/or pus, thereby hampering air exchange and leading to **ventilation/perfusion mismatch**. Symptoms include cough with sputum (phlegm), fever, chills, fast breathing, and chest pain.

Diagnosis is made on the basis of symptoms and signs on auscultation of the chest, blood counts, and X - ray of the chest. Treatment is by antibiotics (oral or intravenous), oxygen, and intravenous fluids. Pneumonia is an important cause of mortality at all ages and the 4th leading cause of death worldwide. According to the World Health Organization, pneumonia is the single largest cause of death in children under 5.

Special Infections of the Respiratory Tract

Covid - 19 pneumonia – About 15% of people with Covid - 19 infection develop pneumonia, while in others, it remains as an upper respiratory tract infection. Pneumonia associated with COVID - 19 infection is a form of bilateral interstitial pneumonia. This often happens in people with long - term COVID - 19 after the **initial infectious phase.**

Tuberculosis (TB) – This is a chronic infection caused by the bacterium **Mycobacterium tuberculosis** (**MTB**). Tuberculosis is primarily an infection of the lungs but can attack any part of the body.

Tuberculosis is a major public health problem in India, which has a disproportionately large burden of tuberculosis cases in the world. In 2020, the Indian government launched the ambitious National TB Elimination Program (**NTEP**) – which aims to eliminate the infection by 2025. NTEP was earlier known as the Revised National Tuberculosis Control Program (RNTCP). It has four strategic pillars - "**Detect - Treat - Prevent - Build (DTPB)** is discussed in Chapter 4. TB is spread when a person has an active infection in the lungs, coughs, or spits sputum. The infection becomes airborne and can affect others in the vicinity.

Symptoms of TB are cough, low - grade fever, weight loss, night sweats, blood - tinged sputum, chest pain, fatigue, etc. TB disease can be fatal if not treated in time. TB is more dangerous in people with HIV/AIDS and those with low immunity.

Tests for tuberculosis are chest X - ray, sputum examination for tubercular bacteria by microscopy, tuberculin skin test, and reverse transcription polymerase chain reaction (RT - PCR) in sputum or other body fluids to look for genetic material of MTB. Vaccination with **BCG** (bacillus Calmette Guerin) to prevent tuberculosis in the individual is done in childhood itself.

Lung TB is treated by 3 - 4 specific antitubercular drugs given together for at least 6 months. Providing **good nutrition** to boost immunity is also important. Sometimes, the TB bacteria become resistant to commonly used TB drugs - multidrug - resistant TB or MDR TB. This is a dangerous situation that has to be treated aggressively with other drugs.

Other diseases of the Respiratory System

Asthma – Asthma is a chronic disease affecting persons of all ages. Genetic predisposition and environmental factors play a significant role in its causation. It is caused by the 'hyper - reactivity' of the airways (bronchi). In response to allergens, respiratory air passages contract and become narrow. Swelling of the mucosa also occurs. This results in episodes of coughing, wheezing, shortness of breath, chest tightness, etc. Allergies may be caused by house dust, bedbugs, moisture, air pollution, airborne irritants like chemicals, paints, environmental allergens, volatile substance evaporation, and smoking.

According to the World Asthma Report, 6% of children and 2% of adults in India are suffering from this disease. Investigation includes a chest X - ray, allergy tests, and spirometry. **The peak expiratory flow meter** measures how fast the patient can breathe out. Treatment is by using bronchodilator medicine by inhalation, which helps dilate the air passages. If it is a severe asthma attack, **steroids** and anti - inflammatory drugs are given. Acute symptoms may necessitate hospitalization, oxygen inhalation, intravenous fluids, nebulized bronchodilators, and even ventilation.

Pleural cavity disease

Pleural effusion and empyema – The lungs are lined on the outside by a membrane that also lines the inner surface of the chest cage called **Pleura**.

Between the two layers of the pleura is a thin pleural cavity filled with fluid that acts as a lubricant during lung expansion and contraction. The pleural cavity may get infected, and excessive fluid (pleural effusion) or pus (empyema thoracic) may accumulate in it, which causes a collapse of lung tissue and breathlessness.

Accumulation of fluid in the pleural cavity, i.e., pleural effusion, may also be non - infective, as happens in liver cirrhosis, pulmonary embolism, malignancy, pleural mesothelioma, trauma, nephrotic syndrome, or congestive heart failure. Infectious pleural effusion, previously called pleurisy, is usually diagnosed as bacterial or tuberculosis after appropriate testing. Empyema or collection of pus in the pleural cavity usually occurs as a complication of underlying pneumonia. Pleural fluid or pus must be either aspirated or drained, sometimes with a long - term pleural drainage tube and a bag. Pleural fluid is tested biochemically, bacteriologically, and by RT PCR for tuberculosis in order to institute appropriate treatment.

Pneumothorax – In this condition, air fills the pleural cavity between the two folds of the pleura, i.e., the space between the lung and the chest wall. Causes of pneumothorax include underlying pneumonia, penetrating chest trauma, emphysema, kerosene poisoning, underlying chronic lung disease, or during drainage of empyema. Pricking pain and **acute shortness of breath** are felt. In pneumothorax, air in the pleural cavity builds up pressure and compresses the lung tissue.

Tension pneumothorax is a very serious condition in which the volume of pneumothorax increases with each breath, and the underlying lung collapses like a deflated balloon called **atelectasis**. This emergency situation is managed and treated by immediate pleural puncture, intercostal drainage, oxygen, ventilation, and treating the underlying cause of pneumothorax.

Bronchiectasis – This refers to permanent thickening, destruction, and dilatation of a part of the bronchial tree, which usually occurs due to infection, pneumonia, whooping cough, asthma, cystic fibrosis, or chronic blockage by mucus plug, etc. The dilated bronchioles become the site of pus collection and recurrent purulent infections. This condition may also be caused by immunodeficiency disorders, such as HIV, some genetic diseases, and COPD. Symptoms are cough with copious expectoration, which may be blood - tinged, wheezing, pain in the chest, shortness of breath, and weight loss.

Investigations include an X - ray of the chest, CT scan of the thorax, culture of sputum, bronchoscopy or bronchogram, etc. According to cultural reports, treatment of antibiotics is usually required on a long - term basis. Respiratory exercises and **postural drainage** exercises, i.e., lying/sitting in such a position as to drain secretions from the airways, are emphasized. Pulmonary rehabilitation may be required.

Cystic Fibrosis (CF) – This is a **monogenic hereditary disorder** transmitted by **autosomal recessive** inheritance. It is very common in Western countries - 1 in 3000 in white Americans. In India, it is probably much less common with calculated incidence in one study of 1 in 40,000.

In India, the most common mutation causing CF is delta F508 **gene mutation.** CF is actually a **multisystem disorder** present from birth with involvement of lungs, pancreas, and other exocrine glands and leading to recurrent lung infections, malabsorption, and involvement of other systems – such as endocrine, hepatobiliary, and reproductive. The basic defect in cystic fibrosis is the failure of chloride conductance, which leads to dehydration of secretions, making them too **viscid.**

This causes difficulty in passing the **meconium** of the newborn (greenish material in the newborn intestine) at birth, abnormal sweat chloride test, abnormal pancreatic secretions, and lung mucus.

There is a failure to thrive due to repeated respiratory infection and colonization by a bacterium, commonly *Pseudomonas aeruginosa*. Ultimately this leads to chronic respiratory failure and low life expectancy of only up to 30 - 40 years.

Obstructive Lung Disease or **Chronic Obstructive Pulmonary Disease** (COPD) is an umbrella term for some progressive lung diseases, such as **chronic bronchitis** and **emphysema**, which represent the two ends of the spectrum. The term emphysema refers to the breakdown of the walls of thin air sacs or alveoli, which are at the end of the bronchial tubes.

Permanent dilatation of these air spaces causes an increase in lung volume. The major cause of COPD is smoking and exposure to irritating gases and particulate matter. Major symptoms include chronic cough with sputum production, perpetual shortness of breath especially on exertion, wheezing, and tightness in the chest. The symptoms of COPD progress gradually over time, making it harder to breathe. COPD is the most common cause of **Cor Pulmonale,** in which the heart also gets affected on account of chronic lung disease.

Restrictive Lung Disease is a group of diseases characterized by a decrease in the elasticity of the lungs. The lungs **become stiff** and are not inflated easily, so the ability to expand during inhalation is lost, and the amount of air taken in during inhalation is reduced. The distinction between restrictive and obstructive diseases is that in obstructive lung diseases, air passages are blocked or narrowed; in restrictive lung diseases, there is a loss of compliance as tissues of the lungs are thickened and stiff.

There may be a visibly reduced expansion of the chest cage due to restriction in the lung to inflate. There is a decrease in the **total lung capacity**, i.e., the total air volume that the lung can hold. Examples of restrictive lung disease are hyaline membrane disease of the newborn, idiopathic pulmonary fibrosis, asbestosis, sarcoidosis, and severe obesity.

Interstitial Lung Disease (ILD) This is a type of restrictive lung disease. Interstitium is the space between the cells of an organ or tissue. **Scarring (fibrosis)** and inflammation occur around the alveoli. ILD is also known by the name **diffuse parenchymal lung disease (DPLD)**. As a result, stiffness in the lungs hampers the exchange of oxygen into the bloodstream.

Once lung scarring occurs, it is generally irreversible. Lung damage from ILD gets worse over time. The etiology is unknown, so ILD is considered an **idiopathic** disease. **Secondary** ILD occurs due to disorders of connective tissues, autoimmune diseases, sarcoidosis, exposure to hazardous inorganic compounds (silica, asbestos, beryllium, printing chemicals, etc.), antibiotics, chemotherapy, arrhythmia, drug abuse, Covid - 19, other specific types of pneumonia, TB, a malignant cancer of lymphatic system, etc. Dry cough, shortness of breath, chest discomfort, extreme tiredness, and loss of weight are troubling phenomena in this disease.

The symptoms of ILD get multiplied by complications like pulmonary hypertension, right - side heart failure, and cor - pulmonale.

Ultimately, respiratory failure sets in, causing death. The life span of the patient is limited to 3 - 5 years. Investigations are chest X - ray, CT scan, genetic testing, trans - bronchial biopsy, and biopsy by surgical intervention. Treatment is by oxygen therapy, corticosteroids, immunosuppressant drugs and pulmonary rehabilitation.

Pulmonary Vascular Disease

Pulmonary embolism – Embolism is a condition wherein the blood clot or other material, such as air, fat, etc., is carried by the blood from one location to another. When this blood clot blocks a pulmonary artery or its branches, this condition is known as pulmonary embolism. We have already learned that blood is composed of 45% solid material and 55% fluid plasma. Thus, **embolism** is a disorder when some solid material blocks the flow of blood – the foreign solid material is called an **embolus**.

The clumping of liquid flowing blood into clots, i.e., in a solid state, is called a thrombus, and the formation of the clot is called **thrombosis.** Thrombosis may occur in deep leg veins in a long air journey when the legs are static, and there is relative dehydration. Another example is post - operative immobilization, which predisposes to thrombus formation in the leg veins. The thrombus travels to the right atrium, ventricle, and then to the pulmonary artery, which gets blocked. This is the reason why patients are urged to keep moving the legs after surgery so that stasis in the leg veins and, therefore, thrombus formation does not occur.

Symptoms are shortness of breath, pain in the chest, coughing up blood, swelling in the legs due to blood clots, oxygen depletion, fast heart rate, mild fever, etc. Different types of emboli may manifest in pulmonary embolism, such as fat embolism, fluid embolism, amniotic fluid embolism (fetal disease), air embolism, etc.

A sudden massive pulmonary embolism can result in sudden death. The most widely used tests for pulmonary embolism are **computed tomography of pulmonary arteries (CTPA)** and **ventilation - perfusion (V/Q) scans**.

Pulmonary Arterial Hypertension (PAH) - In this condition, the blood pressure in the pulmonary arteries remains increased, often due to obstruction in small arteries of the lungs. Causes could be pulmonary embolism, COPD, obstructive sleep apnea, congenital heart disease like ventricular septal defect, valvular heart disease, etc. Sometimes, it is idiopathic, i.e., the cause is not known. Increased pressure in lung vasculature causes strain on the right side of the heart, which ultimately fails, resulting in right - sided **heart failure** – also known by the name **cor - pulmonale. Symptoms** are shortness of breath, dizziness, raised venous pressure in the neck veins, tender enlargement of the liver, swelling of feet, etc. The disease is controlled by medication and oxygen therapy.

Pulmonary Edema – In this condition, fluid from lung capillaries leaks out into air sacs or alveoli. This happens due to back pressure build up in the pulmonary circulation as happens in congestive heart failure or some other causes like valvular heart disease etc.

Symptoms are sudden severe breathlessness, orthopnea (breathlessness on lying flat) wheezing, coughing, frothy / bloody sputum, chest pain and fatigue. This disease is treated by oxygen therapy and medications.

Pulmonary Hemorrhage – Bleeding into the lung tissue is called pulmonary hemorrhage. Causes include pneumonia, TB, cystic fibrosis, bronchiectasis, embolism, injury, tumors of the lung, etc. Blood - stained expectoration may occur **(hemoptysis)**, i.e., coughing up sputum with blood. Other causes include autoimmune diseases and **Goodpasture syndrome**. Symptoms – persistent coughing with hemoptysis.

Tumors or neoplasms of the lung

Benign Tumors

Hamartoma – These are local malformations of the lung with an abnormal mixture of cells and tissues, which grow in a disorganized way. Most hamartomas are benign and are present from birth. They may cause morbidity by various mechanisms like infarction (death of tissue due to obstruction of blood supply), infection, hemorrhage, anemia, pressure, and neoplastic transformation.

Pulmonary Sequestration – This refers to a condition wherein dysplastic nonfunctional lung tissue develops outside the lungs. There is no communication with the trachea - bronchial tree, and this tissue has an anomalous blood supply.

Congenital Pulmonary airway malformation (CPAM) – This was previously known as congenital cystic adenomatoid malformation (**CCAM**). This is a rare developmental anomaly of the lower respiratory tract. Natural pulmonary functioning is impaired. It may get infected. Symptoms like cough, hemoptysis, fever, chest pain, shortness of breath, respiratory distress, and rapid breathing may occur.

Malignant Lung Tumors or Cancer of the Lung - This is the leading cause of cancer - related mortality in the United States. In India, lung cancer is 2nd to oral cancer as a cause of death due to cancer in men, while women are more prone to breast, cervix, and ovary cancer. It is strongly related to tobacco chewing and smoking.

There are two main types of lung cancer – small cell and non - small cell lung cancer. These two types are treated differently.

Small Cell Lung Cancer – Small cell lung cancer is a rare lung cancer that typically occurs in long - time smokers. It is a fast - growing, deadly cancer that spreads early to lymph nodes, bones, brain, liver, and adrenal glands. Smoking is the major risk factor. Symptoms are coughing, shortness of breath, phlegm, chest pain etc. Diagnosis is made by imaging followed by biopsy. Treatment is by chemotherapy, radiation, and surgery, but the outlook is poor.

Non - small Cell Lung Cancer – This is a group of lung cancers that develop in the epithelial cells of the lungs – adenocarcinoma or squamous cell carcinoma of the lungs. Both smokers and nonsmokers may be affected. Symptoms are shortness of breath, weight loss, cough, and hemoptysis.

Large Cell Lung Carcinoma (LCLC) – This lung cancer is a form of non - small cell lung cancer that arises from epithelial cells and grows quickly and aggressively. This type of lung cancer can be found anywhere in the lung, but most often in the lung periphery. LCLC cannot be classified into other specific groups. Similar symptoms occur as in other types of lung cancer – frequent coughing, weight loss, pain in the chest, blood in the sputum, etc.

After spreading to distant organs, symptoms pertaining to that organ occur. Surgery is the best treatment for lung cancer in the primary stage. Surgery is done according to stage viz: partial surgery of the lung that is lobectomy, segmentectomy, wedge - resection, or pneumonectomy (lung removal surgery). In most cases, patients are diagnosed at a stage when surgical intervention becomes difficult to perform. Thus, adjuvant therapy (chemotherapy and radiotherapy) is done to add 1 - 2 years of life. Molecular and genetic tests, viz Ros, ALK, and EGFR, and targeted therapy offer a new gleam of hope. Now, this therapy bestows longevity to patients.

Other types of lung cancer – Other types of lung cancer include neuroendocrine carcinoid, pleural mesothelioma, fibroma, sarcoma, etc. Symptoms and treatment of all these types of cancer are similar, as detailed above.

Tests for Respiratory Diseases:

Fluid test – Samples of blood, sputum, **bronchoalveolar lavage (BAL)** fluid, or pleural fluid is taken for microscopic examination of viral or bacterial infection in the respiratory tract. These may be examined for macroscopic appearance, cell count, malignant cells, protein, sugar, culture, and polymerase chain reaction for diagnosis of infection.

Bronchoscopy – An endoscopic device or bronchoscope is inserted through the nose or mouth into the airways for visualizing and evaluating the pathology in the bronchus, bronchi, bronchioles, etc.

Real time photographs and videos are taken and sometimes a small tissue sample is also taken out **(biopsy).**

Imaging by X - ray, Ultrasound, CT scan, and Magnetic Resonance Imaging – Requisite diagnosis of many pulmonary diseases viz; pneumonia, pulmonary edema, pneumothorax, pleural effusion, or cancer can be made by all imaging modalities – ultrasound of the chest, X - ray, CT scan and magnetic resonance imaging (MRI), etc.

Imaging may be used to guide procedures like thoracocentesis, biopsy, etc.

Pleural drainage of accumulated fluid is also done by an aspiration needle and catheter, which is called **intercostal drainage**. Fluid is examined for appearance and sent for cell count, microscopy, protein, sugar, bacterial culture, polymerase chain reaction etc.

Broncho - alveolar lavage is done to obtain fluid, which is then tested for infection, malignant cells, etc.

Pulmonary Function Tests (PFT) – Pulmonary functions are tested by the apparatus known as **a spirometer, which is also called a** pneumograph. The function of the lung is assessed during the breathing in and breathing out process. It is especially useful for asthma and COPD.

The volume and Capacity of the lungs are measured as follows –

Tidal volume (VT) – Volume of air inhaled in the lungs and exhaled out of the lungs during normal breathing = tidal volume of the lungs.

Inspiratory reserve volume (IRV) – The **maximum volume** of air inhaled in the lungs with full strength during breathing exercises.

Expiratory reserve volume (ERV) – the **maximum** air exhaled out of the lungs with full strength

Residual volume (RV) – the residual air left after exhaling out with full strength

Vital capacity (VC) – the maximum air exhaled out of the lungs with full strength, after the maximum air inhaled by the lungs

Total lung capacity (TLC) – This is the vital capacity + residual volume i.e. **VC+RV**

Inspiratory capacity (IC) – maximum volume of air that can be inspired after reaching the end of a normal, quiet expiration. i.e. sum of tidal volume and inspiratory reserve volume

Functional residual capacity (FRC) – the volume of the residual air after the exhaled - out air

Peak Flow Meter – A small handheld device called peak flow meter helps to monitor asthma. The patient breathes in deeply and then breathes out forcefully and rate of flow of air is measured.

Ventilation - Perfusion Scan: This test is performed by **scintigraphy technology**. Pulmonary ventilation (V) and Perfusion (Q) scan, also known as lung V/Q scan, is a nuclear test that uses the perfusion scan to delineate the blood flow distribution and the ventilation scan to measure airflow distribution in the lungs. Ventilation perfusion mismatch is identified. The most common clinical indication for a V/Q lung scan is to assess the likelihood of pulmonary embolism (PE), pneumonia and COPD.

To conclude, our respiratory system provides us with our *"pran - vaayu"* - the life - giving breath. Paul Kalanithi, a renowned neurosurgeon, captured the essence of this in his powerful memoir, "When Breath Becomes Air." Kalanithi was diagnosed with lung cancer during his residency in California. His book offers an intimate and heart - wrenching account of grappling with the relentless progression of his illness, especially the torment of air hunger in its advanced stages. Despite the full functionality of his heart, brain, and kidneys, the inability of his lungs to oxygenate his body ultimately led to systemic failure. His story is a profound reflection on life, death, and the fragility of breath, as it ebbs away - until breath truly becomes air.

Chapter 33

Sleep Hygiene and Sleep Disorders

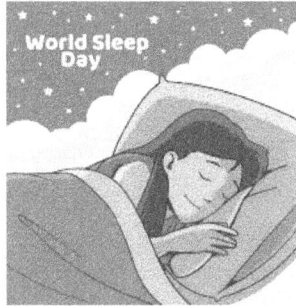

World Sleep Day

Learning Objectives:

- Healthy sleep *vis a vis* disturbed sleep
- Sleep disorders-sleep apnea, insomnia, narcolepsy, somnambulism
- Tests for sleep disorders

Sleep is a state of rest essential for all animals and humans, allowing the body and mind to rejuvenate and heal. The natural rhythm of sleeping and waking often follows the cycles of sunrise and sunset. In our everyday lives, we may experience periods of disturbed sleep, such as brief naps, tossing and turning, or frequent awakenings, which differ from sleep disorders. Disturbed sleep may occur due to external factors like noise, bright lights, or other disruptions, but it does not necessarily indicate a medical condition. For instance, some people require a quiet environment for restful sleep, while others can doze off with background noise like a TV or radio.

This variation may be the result of behavioral conditioning from childhood. Achieving healthy sleep involves maintaining good habits, such as eating a balanced diet, regular exercise, engaging in daily activities, avoiding substance abuse, and limiting the use of electronic devices before bedtime.

The saying "early to bed and early to rise makes a person healthy, wealthy, and wise" reflects the importance of maintaining a consistent sleep routine.

On the other hand, genuine sleep disorders may be linked to underlying health issues or prolonged anxiety, requiring proper diagnosis & treatment.

Sleep Cycle: There are **five stages of normal sleep**, namely – awake state, N1, N2, N3, and rapid eye movements (**REM**) sleep. Stages N1 to N3 are non - rapid eye movement (**NREM**) sleep. Progression from N1 to N3 and REM sleep is progressively deeper sleep. REM sleep lasts for about 90 minutes and may be associated with dreams. These stages make up one sleep cycle, usually lasting 80 - 100 minutes. Typically, an individual would go through **4 - 6 sleep cycles in one night**.

Snoring during sleep is common and occurs when the throat muscles relax, causing the tongue to fall back and partially obstruct the airway. This is more prevalent in people who are obese. Temporary factors such as a swollen nasal mucosa during a common cold or enlarged tonsils and adenoids in children can also obstruct air passage, leading to disturbed sleep. In such cases, a child may breathe through an open mouth, snore, and wake up suddenly during sleep. These children often experience a dry mouth and throat upon awakening.

Obstructive Sleep Apnoea (OSA) is a condition characterized by repeated episodes of breathing cessation during sleep, which can occur sporadically or frequently throughout the night. People with OSA typically experience loud snoring, gasping or choking during sleep, waking with a dry mouth and throat, excessive daytime sleepiness (hypersomnia), irritability due to sleep deprivation, morning headaches, and high blood pressure. Factors that exacerbate OSA include obesity, metabolic syndrome, advanced age, drug abuse, and certain genetic conditions.

OSA becomes a pathological concern when it leads to poor oxygenation of the blood, known as **hypoxemia**. This can trigger nocturnal spikes in blood pressure, which may persist during the day, making OSA a recognized cause of secondary hypertension. A diagnostic test for OSA is **nocturnal polysomnography**, which monitors oxygen levels, heart rate, respiratory volume, and brain activity via electroencephalography (EEG) during sleep.

Daytime sleepiness from OSA can increase the risk of accidents, especially during tasks requiring concentration, such as driving, piloting, or operating machinery.

Treatment options for OSA are i) the use of a mechanical respiratory device that uses **continuous positive airway pressure (CPAP)** to keep the airway open during sleep wearing a nose mask, ii) a mouth piece to thrust the lower jaw forward during sleep and iii) surgery. Nose block is prevented using various nasal drops and lubricants like glycerin drops in the nose.

Obesity hypoventilation syndrome (OHS) – This is also called **Pickwickian syndrome**. This is a triad of obesity with a body mass index (BMI) of ≥30 kg/m2, hypoventilation with high carbon dioxide and hypoxemia while awake, and sleep - disordered breathing without an alternative explanation. It is a kind of central hypoventilation, i.e., **diminished ventilatory drive** and capacity related to obesity. There may not be features of upper airway obstruction.

Insomnia is a very common sleep disorder characterized by difficulty falling asleep or trouble staying asleep for short or long periods, which may persist for days, months, or longer. It is categorized into three stages based on severity: transient insomnia, acute insomnia, and chronic insomnia. Despite being in an environment conducive to sleep, individuals with insomnia often struggle to sleep, leading to daytime tiredness and fatigue. Some people resort to sedatives, which may become habit - forming. Treatment often includes abstaining from sedatives, light exercises, and cognitive behavioral therapy. Chronic insomnia may be associated with physical, mental, and psychological conditions such as cardiovascular diseases, menopause - related disorders, depression, neurosis, psychosis, or schizophrenia. Testing for chronic insomnia and **REM sleep disorder** can be done through a multiple sleep latency test. **Melatonin** is a non - habit - forming sleep - inducing drug that is often recommended.

REM sleep disorder is diagnosed when a person, while dreaming, engages in abnormal or violent actions during sleep. In this condition, the sleeper may act out their dreams with vivid physical movements, such as thrashing arms, kicking, or shouting. The dream is often remembered upon waking.

REM sleep disorders are sometimes linked to neurological conditions like Parkinson's disease, dementia, and multisystem atrophy (failure of sensory and motor organs). Management includes ensuring safety by padding the floor, removing harmful objects from the room, and installing window grills to prevent accidents.

Somnambulism, or sleepwalking, is when an individual performs actions while asleep. It primarily occurs during non - REM sleep, specifically during N3 sleep, and is more common in children. There is usually little or no recall of the event. In some cases, sleepwalking happens during deep sleep, and people may perform activities such as climbing out of windows, driving, or even engaging in criminal behavior like assassination. Actions proven to have been done during somnambulism are typically not considered criminal offenses. The Bollywood film *Neelkanth* explores the story of a woman who walks in her sleep, searching for something she remembers from a past life. In Shakespeare's *Macbeth*, Lady Macbeth, overwhelmed with guilt over the murder of King Duncan, falls into a state of hysterical somnambulism, which leads to her suicide.

Narcolepsy is a sleep disorder in which the person has a strong, uncontrollable urge to sleep during daytime. The periods of daytime sleep are short (about 15 to 30 minutes). Once awake, the person is rested and ready to resume activities. However, this can happen several times during the day, which is why narcolepsy is so disruptive. The cause of narcolepsy is not well understood but may involve genetic and autoimmune factors. About a fifth of patients also have **cataplexy,** which is a sudden loss of muscle tone, causing the patient to fall.

In conclusion, the belief that one may be more creative by staying awake at night and sleeping during the day is misleading. While some may find the quiet of the night conducive to productivity, being nocturnal is generally harmful to human health. Early morning hours, from around 3 a.m. onward, are often regarded as the most productive and creative. Many cultures emphasize the importance of healthy sleep. In *Ayurveda*, sleep is described as *Nidra Bhootadhaatri* (निद्रा भूताधात्री), meaning "sleep, like a mother, nurtures and cares for all beings," preparing them for the day's tasks. Sleep is essential for good health, acting as an anti - inflammatory, rejuvenating, and healing both body and mind.

Chapter 34

Rheumatism – Arthritis and Rheumatic Disorders

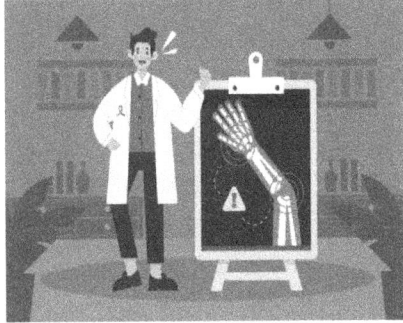

Learning Objectives:

- Common symptoms of arthritis like pain, swelling and inflammation in bones, joints, muscles, connective tissues etc.
- Bone, joints and cartilage disorders - osteoarthritis, osteoporosis, rheumatoid arthritis, juvenile idiopathic arthritis, Sjogren syndrome, systemic lupus erythematosus
- Tests and treatment for rheumatic disorders

Rheumatic disorders or rheumatism are a group of diseases in which pain, swelling, and inflammation in the joints and connective tissues occur. These symptoms may have a relapsing and remitting course over time. The study of rheumatism is called **Rheumatology**. Rheumatic diseases usually affect joints, tendons, ligaments, bones, and muscles.

Arthritis – Arthritis is an acute or chronic inflammation affecting one or more joints, characterized by symptoms such as joint pain, stiffness, tenderness, redness, swelling, and reduced mobility or rigidity in the tissues surrounding the joints.

The causes of arthritis are varied and may include injury to the joint cartilage during physical activities or heavy work, excessive pressure or load on the joints, obesity, genetic predisposition, autoimmune conditions, and infections.

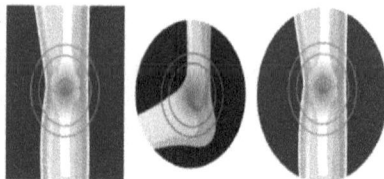

Infectious Arthritis or acute suppurative arthritis is a very painful condition of joints. It is usually due to bacterial infection in one of the large joints. There is fever, intense pain, redness, swelling, and immobility of the affected joint.

Arthrocentesis (tapping or aspiration of the **joint fluid** or pus) may be required for examination. The aspirated fluid is seen under the microscope for pus and other cells. It is sent for bacterial culture to identify the exact causative micro - organism.

Treatment is usually intravenous, followed by oral antibiotics. A more chronic bacterial infection is **tubercular arthritis**, which is treated by specific antitubercular drugs for 18 months. TB in joints is recognized by special features in the X - ray and certain tests like PCR in the joint fluid.

Rheumatic Arthritis – This type of arthritis is not an actual infection of the joints but rather an **autoimmune** disorder triggered by a bacterial infection, specifically by **group**

A beta - hemolytic streptococcus, which commonly infects the throat. The body subsequently produces antibodies against this organism, but due to 'antigen mimicry,' these antibodies mistakenly attack the body's own tissues, including those in the joints, heart, and brain.

The arthritis associated with this condition is typically of a 'fleeting' nature, moving from one joint to another. The most severe impact is often on the heart, where it can cause permanent damage to the **heart valves, leading to chronic rheumatic** heart disease (RHD), which was once the most common type of heart disease in young people in India.

Osteoarthritis – Osteoarthritis is an extremely common degenerative disease, typically affecting the knee joints due to chronic 'wear and tear' of the cartilage.

This condition is most common in middle - aged or elderly individuals, especially those who are overweight. The degenerative process is accelerated by years of increased pressure on the cartilage, as seen in activities like climbing steep stairs, prolonged squatting, obesity, or neglecting knee injuries. Symptoms include pain, redness, swelling, stiffness, joint instability, and eventual **deformity**. When flexing or extending the joints, a crackling sound or sensation known as '**crepitus**' may occur.

The cartilage in our joints acts similarly to a rubber washer in household taps or a gasket in a pressure cooker - if the surfaces rub against each other excessively, the cartilage wears down. Overuse of joints, as in the case of athletes or those who frequently squat, combined with excessive body weight, leads to added strain on the joint cartilage, resulting in osteoarthritis.

In osteoarthritis, persistent pain and inflammation in the knee joints are common, often worsened by concomitant osteoporosis, which leads to a loss of bone density, particularly at the joint ends. The thinning of the cartilage reduces the joint space between bones, leading to severe joint damage, commonly affecting the knee. Imaging tests like X - rays or MRI scans typically reveal the extent of cartilage deterioration.

Current treatments for osteoarthritis focus on pain management, reducing inflammation, and delaying joint damage. These include exercises to strengthen the muscles around the knee joint, painkillers, anti - inflammatory injections, and joint replacement surgery.

Regular exercise and calcium supplements may delay the need for surgery, but once the cartilage is severely damaged, knee replacement surgery often provides significant relief, allowing pain - free joint movements and improved mobility.

Rheumatoid Arthritis – This is a chronic autoimmune disease which causes inflammation mostly of small joints of the hands, wrists, ankles, knees etc. It is more common in females. The body's immune system attacks its own cells and tissues. Genetic and ecological reasons may also trigger this disease. The patient may have remissions and relapses – a chronic undulating course – swelling, inflammation and pain starting from any joint or several joints together.

Blood test is specially done for three molecules in the blood - sample viz: **Rheumatoid Factor, C Reactive Protein** and **Anti - cyclic citrullinated peptide** (anti - CCP). Treatment is by pain killers, steroids and other anti - inflammatory drugs for relieving pain and swelling. Now the treatment is done by innovative biologic and targeted therapy which are proving highly effective in the treatment of rheumatoid arthritis.

Juvenile Idiopathic Arthritis (JIA) – Formerly known as juvenile rheumatoid arthritis, it is the most common type of arthritis in children under 16. The disease is triggered by autoimmunity, where the body's immune system mistakenly attacks its own cells and tissues.

While the exact cause is unknown, a combination of genetic and environmental factors is believed to contribute. Symptoms include persistent joint pain, redness, swelling, and stiffness, often affecting large joints like the knees, ankles, and wrists. The disease can have periods of flare - ups followed by periods of remission.

JIA has several subtypes, with the most common being **polyarticular** (affecting five or more joints), **pauciarticular** (affecting fewer than four joints), and **systemic** JIA. The systemic type is more severe, characterized by high fevers, rashes, and enlargement of the liver and spleen. Complications from JIA can include stunted physical growth, joint damage, and eye inflammation, especially **uveitis.**

Treatment for JIA is aimed at reducing inflammation and pain, preventing joint damage, and improving joint function. This may include medications like nonsteroidal anti - inflammatory drugs (NSAIDs), disease - modifying anti - rheumatic drugs (DMARDs), and biologic agents, along with physical therapy to maintain mobility and strength.

Psoriatic Arthritis – Psoriasis is a form of chronic autoimmune skin and nail disease whereby red scaly and troublesome itchy plaques with silvery scales may be visible on the skin. These may flare up intermittently.

There may also be thickening, discoloration and pits on the nails. Psoriasis may be accompanied by arthritis with pain, stiffness and swelling in several joints of the body.

Spondylitis & Ankylosing Spondylitis – These terms refer to chronic inflammation of joints of the spine or vertebral column. It is more common in males and starts at a young age. Chronic pain and stiffness of the back occur, and spine flexibility may be reduced with forward bending.

Other symptoms may be neck and shoulder pain, pain and stiffness of ribcage, hips and thighs, and foot and heel pain. The exact cause is not clear, but is believed to be autoimmune related to genes, being more common in people with **positive HLA - B27 antigen** (test done through a blood sample). Infection, injury, and age - related wear and tear may also trigger Spondylitis and Ankylosing Spondylitis.

Gout – This presents severe attacks of inflammation, pain, swelling, and redness in one or more joints – most often in the big toe. This condition is caused all of a sudden when uric acid increases in the blood and is deposited in the joints. Uric acid crystals in and around the joints cause acutely painful and tender joints. Uric acid stones may form in the kidneys. Attacks may be precipitated by meals high in purine – such as meat. This disease is controlled by medicines that reduce the level of uric acid. Acute and chronic gout are part of metabolic syndrome. In this disease, the quantity of protein in the food should be restricted.

Reactive Arthritis – Reactive arthritis is a condition caused by certain infectious diseases viz; Lyme's disease, Chlamydia, Salmonella, Shigella, Campylobacter, Chikungunya etc.

Palindromic Rheumatism – This is a form of painful arthritis wherein inflammation flares up and remits at intervals. Lasting damage to joints does not occur.

Diseases of bone

Osteomyelitis – This is usually a bacterial infection of bone. Infection is difficult to treat and requires prolonged intravenous therapy with antibiotics to which the bacterium is susceptible. Tuberculous osteomyelitis also occurs occasionally and requires treatment with anti tubercular drugs for at keast 18 months.

Osteopenia, Osteoporosis & Osteomalacia – Osteopenia or osteoporosis is a reduction in bone density i.e sparsity in the bone mineral due to which the bones in the hips, wrists, spine or any other bone may be fractured even by minor injuries. Osteopenia is caused by a deficiency of calcium and phosphorus. Osteomalacia is caused by the deficiency of vitamin D in adults, which leads to soft bones. The treatment of these diseases is by calcium, vitamin D, bisphosphonate, physical exercises, physiotherapy, etc. Women in childbearing age, lactating women and elderly frequently suffer from osteoporosis.

Rickets – This is a disease of growing bones, therefore seen in children. Chronic deficiency of Vitamin D leads to the widening of the ends of bones. Later, there are bony deformities like **knock knees** and **bowlegs**. Rare inherited problems can also cause rickets. Treatment includes exposure to sunlight, and supplements of Vitamin D, phosphate, and calcium. Remodeling of bones and correction of deformities may take years. Corrective surgery may be required.

Diffuse Connective Tissue Diseases – These are a group of diseases also called **collagen vascular diseases**. They are autoimmune in nature often associated with arthritis. Some of these are briefly described below.

Systemic Lupus Erythematosus (SLE), or lupus – is an autoimmune disease of unknown origin, where genetic and environmental factors are believed to play a significant role. It is a multisystem disorder with a relapsing and remitting course, affecting more women than men.

Common initial or relapsing symptoms include nonspecific fever, arthralgia (joint pain), fatigue, and weight loss. A characteristic **butterfly - shaped rash** on the face, triggered by sun exposure, is often observed.

The kidneys are frequently affected, with acute nephritic illness presenting as high blood pressure and blood in the urine. Nephrotic syndrome can develop, leading to excess protein in the urine, low blood protein levels, high lipid levels, and body swelling. Kidney failure, both acute and chronic, may also occur, accompanied by elevated blood urea levels.

The nervous system can also be affected, resulting in neuropsychiatric symptoms, while chest involvement can lead to pleural effusion and pericarditis, causing chest pain. SLE can cause a reduction in red blood cells, white blood cells, and platelets.

The disease follows a fluctuating course, with periods of improvement and worsening. Management includes improving quality of life through sun protection, a healthy diet, anti - inflammatory medications, and steroids to control inflammation and organ damage.

Sjogren Syndrome – This is an autoimmune disease with genetic and environmental factors playing their role. It is more commonly found in females. The immune system attacks the glands that make saliva and tears.

Symptoms include **dry mouth** and **dry eyes** because of inflammation of the lacrimal and salivary glands. This disease aggravates with symptoms like dry skin with rashes, persistent dry cough, vaginal dryness, numbness in limbs etc.

Other parts of the body may also be affected, causing fatigue and joint and muscle pain. Similarly, the thyroid glands, lungs, kidneys, and nervous system are gradually affected. The risk of lymphoma – a malignancy of lymph nodes, is increased and tested by biopsy. Samples of saliva, tears, and blood are tested.

Scleroderma or Systemic Sclerosis – Again, this is an autoimmune disease especially affecting women. There is tightening and hardening of the skin due to too much **collagen** – a protein found in connective tissue. Blood vessels, esophagus, internal organs may also be affected.

Raynaud's phenomenon is a peculiar sensitivity to cold resulting due to excessive constriction of blood vessels in the fingers and toes. This phenomenon may precede the other symptoms of this disease.

Polymyositis & Dermatomyositis – These diseases are associated with inflammation of muscles. In dermatomyositis a skin rash is also present, while in polymyositis there is muscle weakness without skin rash.

The cause of these conditions is unknown but may be related to immune dysfunction. Malignancies of internal organs like lung may be associated.

Bechet's Disease – This is an inflammatory disease of blood vessels of unknown etiology. It is characterized by recurrent genital and oral **ulcerations**, eye inflammation (uveitis), and systemic vasculitis.

Extra - articular Disorders –Inflammation of soft tissues around joints – bursae, ligaments and tendons can result from repeated stress, irritation and injury. Pain, stiffness and swelling are the usual symptoms.

Rheumatic disorders often involve autoimmune processes, and diagnostic tests typically include antibody testing to confirm the diagnosis. Imaging studies like X - rays, CT scans, and MRIs help assess the extent of joint and tissue involvement. Inflammatory markers, such as hematocrit, ESR, CRP, and anti - CCP, are also used to monitor disease activity.

Treatment for rheumatic disorders generally involves a combination of reassurance, compassionate care, pain relievers, and anti - inflammatory medications. Corticosteroids and immunosuppressive drugs are often prescribed for autoimmune conditions. Recently, biologics and targeted therapies have shown significant promise in improving patients' quality of life.

In conclusion, rheumatic disorders are prevalent, affecting a significant portion of the population. Many of these conditions are immunological in nature, often with a relapsing and remitting course.

While a permanent cure remains elusive for many, advances in medical treatments, including pain management, anti - inflammatory drugs, and targeted therapies, have greatly improved outcomes for patients. **Rheumatologists** now play a key role in the specialized care of individuals with both acute and chronic rheumatic diseases.

Chapter 35

Cancer - Causes and Treatment

Learning Objectives:

- Cancer results from uncontrolled cell growth
- Cancer is caused by environmental carcinogens and genetic changes (mutations and polymorphism)
- Proliferation of cancer may occur in various organs of the body
- Modes of cancer spread in the body
- TNM staging of cancer and grading of cancer
- Modalities of cancer treatment - surgery, radiation, chemotherapy (treatment by medicines), targeted therapies, emerging new dimensions

---

Cells are the fundamental building blocks of life in the human body, with millions continuously dividing to create new ones. Each cell has a finite lifespan, and millions naturally die each day through a process known as 'programmed cell death' or **apoptosis.**

Oncology, the science of cancer, has demonstrated that when apoptosis is hindered, old cells grow uncontrollably, accumulating in a particular area and forming a tumor or cancer.

Cancer can also arise from disruptions in another vital process: mitosis, the division of cells. Under normal conditions, mitosis ensures that worn - out cells are replaced by healthy ones. In cancer, however, this process accelerates and becomes unregulated, leading to unchecked cellular growth. Genetic mutations in the DNA of specific cells, tissues, or organs cause this uncontrolled cell division. Cancer is a complex and deceptive disease, often triggered by a combination of environmental factors, ecological influences, and genetic predispositions.

The decline in the body's immunity allows external factors to contribute to cancer's progression. Diagnosis typically involves a **biopsy,** where a sample of the tumor is examined under a microscope.

Further diagnostic refinement is achieved using molecular markers through **immunohistochemistry (IHC).** Globally, approximately 200 to 400 people per 100,000 suffer from cancer in their lifetime, with around 10 million (or 1 crore) cancer patients worldwide at any given time.

Tumors are of two types. There are **benign** tumors (non - cancerous) and **malignant** tumors (cancerous). Benign tumors are less rapidly growing, well confined usually inside a capsule and more easily treatable, whereas malignant growth of pathogenic cells goes on exponentially.

Abnormal cells infiltrate directly into neighboring healthy tissues of the body or spread through blood into liver, lungs, bones, brain etc. and through lymphatics into regional lymph nodes. The load of cancer cells in the body is increased and other organs get affected. This potential of the cancer cell to spread throughout the body called **metastasis** deprives the normal body organs of nutrition, leading to deterioration of health day by day, and untimely death.

Causes of Cancer – Any disease in the body is the result of interplay of many factors. For example, many heavy smokers despite the exposure of this environmental carcinogen do not develop lung cancer because they are genetically protected and do not have predisposing genetic constitution. **Cancers occur as a result of genetic change (mutation) in DNA** in a particular cell, tissue or organ.

Factors causing mutations in cells and leading to cancer are:

1. **Aging** – The likelihood of cancer increases with age due to various changes or mutations in DNA. In some cases, even minor mutations in genes can increase the risk of cancer. For example, mutations in oncogenes like single - nucleotide polymorphisms (SNPs) can increase the likelihood of cancer in any generation.

2. **Radiation and Radioactive Substances** – Exposure to radiation such as infra - red, ultraviolet (UV) radiation from the sun, radioactive substances or carcinogens like radium, uranium, thorium, various types

of radiation viz; X - rays, gamma rays, certain high frequency radio waves, radioactive waste material leakages and nuclear bomb, etc. can damage DNA in the body, leading to mutations in genes.

3. **Infection** – Many cancers are linked to known infectious agents. Human papillomavirus (HPV) can cause cancer in cervix, skin, mouth, and throat etc. Human immunodeficiency virus (HIV) can lead to Kaposi's sarcoma. Hepatitis B and C virus can cause liver cancer, Hepatitis C virus can also cause lymphoma and Epstein Barr virus is the cause of nasopharyngeal cancer.

4. **Chronic Irritation** – Some cancers such as oral cancer can result from chronic irritation from ill - fitted dentures etc. Tobacco is also a cause of chronic irritation resulting in cancers of the lung, esophagus and oral mucosa.

5. **Oncogenes** – Certain predetermined **proto - oncogenes** develop in the body **de novo** which when exposed to peculiar environmental stimulus transform or mutate into **oncogene** leading to unbridled division in cells, ultimately transforming into malignancy.

   Examples of **proto - oncogenes** are *PDGF, Cer - B2, Hras, Kras, bcr - abl, cyclin D, N - myc*, etc. The emergence of unpredictable mutations in proto - oncogenes (genes involved in regulating cell growth) can promote uncontrolled cell division, leading to cancer.

   On the other hand, there are **tumor suppressor genes** also like *p53, Rb, BRCA1/2* etc. that prevent tumor progression and development. When tumor suppressor gene malfunctions, mutation in cells causes cancer.

6. **Certain other environmental causes** – Obesity has been linked to several cancers like breast, uterine, liver, kidney, colorectal, esophageal, gallbladder and pancreatic cancer. About 4 - 8% of cancers can be ascribed to obesity. Excessive consumption of tobacco, alcohol etc. for a long time may trigger cancer. Industrial exposure to asbestos and several chemical carcinogens can cause lung and skin cancers.

However, the exact cause of many cancers is still not known and there may be some common causes of cancer.

How Cancer Grows and Spreads – Cancer or malignant tumor thrives and spreads in the body. Taking abundance of nutrition, oxygen and energy from the body, it initially grows slowly and after a certain stage, the malignancy grows sharply, and rapidly. As the tumor grows, it creates a cluster of cells, similar to a lump. Rapidly growing tumors trigger **angiogenesis** i.e. the formation of new blood vessels inside the tumor mass, which increases the density of tiny blood vessels called capillaries.

This leads to reinforcement of malignant growth due to increased oxygen and nutrient supply. Cancer cells are loosely attached to each other (exfoliating) thus easily travel into blood and lymphatic streams to spread. The spread of a solid or localized tumor to another location is called **metastasis**. In this process, cancer cells from the primary or original tumor break away and travel through the bloodstream or lymphatic vessels to other parts of the body. Body's immune system is also compromised because of involvement of other organs and lymphatic system. Certain predisposing **genes promoting tumor metastasis** are *PTGS2, EREG, MMP1* and *LOX*. Doctors determine the stage of cancer by the size of primary tumor, examination of the regional lymph node enlargement and spread to distant organs.

Cancer can spread in many ways:

1. **Direct Local Extension** – Cancer in a specific organ often spreads like a crab's pincer, grasping the surrounding tissues (locally invasive) and not sparing adjacent organs.

2. **Via Lymphatic Channels** – Often, cancer of a specific organ can spread to nearby lymph nodes through the lymphatic system and into a distant lymph node basin.

3. **Through Bloodstream** – Occasionally, cancer of a specific organ can spread to other parts of the body through the bloodstream. Malignant tumor present at a primary site may have a small break - away portion which dislodges and gets organized at another site. This is called **secondary** or **metastatic** tumor. This spread is by the process of **embolization** or lodging of an embolus or clump of cancer cells travelling through the bloodstream. Solid tumors can commonly spread to the liver, lungs, bones, brain etc.

Types of Cancer

Cancer is not a single disease; there are approximately 150 different cancers arising from different cells, tissues or organs in the body.

The main types of cancer are:

1. **Carcinoma (Solid Tumors)** – Carcinoma is a type of cancer that originates in the epithelial cells which line the body's external and internal surfaces called skin and mucosa. Carcinomas can affect the skin, breasts, mouth, vocal cords, and more. **Squamous cell carcinoma** arises from the skin's outermost layer and the lining of the mouth, tongue, larynx etc. **Adenocarcinoma** originates from the inner lining of various organs or tissues, such as the lining of breast glands, gallbladder, pancreas, stomach, large intestine, prostate and lungs.

2. **Sarcoma** – Sarcoma is the second type of solid tumor. It begins in connective or supportive tissues (muscles, bones, cartilage, blood vessels, and fat cells). Major types include osteosarcoma (bone cancer), angiosarcoma (blood vessels cancer), gastrointestinal stromal tumor (GIST), liposarcoma (fat cells cancer), Kaposi's sarcoma, chondrosarcoma (cartilage cancer), fibrosarcoma (fibrous tissue and tendons) and more.

3. **Blood Cancer (Hematologic Cancer)** – This type of cancer occurs in cells responsible for making blood. The blood formation takes place in the bone marrow and the malignancies arising from bone marrow are also known as **leukemias** or myeloproliferative disorders. It includes **acute lymphoblastic leukemia** (ALL), **acute and chronic myeloid leukemia** (AML and CML) and **chronic lymphocytic leukemia** (CLL), among others.

When plasma cells (immune cells) are infected with cancer, it is called multiple myeloma, also other names viz; Kahler disease, myelomatosis and plasma cell myeloma. When RBCs are affected by cancer, it is called **polycythaemia** vera.

4. **Lymphoma** – Lymphoma affects the cells of the lymphatic system. Lymph nodes, spleen, tonsils, bone marrow, intestines etc. are involved.

The major types are Hodgkin's and non - Hodgkin's lymphoma. Treatment is done through chemotherapy, targeted therapy and bone marrow transplant.

5. **Skin Melanoma** – This is also a type of solid cancer. When melanocytes (cells that produce melanin pigment) in the skin undergo uncontrolled division or unimpeded mitosis, it results in skin **melanoma.** It can sometimes develop in the mucosal lining of the mouth and anus as well. This disease is more common among fair - skinned individuals and is often associated with exposure to ultraviolet radiation from the sun. Suspicion arises from the appearance of new moles, changes in skin color or irregular growth or itching of a mole. It spreads into draining lymph nodes. Melanoma is an **aggressive** cancer.

Cancer Prevalence in the World – The global cancer landscape varies significantly across different countries, including India. In developed nations, non - communicable diseases such as obesity, diabetes, and high blood pressure are rising alongside cancer. Globally, around 200 to 400 out of every 100,000 individuals are affected by cancer annually. Among the most prevalent cancers, **lung cancer** (17.6%) is the leading type in men, while **breast cancer** is the most common in women, with about 1 in every 12 to 20 women developing it over their lifetime. Prostate cancer is particularly common among non - smoking men. Additionally, stomach cancer, oral cancer, and cervical cancer are other frequently diagnosed cancers worldwide.

Cancer Prevalence in India is monitored through population and hospital based Cancer Registries maintained by the Department of Health Research, Indian Council of Medical Research (ICMR), and the Ministry of Health, Government of India, under the National Centre for Disease Informatics and Research (NCDIR). Approximately 1.5 to 2 million new cancer cases are diagnosed in India annually. The most prevalent cancers in Indian men are lung, oral, and prostate cancers, while breast, oral, and cervical cancers are most common among Indian women.

Tobacco Use in India is notably high, with around 35% of men and 15% of women using tobacco. Many young people, particularly those aged 16 - 18 years, become addicted to tobacco in various forms.

Tobacco consumption significantly contributes to cancers in multiple organs, including the mouth, throat, esophagus, lungs, stomach, urinary bladder, and pancreas. In India, tobacco use accounts for approximately 40% of the country's total cancer burden.

Challenges in Cancer Diagnosis and Treatment – According to the Indian National Cancer Research Program, around 15% of cancer patients in India are unable to receive timely and appropriate diagnosis, treatment, and rehabilitation due to factors such as poverty, geographical distance, and limited healthcare resources. While the Government of India has established large institutions in several cities to address cancer care, these centers are overwhelmed by the increasing demand for cancer treatment. A significant number of cancer patients are unable to access treatment during the early stages of the disease. This delay in diagnosis allows the cancer to progress, often leading to advanced disease stages. Patients in such conditions face helplessness, wandering from one facility to another, hoping for effective treatment.

For those with advanced cancer, palliative care becomes essential to alleviate pain and provide dignified end - of - life care. However, there is a lack of skilled palliative care services in many regions, further depriving these patients of the support they desperately need during the final stages of their illness.

Diagnosis of cancer

Biopsy is the definitive test for cancer confirmation, as treatments cannot proceed without it. This involves removing tissue from the affected organ, usually performed by surgeons or cancer specialists, and involves minimal surgery.

In **incisional biopsy**, a small piece of tissue is taken from the edge of the tumor or growth. In **excisional biopsy,** a small lesion is entirely removed and sent for microscopic examination. Biopsies from areas such as the respiratory tract, esophagus, stomach, or colon are often done using an endoscope.

For organs like the breast, liver, kidney, or other lumps in the body, a special needle that can cut a core of tissue (**core biopsy**) is used.

Sometimes, the biopsy is done with the guidance of ultrasound or CT scans for precision.

The biopsy sample is preserved in formalin and embedded in paraffin blocks. Thin slices of the tissue sample are prepared for microscopic examination, which involves histopathology (microscopic study of tissues), immunohistochemistry (IHC), or molecular tests like **FISH** (Fluorescence in situ Hybridization).

Biopsy is not harmful, and there should be no anxiety if performed by an expert. The type and grade of the tumor are identified through histopathology, which uses various stains to assess how much the cells differ from their normal structure, indicating the tumor's severity.

Cytology is of two types: **aspiration** and **scraping**. Cytology is different from biopsy. In biopsy a small piece of tissue or tumor is taken out for detailed study alongside normal tissue, while in cytology loosely bound exfoliating cells that stick to the needle or scraped off are stained and examined.

A thin - hollow needle inserted in the tumor or mass is gently swirled and moved up and down for collecting fluid from the tissue – in this process some tumor cells are also drawn out and are identified by pathologist through the microscopic examination. Accuracy of cytology is less than histopathology but gives results quickly. Cytology is also known as **fine needle aspiration cytology (FNAC).**

In women cancer of the cervix is very common and the technique of cytology is very useful by taking a scrape from the mouth of the uterus (cervix) which is smeared on a glass slide and stained and examined under the microscope. This popular technique is called **Pap smear** and is used in screening for cancer cervix. Now a days cervix cancer screening program is being conducted world over in the female population above 30 years of age.

The cells in the sediment are studied through Pap test. Fluid accumulated in the abdominal peritoneal cavity, thoracic pleural cavity and other places are centrifuged and examined in various cancers.

Endoscopy is a state of art **fiber - optic technology** equipped with an illuminating source. It is employed to visualize inside orifices and body cavities like oral cavity for esophagus, stomach and duodenum, through anus for rectum and colon and through the respiratory passage into trachea and bronchus. These body cavities are lined by mucosa and gross pathological changes in this lining are recognized by the endoscopists. The lining can be directly visualized or projected on a screen. Inbuilt operating channels in the endoscopes are used for minor surgical procedures and biopsy. The biopsied materials are sent to laboratory for histopathology.

Imaging Techniques include plain X - rays, contrast enhanced X - rays, computerized axial tomography X - ray (**CAT scan**), ultrasound and Magnetic Resonance Imaging (MRI). Bone involvement, soft tissue changes in various images of cancer and contrast enhancements of these images are done in radio diagnosis setups in a big way these days.

The spread of cancer in the nearby organ or distant parts of the body is screened by various imaging techniques. The detailed study of spread of cancer deciphers the stage of tumor. Screening and detecting early cancer and staging it in the breast (**mammogram**), thyroid, prostate etc., are possible by the new evolving special techniques of imaging.

Positron Emission Tomography (PET scan) is a biological technique of **scanning of entire body**, which provides appropriate information about the spread of almost all types of cancer. It is a sophisticated scan technique in which radioactive chemical or **radiotracer fluorodeoxyglucose** (**FDG**) is injected into the bloodstream, which is selectively absorbed by cancer cells wherever they are located in the body. The positron emission from this tracer is recorded by the whole - body CT scan. This helps in identifying a hidden tumor in the body and the stage of cancer accurately.

Cancer Staging or **Tumor, Node, Metastasis (TNM)** staging or the level of cancer progression is determined based on the size and spread of solid tumors. Staging is essential for deciding the treatment plan.

The location and size of the tumor, lymph node involvement and the spread of cancer in other parts of body are determined and reported as **TNM staging system**. Here, **T** refers to size of the primary/original tumor, **N** refers lymph node involvement and **M** refers metastasis or spread of cancer.

Staging ranges from 1 to 4, with Stage 0 being used for precancerous conditions (carcinoma *in situ*) where cellular changes indicate the beginning of cancer.

Stage 1 represents localized cancer with a tumor size of up to 2 cm. **Stage 2** is characterized by localized cancer in a single organ with a tumor size larger than 2 cm but smaller than 5 cm. **Stage 3** signifies localized cancer with a tumor size greater than 5 cm. **Stage 4** indicates that cancer is no longer localized and it has spread to other parts of the body through blood, lymph or direct extension to distant organs. The TNM staging methodology is recognized and approved in medical science by the organizations like **AJCC** (American Joint Committee on Cancer) and the **UICC** (Union for International Cancer Control). Staging determines the pathway towards cancer treatment and also provides the clue to the life expectancy of the patient. A detailed clinical examination of the patient and various tests are conducted to determine the stage towards which cancer has progressed.

Cancer grading indicates how abnormal cells and tissues of organ - cancer (prostate cancer, ovary cancer etc.) have become in comparison to healthy cells of that part of the body. Cancer cells looking more closely like healthy cells may be indicative of low - grade tumor.

Grading of the cancer cells is done under microscopic examination according to what extent the morphological changes in the cells have taken place. viz,

Grade 1 – cancer cells that nearly resemble normal cells and not growing rapidly; **Grade 2** – cancer cells not looking like normal cells but growing faster than normal cells; **Grade 3** – cancer cells not much looking like normal and growing aggressively and **Grade 4** – cancer cells not resembling at all to the origin and dividing very rapidly.

Breaking the news about cancer requires confirmed clinical findings and test reports and is a sensitive and responsible task. The doctor must convey the diagnosis while maintaining the confidence and morale of both the patient and caregivers.

Effective cancer treatment depends on encouraging everyone involved to fight the disease with optimism.

The process of delivering this life - altering news is often guided by international protocols such as **SPIKES**, which provides a step - by - step framework to handle this challenging discussion with empathy and care:

S - Setting and Support: Ensure the news is broken in a private setting, offering both physical and emotional support to minimize the patient's and caregivers' distress.

P - Perception and Planning: Understand the patient's and caregivers' perception of the situation, including their financial, emotional, and physical capacity, to offer pragmatic and affordable treatment options.

I - Invitation or Information: Invite the patient or caregivers to ask questions and provide detailed information about the diagnosis and treatment options.

K - Knowledge: Share medical information and knowledge about the patient's condition clearly and truthfully, ensuring the patient understands their situation.

E - Empathetic Responses: Show empathy, listen to concerns, and acknowledge their emotional reactions.

S - Summarize or Strategize: Summarize the key points and strategize the treatment plan, providing options and outlining the prognosis.

The **SPIKES protocol** is crucial in ensuring that the difficult task of breaking cancer news is done with sensitivity, support, and a clear path forward for treatment and care.

Cancer Screening is a population - based expensive exercise which is undertaken by various governments and health organizations in order to detect common cancer types during early stage or pre - cancerous stage. Screening is the presumptive identification of unrecognized disease by the application of tests or examination applied *en masse* and rapidly.

Notably, various cancer types do not have any symptom in its early stage, for example women may be harboring a painless lump in the breast, smokers may have a lesion in the lung or mouth.

Certain types of clinical examination and tests like mammogram of breast, Pap test of cervix is done on the entire population of the region in certain age group to detect early stages or incipient stages of cancer. This is an epidemiological exercise in **down staging** the disease in the entire population. Treatment is more effective, less expensive and far less mutilating if instituted while primary pathology is still early. This public health exercise is a significant measure in saving the costs to governments and the patients as well. Cancer types occurring in a particular society with high incidence are chosen for screening. Breast cancer in Caucasian women, colon cancer, prostate cancer and lung cancer are some of the cancers for which various countries of the world run screening programs.

Cancer Care and Treatment is an enormous management involving highly technical and expensive infrastructure and manpower. About 150 types of cancer affect human beings in various propensity requiring multimodality treatments like surgery, chemotherapy, radiotherapy, immunotherapy, palliative treatments and rehabilitation etc. The science of oncology embedded with specialist ramifications like surgical oncology, medical oncology, radiation oncology, oncology nursing, palliative care and hospice and oncology emergency has become extremely useful in promoting total cancer care. **Tumor boards** constituted of specialists in cancer hospitals ascribe and assign the treatment algorithm for often long drawn and multi - modality cancer treatment. Treatment of different types of cancer proceeds on the staging, histopathological morphology and grading, molecular and genetic profile of the cancer type. Besides, the treatment process starts after taking into consideration various characteristic features of the patient and their family like their values, belief system, expectations, living environment and available resources with the providers. Highly expensive molecular, targeted, genetic and immunological therapies have been invented recently and affordability has become a major predictor in prescribing these treatment methods especially when the outcome of the disease and life expectancy is unpredictable. About 40% of cancers originate from the use of tobacco, so quitting tobacco is definitely a distinctive and momentous lifestyle change. Thus, lifestyle changes ought to be advised and even imposed in certain types of cancer for example quitting tobacco is necessary when treating lung and oral cancer. Rarely, certain cancers being hereditary, the treatment is carried on the basis of genetic or family history of the patient.

The detailed data of genetic cancer is collected and confirmed on the basis of various lab testing for example in young women with both side breast cancer, *pari pasu* ovary cancer, family history of breast cancer, triple negative type cancer may have gene *BRCA 1 and 2* positive tests. Now a days whole gene sequencing by Next Generation Sequencing (NGS) of DNA to study the entire human genome is also done in certain cancers. NGS determines highly specific and **personalized cancer treatment** which is targeted towards offending gene constitution. Treatment modalities for different cancer types can be a lone modality or a combination of certain modalities into different sequences.

Surgery is done to remove cancer from a certain specific organ and surrounding affected tissues such as lymph nodes. Cancer is mostly removed or excised with a margin of normal looking tissue, and this is called **wide local excision**. When tissues farther away from the cancer are also removed, it is called a **radical excision**. For example, total breast removal for malignant lump is called **mastectomy.** Surgical removal of only a certain part of malignant lump in the breast and preserving the remaining breast is called **breast conservation surgery**.

Reconstructive surgery was done to construct a new chest mound mimicking the breast from the nearby tissue after removing the entire breast. Complete breast reconstruction to adjust size and shape of breast with areola and nipple has evolved into a new *genre* of surgical speciality called **oncoplastic breast surgery**. With the development of better and efficacious hormonal and targeted therapies and highly focused radio therapy, larger numbers of patients are offered breast conservation and oncoplastic breast surgery. Two decades ago, mostly total breast removal or mastectomy was offered. The removed and widely excised part of the breast is marked with ink on its outer surface for examination for cancer cells through histopathology. A detailed histopathological and molecular examination is done and breast cancer now a days is labelled as 5 different types described in the chapter on breast cancer. Even after surgery, cancer may recur in the same place or in another distant area. With a view to checking or preventing such a recurrence chemotherapy, appropriate hormonal therapy, radiation therapy etc. is undertaken. The above illustration of surgical treatment in breast cancer is a prototype of surgical treatments performed in various cancer types of other organs in the body.

With the advent of new surgical technologies **minimally invasive surgery** has achieved a new milestone in the arena of surgical oncology. Surgery of abdominal cancer especially that of esophagus, colon, prostate etc. are done using laparoscope by making small holes in the abdominal wall with less pain and speedy recovery.

Robotic Surgery is a multiple combined endoscopic - laparoscopic innovative technology in which robot performs surgery, wherein specialist surgeon commands the robot through computer console kept at a distance. Robotic Surgery is recognized for even more precision in surgery and ability to operate with convenience in various **nooks and corners** of the human body which would be otherwise inaccessible. Surgical robots are fitted with as many numbers of laparoscopes, cameras and sensors as can be driven skillfully. The laparoscopes are fitted with a variety of operating tools. After adequate anesthesia and abdominal cavity insufflation to create operating space in the abdomen, these cameras and tools fitted laparoscopes are inserted inside the abdomen (docking). The organ which is to be operated on is located and focused. One operator stays near the patient to assist in making small holes in the body through skin and abdominal wall to put in the camera, the scopes and the instruments all of which follow the command from **console unit**. The console is placed usually in the same room 4 - 5 meters away from the main operating surgeon sitting on a multi - functional mobile stool. Once the camera starts sending images of the concerned organ or area inside the body the surgeon - in - chief performs the actual surgery using finger ports and pedals in the console unit which activate various laparoscopes and its instruments. Now this technique is used for the surgery of prostate gland, colon and rectum etc.

Radiation Therapy is used to treat localized cancer at a specific site in the body using high - energy radiation beams directed at cancerous tissues, cells or tumors. It aims to destroy cancer cells while sparing adjacent healthy tissues using focused beams of high - energy radiation, such as cobalt, linear accelerators, gamma rays and more. Radiation therapy is employed in various cancers, including brain, breast, cervix, esophagus, prostate gland, rectum etc. Cancer affected organs and surrounding tissues are treated by dose regulated irradiation. The objective of this therapy is to protect the function of the affected organ and have the least amount of radiation dissipating into normal surrounding tissue.

For this, protective lead shields are specially designed for each patient.

There are two primary types of radiation energy:

External radiation administered from a suitable distance is called **external beam radiation** or **EBRT** or **teletherapy** and,

Secondly radiation delivered from the close proximity of the cancer affected organ called **brachytherapy**.

Each day a fraction of the total dose is delivered to reduce the toxicity. Generally, 15 - 30 doses are prescribed in most cases.

Chemotherapy was discovered during World War II when several successful experiments were conducted with **mustard gas** in treating cancer. Dr Sidney Farber observed remarkable benefits in children suffering from **leukemia** or **white blood**, as was seen in 1947 in patients with acute lymphoblastic leukaemia who had temporary but definite relief with an agent called **aminopterin**.

Later Dr Farber discovered other agents to treat cancer – actinomycin D for Wilm's tumor in children at Dana - Farber Cancer Institute in Boston, USA. New anti - cancer drug discoveries take place frequently bringing in more efficacious and less toxic chemotherapeutic agents and properly researched pharmaceutical agents. Chemotherapy is a systemic therapy, using oral and intravenous medications to treat cancer. It has proven to be an increasingly effective method for cancer treatment, especially for blood and pediatric cancers. Cancer drugs undergo rigorous testing through drug trials to ensure their efficacy and the fear that these are some toxic chemicals should be allayed. Chemotherapy is administered at different time intervals. Some side effects of chemotherapy are tolerated well after proper counselling of the patients and caregivers about the possible side effects and benefits of the chemotherapy.

The side effects include loss of appetite, hair fall, nausea, vomiting, muzzy head, constipation or diarrhea, dryness and ulcers in mouth, weakness, tingling and aching feet, anemia and low white blood cell and platelet counts. These side effects are also treated with marrow hormone injections which build up the RBC, WBC and platelets. Chemotherapy drugs destroy and kill rapidly dividing cells in the body.

Thus, chemotherapy along with destroying cancer cells also kills hairs, nails, mucosa and blood cells because these are also somewhat rapidly dividing cells. Chemotherapeutic drug administration regimen involves pulse therapy usually at 3 weekly intervals. This 3 weekly interval or pulse therapy is given to allow the normal cells to recover and achieve a bigger differential kill of the more rapidly dividing cancer cells.

Administering chemotherapy before surgery or radiotherapy is called **neo adjuvant** chemotherapy, if it is administered afterwards – it is called **adjuvant** therapy, but whenever it is administered along with radiotherapy it is called **concomitant** therapy.

Immunotherapy is based on the principle that if the immune system of the patient is strengthened, the body will cast off cancer. Immunotherapy capacity builds the patient, and the cancer cells will be phagocytosed (eaten up by body's scavengers - the WBC). This therapy is undertaken for enhancing the body's natural defense mechanisms against cancer. It is an emerging approach with a few epoch - making achievements in cancer treatment and includes methods such as immune checkpoint blockade and biologic therapy. It shows significant promise in treating cancers like chronic myeloid leukaemia, multiple myeloma, kidney, lung, prostate, rectal, thyroid and urinary bladder cancers, among others. Additionally, combination therapies involving **immuno - modulation** and gene therapy are being researched for their effectiveness in cancer treatment. In immune modulation the immune system of the body is strengthened.

Hormone Therapy – is used to treat cancers that are hormone sensitive, such as breast, prostate and thyroid cancer. It involves opposing those hormones that fuel cancer growth, either by introducing necessary hormones into the body, blocking existing hormones or altering hormone behavior. Hormone therapy like chemotherapy is also a systemic therapy administered orally or through injections.

The cancerous tissue removed especially from breast cancer is tested for presence of hormone receptors. Anti - estrogens for breast cancer and anti - androgens for prostate cancer are frequently prescribed agents. Thyroid hormone therapy is prescribed to stop recurrence of thyroid cancer and substitute the need of thyroid hormone.

Targeted Therapy aims to block specific molecules or pathways involved in cancer growth and spread. They prevent the growth of new blood vessels, activate and strengthen the immune system, changing the behavior pattern of proteins produced by cancer cells, blocking the signals responsible for growth of cancer cells, targeting toxic effect of cancer drugs and channelizing them to destroy only cancer cells. In this process of targeted therapy, **messenger ribonucleic acid** or **mRNA** is directed to a certain target for preventing the growth and development of cancer cells. Targeted therapies have shown success in treating cancers like chronic myeloid leukaemia, multiple myeloma, breast, kidney, lung, prostate, rectal and thyroid cancers among others. These therapies are designed to kill cancer cells while minimizing damage to healthy cells. They are typically administered orally but sometimes through injections.

Concomitant targeted therapy along with immunopotentiation and gene therapy is also under trial for some cancers.

Gene Therapy – Gene therapy is an emerging field in cancer treatment and early trials are underway. It involves modifying or enhancing cells, typically using genetically engineered viruses or viral particles, to attack cancer cells more effectively. Gene transfer is used to deliver new genetic material into cancer cells, which may trigger apoptosis (cell death) or inhibit their growth. Gene therapy is currently being explored as a treatment for lung, pancreas and prostate cancer among others.

In this process of therapy largely three methods are applied viz.

- **Gene Therapy Through Immuno - therapy** wherein immune system is invigorated by means of administering the vaccine containing modified cells and viral particles. This therapy is carried out in resemblance with methods as applied in immuno - potentiation.

- **Oncolytic Viral Therapy** wherein viral particles being administered through vaccine like material replicate and inhibit growth and development of cancer cells.

- **Gene Transfer Therapy** wherein new genes are transfected into cancer cells which are inhibited and destroyed.

Bone Marrow Transplantation is an effective but highly demanding and cumbersome method of treatment. Bone marrow transplant requires infrastructure with an expert team of doctors and highly specialized barrier nursing care, for which special bone marrow transplantation suites are created. Diseases like leukaemia, lymphoma, myeloma, aplastic anemia etc. are treated successfully where bone marrow or **stem cells** of the blood is replaced or transplanted from the same person(**autologous** transplantation) or from another matched donor (**allogenic** transplantation).

This is a complex procedure in which at first **intensive chemotherapy** is given to destroy all types of cancer cells in the body. Afterward, bone marrow is transplanted establishing a new series of blood producing cells in the body.

Cryotherapy – In this treatment modality, cancer cells are destroyed by freezing them – thus probes are frozen at extremely low temperature for killing cancer cells (rapidly cooling and thawing the cells). This may be suitable only for a small, localized surface or skin tumor.

Radiofrequency Ablation or **RFA** is a treatment modality wherein cancer cells are destroyed by high frequency radio waves. RFA is also suitable only for a small, localized surface or skin tumor and sometimes used for liver tumors.

Palliative Care and Hospice means providing consistent and compatible relief to the patient suffering from terminal stage of cancer. When all the available methods of cancer cure and life prolongation become unproductive, the patient is provided with palliative care to **add some life to remaining days**. All governments and health care providers should develop palliative care facilities. Palliative care involves comfortable boarding, eminent pain relief, oxygen, respiratory or ventilatory support in case of breathlessness and treatment of psychiatric disturbances. In some cases, in order to alleviate pain or an obnoxious foul smelling growth palliative surgery is done.

Palliative radiotherapy is given for severe pain localized to one or two areas in bones. Another special modality of palliative chemotherapy is called **metronomic chemotherapy** in which certain low doses, less toxic preferably oral chemotherapy is administered.

Treatment is done with the aim of improving quality of life. **Palliative therapy** entails in its scope such methods and means which may console the distressed patient. Now special counsellors for emotional, psychological and spiritual empowerment of patients are available for their mental and spiritual upliftment and transcendence.

For relief pain - relieving medications, herbal remedies, local anesthesia, regional nerve blocks are provided. Most effective pain - relieving agents are derived from 2 natural plants – **opium and cannabis**. *Delta and Kappa Opioid receptors and CNB 1 & 2 Cannabinoid receptors* are present in the human body.

Indigenous preparations and pharmaceutical agents are available for both these sources for pain treatment and mood elevation. Now a days patients suffering from terminal diseases like cancer are permitted **passive euthanasia** for a **DNR** or '**do - not - resuscitate**' or **withdrawing life support system** consent with due diligence.

Diet - As for dietary recommendations for cancer patients, it is exemplified that some people have successfully treated cancer by controlling their diet, avoiding certain foods, and fasting heartfully abiding by the rules of do - s and don'ts. To some people abstinence may sound controversial but scholars and saints have reiterated that abstinence not only prevents uncontrolled cell growth and unnecessary DNA damage but maintains biological clock by promoting equilibrium in the process of apoptosis.

Cancer primarily thrives on carbohydrates and glucose. With this reasoning, some physicians advise cancer patients to completely eliminate sugary sweets and carbohydrate - rich foods like wheat and rice. Even milk and dairy products, poultry and bakery products may be prohibited for cancer patients. Beneficial foods include seasonal fruits and vegetables, turmeric, neem, wheatgrass, alkaline foods like bottle gourd, ridge gourd, pumpkin, jackfruit, lentils, etc.

India since the beginning of human civilization propounded the science of interval fasting which not only maintains the wellbeing of our physical system but develops spiritual enrichment as well. It is believed that many serious diseases like cancer may not appear in the body.

In conclusion, cancer is a broad term encompassing various malignant disorders that affect the blood and numerous organs in the body. Common cancers include breast and uterine cervix cancer in women, prostate cancer in men, and lung and oral cavity cancers, particularly in smokers.

Cancer results from the uncontrolled division of cells, often triggered by genetic mutations. Tobacco stands out as the leading environmental cause of cancer, contributing to around 40% of cases in India, including cancers of the lips, oral cavity, lungs, esophagus, and urinary bladder.

Environmental factors like tobacco exposure can activate oncogenes, leading to the malignant transformation of cells. As part of the global non - communicable disease burden, cancer rates are rising and necessitate early detection, often through screening. Its treatment usually involves a combination of surgery, chemotherapy, and radiotherapy, making timely intervention critical.

Chapter 36

Breast Disorders & Cancer

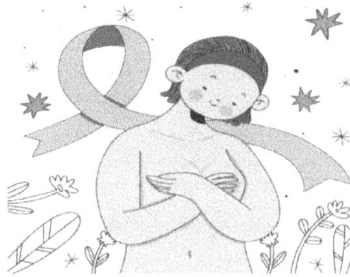

Learning Objectives:

- Breast development

- Importance of breast self-examination

- Breast size changes, dimpling, nipple retraction, nipple discharge, breast pain, or mastalgia

- Screening and mammography to identify breast cancer

- Early signs of breast cancer, breast cancer diagnosis, and its molecular sub-types viz; hormone receptor-positive, HER2-positive, Triple-negative, etc.

- Methods to treat breast cancer

The breast, or 'mamma,' is unique to mammals, forming along the milk line from the axilla (armpit) to the groin during fetal development. While humans develop one pair of functional breasts, several pairs of breasts form in certain animals like pigs and dogs. In humans, the breast extends from below the clavicle to the armpit and across to the sternum.

The mammary ridge thickens in girls during puberty, and the breast further develops during pregnancy, producing milk after delivery. This cycle repeats with each pregnancy.

Breasts are not only functional for feeding babies but also serve cosmetic and sexual roles, often seen as a source of pride for women.

In men, the breast tissue does not fully develop, though an imbalance in sex hormones may cause **gynecomastia**, - a benign condition with an increase in breast tissue. Male breast cancer, though rare, can occur, accounting for 1% of all breast cancer cases.

Breast cancer remains a significant cause of early mortality in women. Regular breast examinations, ideally once a year, are vital for maintaining breast health. Women should feel comfortable undergoing these screenings during routine doctor visits. Breast cancer screening is standard practice in many Western countries, and early detection plays a crucial role in improving outcomes.

Let us now discuss common pathologies related to breasts:

'Normal' Breast Lumps, Breast Nodularity *vs* **Pain** – The size of the breast and its fullness are regulated in consonance with hormonal changes, menstrual cycle and genetic build. In these cyclical changes, some lumps naturally form in the breast and may lead to misapprehension about breast cancer.

Most often, having larger breasts or feeling lumps or swelling in the breast is not indicative of cancer. These lumps, which sometimes appear harder or larger before menstruation, are usually normal and may occasionally, cause some tenderness and discomfort. This is suggestive of normal cyclical change of the breast and is not a disease. **Painful nodular breast is not a disease**, it is also called **ANDI** or **A**berration of **N**ormal **D**evelopment and **I**nvolution. Thus, feeling of occasional nodularity or pain in the breast during menstruation or pregnancy is a natural phenomenon.

The breasts of women lactate after childbirth. Some amount of breast proliferation pre - menstrually and involution in the post - menstrual period are regular phenomena. A little aberration leads to pain or nodularity or both in the breast of women in childbearing age. Women must consult the specialist whenever their discomfort rises too much. Doctors may advise X - ray **mammogram** to the women above 35 years of age and sono - mammogram for women under 35 years of age.

If a **separate or discrete lump** in the breast is felt, it should be critically examined. Doctors may advise core biopsy if the nodule in the breast is suspected to be malignant.

Breast Pain – Some women experience breast pain or heaviness a few days before their menstrual cycle begins, which is generally normal. This breast pain is referred to as **mastalgia** and usually subsides with the onset of menstruation. If breast pain lasts for an extended period or disrupts a woman's daily routine (such as dressing or sleeping), it is called **pronounced cyclical mastalgia**. It can be relieved with medications like **centchroman** or **danazol**. Vitamin E is not beneficial for this condition. Pain in breast temporally unrelated to menstrual cycle is called **non - cyclical mastalgia**.

Women who are breast feeding, having continuous pain, redness, localized swelling and tenderness with or without fever may be indicative of puerperal **breast abscess**. Milk flow in the milk - duct system may be obstructed leading to abscess. An abscess may also develop in older women and in women who are not lactating which is called **non puerperal breast abscess.** This must be treated with antibiotics, aspiration and sometimes surgical drainage. Milk ducts may be widened near the nipple causing severe soreness and painful nipple – the condition is referred as **duct ectasia** which occurs commonly in women about 35 - 45 years of age.

Tuberculosis of breast and chronic granular mastitis are also painful inflammatory and benign conditions of the breast. Tuberculosis in breast is treated by aspiration of TB abscess and anti - tubercular drugs. Chronic granular mastitis is a troubling inflammatory condition treated variously by corticosteroids, repeated drainage and the Ayurvedic alkaline seton called *kshar sootra*. Pain in the ribs and costal cartilages may also present like breast pain commonly seen in young women with calcium and Vitamin D deficiency —osteomalacia.

Other types of breast lumps – A discrete lump, which is usually not painful, accidently discovered by young women herself and is moveable on finger palpation (like mouse in the breast) is usually a benign lump called **fibroadenoma**. These may be single or multiple, usually 2 - 4 cm in size, sometimes larger also.

After examination, doctors may recommend either no intervention or surgical removal. Another type of lump that can occur, which may be slightly larger in size, is called a **phyllodes tumor**. These can be more dangerous and malignant. Surgical removal of the entire breast may be advised in phyllodes tumor. There are other various and rare types of lumps in the breast like fat necrosis, anti - bioma, hamartoma etc.

Breast Cancer – Breast cancer typically starts with the formation of a lump in the breast, sometimes in the axilla. It may be detected all of a sudden. Breast cancer develops in the cells of lobules (small glands) and ducts (tubes) of the mammary glands. Cancer of the ducts is called **ductal carcinoma** and cancer of the lobules is called **lobular carcinoma**.

Breast cancer cells which do not infiltrate the lining basement membrane of the duct, or the lobule is called **carcinoma *in situ*** – ductal carcinoma in situ (**DCIS**) and lobular carcinoma *in situ* (**LCIS**) respectively. Some key signs of breast cancer include the presence of a **discrete and new painless lump** in the breast that has somewhat thickened skin overlying it.

Nipple retraction or pulled up nipple, **skin thickening and dimpling** and mild tenderness on palpation may be present. Other symptoms of breast cancer can include breast enlargement, changes in breast shape, skin resembling an orange peel – *peau d' orange* and blood discharge from the nipple.

Remember, breast cancer often does not cause pain. Breast cancer can affect women at any age but most commonly presents in women between the ages of 45 and 55. Women who remain unmarried, marry at a later age with delayed first pregnancy or do not breastfeed and obese women have slightly higher risk towards breast cancer. Contact with X - rays (radiation rays) also increases the risk of breast cancer. If a woman's mother or sister had breast cancer, the risk of developing breast cancer is two to three times higher. Genetic factors, such as specific **genes like BRCA1 and BRCA2**, can also contribute to the risk of developing breast cancer.

Women with breast cancer presenting in both breasts either at the same time or one after another, who are younger in age with immediate family member like mother and sister having had breast cancer, or history of ovarian cancer also should be tested for BRCA1 and 2 genes.

Diagnosis and Investigation of Breast Cancer – Detecting a lump or mass in the breast can be done through skillful palpation using the flat of the hand against the chest wall, especially for lumps of 1 - 2 cm or larger. However, smaller lumps may not be easily detected, particularly in obese breasts. For accurate diagnosis, **high - resolution ultrasound** and **X - ray mammography** are commonly used. Women under the age of 35 usually undergo ultrasound, while those above 35 typically have X - ray mammograms. Mammograms are performed in two planes - cranio - caudal (vertical) and medio - lateral (horizontal) - to provide detailed images of the breast tissue.

Radiologists then evaluate these images using the **BIRADS (Breast Imaging Reporting and Data System)** scale, which ranges from BIRADS 1 to 5. A BIRADS score of 1 is normal, while BIRADS 5 signals a high suspicion of malignancy. It is important to note that mammography requires a specialized **low - voltage digital X - ray machine** to accurately detect abnormalities.

In countries with a higher incidence of breast cancer, such as in the West, **screening mammography** is often mandatory every two years for women starting at age 50.

This public health initiative helps detect early - stage cancers even in asymptomatic women, leading to better outcomes and lower treatment costs. Mammography is also useful for pinpointing suspicious areas in large or obese breasts, aiding in precise surgical removal.

The **definitive diagnosis** of breast cancer is made through a **biopsy**. If the tumor is large or has fungated, a knife biopsy may be necessary to remove a small wedge of tissue. However, a more common method is the **core needle biopsy** (Tru - Cut®), where a motorized or catapult - like device is used to extract a small core of tissue (10 - 15 mm x 2 mm) after local anesthesia. The tissue is preserved in formaldehyde and sent for **histopathology** and **immunohistochemistry** (IHC) to determine molecular markers of the cancer. In addition to breast examination, the **axilla** (armpit) is palpated to check for cancer spread to the lymph nodes. Further investigations like **ultrasound, X - ray, CT scan, isotope bone scan,** and **PET - CT scan** are used to assess the spread of cancer to other body parts, a process known as **staging**.

Types of Breast Cancer – Breast cancer occurs in the following **molecular subtypes** with different survival potential. These are treated in accordance with the denoted molecular markers.

- **Luminal A Subtype** – In this type of breast cancer, estrogen receptor (ER+ve) and progesterone receptor (PR+ve) are present and tumor is **hormone dependent**. Human Epidermal Growth Factor type 2 (HER2 neu) is not present. The overall incidence of Luminal A is 60 - 70 percent. However, in older women above 60 years it is 80 - 90 percent. Anti - estrogen drugs, aromatase inhibitors and selective estrogen receptor modifiers (SERMs) are highly effective drugs in treating this subtype. Thus, medications like tamoxifen, exemestane, ormeloxifene, letrozole, anastrozole are effective. This subtype has approximately 80% survival rate with treatment.

- **Luminal - B Subtype** accounts for 10% of total breast cancer cases. All three hormone receptors (ER, PR, and HER2/neu) are positive. Medications like trastuzumab (Herceptin), pertuzumab (Perjeta) and other targeted therapies are effective. Anti - estrogen drugs are less effective. Survival rate is ≈ 70 - 80%.

- **HER - 2 Positive or HER - 2 Enriched** type of breast cancer with HER2 receptor highly positive are seen in 10 - 12 % patients. Drugs like trastuzumab, pertuzumab are used. Overall prognosis is poor and survival rate < 60%.

- **Triple - Negative Breast Cancer (TNBC)** – In this type of breast cancer, all three hormone receptors (ER, PR, and HER2/neu) are negative i.e. no recognizable target or receptor is identifiable. It accounts for 15 - 20 percent breast cancer cases especially when detected at a younger age. Treatment options for triple - negative breast cancer are limited. Genetic testing may be necessary for this type of cancer when it is bilateral, and the family history of breast cancer is positive. BRCA1/2 genes are tested in TNBC. This cancer is mostly treated with chemotherapy drugs such as paclitaxel, platinum, doxorubicin (Adriamycin) and PARP inhibitors. TNBC BRCA gene positive patients are treated with drugs like pembrolizumab, Adriamycin, talazoparib, Olaparib etc.

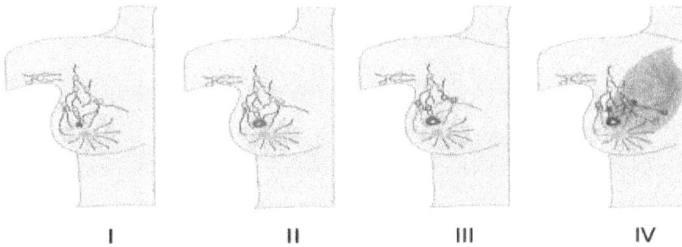

I   II   III   IV

Prognosis of TNBC is poor with survival rate ≈ 40 - 50%.

Breast Cancer Stage denotes size and peripheral spread of the tumor in 4 stages. **T** = tumor size, **N** = lymph node involvement number and size, **M** = metastasis in other body organs. Treatment according to the breast cancer stage may determine survival of the patient. The staging of breast cancer is illustrated as follows. **Stage 1** – tumor in breast is small < 2 cm with no regional spread. **Stage 2** – tumor may be 2 - 5 cm with few regional lymph nodes in axilla. **Stage 3** – tumor between 5 - 10 cm with big regional nodes in axilla and **Stage 4** – tumor is big, involves skin, ulcerates, axillary lymph nodes become large and fixed, or tumor may spread to distant organs like opposite breast, neck nodes, lung, liver, brain, bone etc.

Breast Cancer Treatment Modes– Breast cancer treatment has evolved significantly over the past century. In 1894, **Halsted's radical mastectomy** was the standard procedure, involving the complete removal of the breast, underlying muscles, and all axillary (armpit) lymph nodes. This extensive surgery was the main modality for nearly a century, with a 50 - 60% cure rate. However, advancements in **oncoplastic surgery**, breast conservation, and modern treatment methods have reduced the need for such radical surgery.

Today, breast cancer treatment incorporates a combination of **surgery, chemotherapy, radiotherapy, hormonal therapy,** and **targeted therapies**, allowing for less extensive surgical procedures, especially in early - stage diagnosis.

Surgery remains the cornerstone of breast cancer treatment. A **simple or total** mastectomy involves the complete removal of the breast from the chest wall using a **transverse incision**. When lymph nodes in the axilla (armpit) are also removed, it becomes a **radical mastectomy**.

However, axillary lymph node dissection can now be avoided in many cases using **sentinel node** biopsy technology, which helps determine whether cancer has spread to the lymph nodes without needing full dissection.

For smaller breast cancer size, **wide local excision (WLE**) is performed, where the tumor and a surrounding margin of 1 - 2 cm of healthy tissue are removed. The resulting void in the breast tissue is filled using **oncoplastic breast** surgery techniques, which rotate and reshape the remaining breast tissue. This allows for breast conservation while maintaining an aesthetic appearance. In cases where only the tumor - bearing area and some normal surrounding tissues are removed, the remaining breast tissue is treated with radiotherapy to eliminate any residual cancer cells. This **breast-conserving approach**, combined with radiotherapy, has become a standard option for many patients with early - stage breast cancer.

Chemotherapy has become more targeted, less toxic, and highly effective in the treatment of breast cancer. Typically, chemotherapy is administered in **3 - week cycles** through intravenous infusion, lasting 6 - 10 hours in a **day - care setting**. However, different regimens exist, and specific cancers respond better to certain drugs. Common agents include **taxanes, platinum, anthracyclines (such as doxorubicin or Adriamycin),** and **PARP** inhibitors in certain cases. One of the latest developments, **antibody - drug conjugates (ADCs)** like **Enhertu**, has shown high efficacy in treating certain subtypes of breast cancer.

Radiotherapy, often used as an **adjuvant treatment** following surgery or chemotherapy, helps eliminate residual cancer cells in the breast, axilla, or neck nodes. Delivered in **special shielded suites**, radiotherapy utilizes **gamma rays** or X - rays from sources like **cobalt -** 60 or **linear accelerators**. The radiation works by damaging the DNA of cancer cells directly or by releasing **free** radicals that further induce DNA damage, effectively killing the cancer cells.

Hormonal and Targeted Treatments are tailored based on the molecular subtypes of breast cancer. **Estrogen receptor antagonists** like **tamoxifen** or letrozole are used for hormone receptor - positive cancers. In **HER2 - positive cancers, trastuzumab** has significantly improved patient outcomes.

Additionally, **PARP inhibitors** such as **talazoparib** and olaparib have made a significant difference for patients with **triple - negative breast cancer. CDK 4/6 inhibitors** like **palbociclib** are highly effective in treating hormone receptor - positive metastatic breast cancer.

Breast Self - Examination (BSE) is a vital self - care practice that can help women detect lumps early. Women are encouraged to learn the technique of **self - breast examination (BSE)** and to practice it regularly, especially after menstruation. It is a proactive approach to breast health, and all women over the age of 20 should be aware of it and practice it monthly to detect any changes in their breasts.

A woman should begin **breast self - examination (BSE)** by standing in front of a mirror with her hands relaxed by her sides. Using the flat of her hand, particularly the first three fingers, she should apply gentle but firm pressure against the chest wall, examining each breast one at a time. During this process, she should closely observe any changes in breast size, redness, swelling, or abnormalities like dimpling, thickening of the skin, or lumps. Special attention should be given to the nipples for any signs of bleeding, changes in shape, or direction, and these should be compared with the other breast.

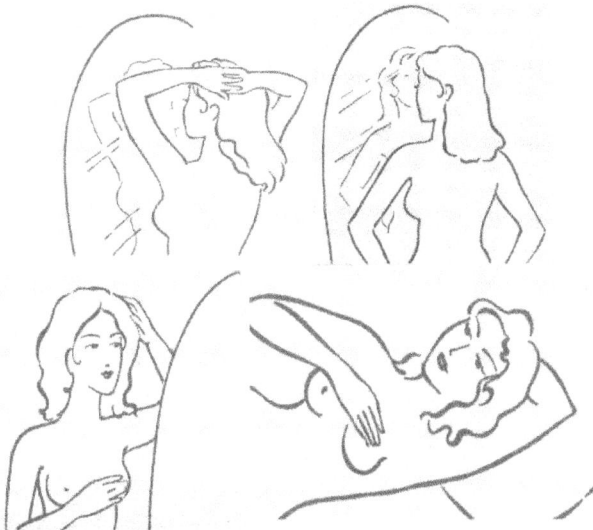

The examination should also be repeated while leaning forward so that the breasts fall away from the chest wall. During this position, the woman should lift each breast and feel it by rolling the tissue against the chest wall.

Another method of examination is while lying down on the bed. In this position, the breast tissue spreads out evenly, allowing for a more thorough check. By performing BSE standing, bending forward, and lying down, any unusual lump or abnormality can be detected early. If any suspicious changes are noticed, it is important to consult a family physician or specialist for further evaluation.

In conclusion, breast health is a significant concern for women, as breasts play a crucial role in lactation, sexuality, cosmetics, pride, and self - esteem. They are prone to various issues, including developmental problems, lactational challenges, breast pain (mastalgia), benign lumps, and breast cancer. Breast cancer remains a leading cause of death among women, with several subtypes identified. Advances in hormonal and targeted therapies have significantly improved survival rates for breast cancer patients. The importance of breast cancer screening cannot be overstated, as it helps detect cancer at earlier stages, improving outcomes through public health efforts. Additionally, innovations in breast conservation and oncoplastic surgery have enhanced the quality of life for those affected by breast cancer.

Chapter 37

Thyroid Disorders

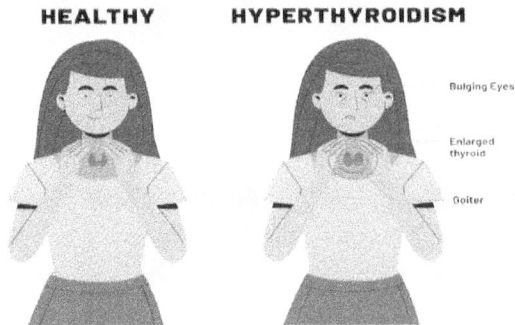

HEALTHY   **HYPERTHYROIDISM**

Bulging Eyes

Enlarged thyroid

Goiter

Learning Objectives:

- Essential functions performed by thyroid gland.

- Role of Iodine

- Thyroid disorders affecting metabolic processes

- Role of pituitary gland in balancing thyroid function

- Autoimmune and genetic diseases of thyroid

The thyroid is a vital endocrine gland responsible for secreting thyroid hormones that regulate numerous bodily processes. Positioned in the front of the neck and resembling a butterfly with two lobes connected by an **isthmus**, the thyroid ensures proper growth and overall function.

Regulation of Metabolism

Thyroid hormones, primarily T4 (thyroxine) and T3 (triiodothyronine), are crucial in controlling metabolic rates, influencing body weight, heart rate, digestive function, and bone and muscle health. These hormones regulate the body's energy usage and are critical for maintaining optimal metabolic activity.

Imbalances, such as low thyroid hormone levels, may lead to fat accumulation, fatigue, and rough skin, while excess hormones may cause accelerated metabolism. Thyroid hormone production relies on iodine from the diet and is regulated by the hypothalamus and pituitary gland. The pituitary gland secretes thyroid - stimulating hormone (TSH), which controls the levels of T3 and T4. The thyroid can become enlarged, resulting in goitre, and this can lead to either an overactive thyroid (hyperthyroidism) or an underactive thyroid (hypothyroidism), each with various causes and symptoms.

Hyperthyroidism is a condition in which the thyroid gland produces an excessive amount of thyroxine, leading to an increase in the body's metabolic rate. Hyperfunction of thyroid is also called **thyrotoxicosis**. Common symptoms include unexpected weight loss, rapid or irregular heartbeat, sweating, and irritability. Older individuals may experience fewer symptoms despite the condition. Diagnosis is confirmed by measuring thyroid hormones (T3, T4), TSH, and thyroid antibodies. Treatment options include anti - thyroid drugs, radioactive iodine, and, in some cases, surgery to remove part of the thyroid gland.

Hypothyroidism is the most common thyroid disorder, where the thyroid gland produces insufficient thyroid hormones. It may occur for unknown reasons, or an autoimmune disorder known as **Hashimoto's thyroiditis**.

A major study in India found hypothyroidism prevalence, including undiagnosed cases and anti - thyroid peroxidase (anti - TPO) antibody positivity, at around 10% of the population. Hypothyroidism slows down metabolism, heart rate, and body temperature, with symptoms such as fatigue, cold sensitivity, constipation, dry skin, unexplained weight gain, puffy face, hoarse voice, muscle weakness, scanty menstrual bleeding, and depression. A severe form, called **myxedema**, causes puffiness of the body.

Congenital Hypothyroidism - A severe form of hypothyroidism present at birth is known as **cretinism**, often caused by iodine deficiency during pregnancy. It results in stunted physical growth and mental retardation. Congenital hypothyroidism, which may be genetic or sporadic, can also be caused by **thyroid aplasia or hypoplasia**. If left untreated, it can lead to permanent physical and mental disability, though early diagnosis through neonatal screening allows for timely treatment.

Grave's Disease is an **autoimmune** disease that primarily affects adult women. It is characterized by the production of autoantibodies through the body's immune system that stimulate thyroid - stimulating hormone (TSH) receptors in the thyroid gland to secrete excess hormones.

These autoantibodies induce **hyperthyroidism** and **goiter** by mimicking the action of its natural ligand, TSH. In this disease, the body's immune system mistakenly attacks the thyroid gland and damages it incrementally. This condition can also be caused by genetic factors and is known as hereditary toxic goiter. There may be protruding eyes **(exophthalmos)** in Grave's disease.

Solitary and Multiple Nodules can form in the thyroid gland, which may be either fluid filled or solid (nodular). The nodules may be benign (non - cancerous) or malignant (cancerous). Some solid nodules can produce excess hormones, leading to toxic nodules or hyperthyroidism. If multiple nodules are present, it is called **multinodular goiter**. Some multi - nodular goiter can become very big. A few decades ago, patients neglected their thyroid enlargement which at times developed into huge multi - nodular thyroid gland enlargement. Such large thyroid gland enlargement or goiters were common in the sub - Himalayan area of northern India. Occasionally, thyroid nodules can be cancerous.

Iodine Excess /Deficiency of Iodine – Thyroid gland produces hormones using iodine. Iodine is present in various foods like strawberries, guava, pineapple, green beans, white beans, tuna fish, cod fish (rohu fish in India), milk, cheese, yogurt and egg yolks. In the past, iodine deficiency was widespread in India, leading to goiter (an enlarged thyroid gland).

Excess iodine intakes may be due to certain drinking waters, animal milk rich in iodine, certain seaweeds, iodine containing drugs and dietary supplements etc. Generally, high iodine intake is well tolerated, but in some people, excess iodine intake may precipitate hypothyroidism, goiter, hyperthyroidism and/or thyroid autoimmunity. Ingestion of over 1.1 mg/day of iodine may be harmful and can lead to acute and/or chronic toxicity.

Deficiency of iodine in the diet can lead to thyroid diseases especially goiter, and was a public health problem in many countries, including India.

To counter this problem, small doses of iodine element are added to the common salt (**iodized salt**) which substantially brings down the incidence of goiter.

In 1962 Government of India launched the **universal salt iodization (USI)** program and banned the sale of non - iodized common salt in states prone to endemic goiter.

According to world statistics data published in 2020, 124 countries have legislation for mandatory salt iodization and 24 have legislation allowing voluntary iodization. Eighty eight percent of the global population uses iodized salt only.

Thyroiditis – This is the inflammation of the thyroid gland which initially causes leakage of thyroid hormones resulting in hyperthyroidism – this is called the **thyrotoxic phase** of thyroiditis. Over a period of time, this inflammation impairs thyroid hormone production, resulting in underactivity or **hypothyroid phase**. When the thyroid hormone levels become normal – this is called **euthyroid phase**. Sometimes, symptoms may remain absent and when symptoms are manifested, they may vary according to the level of inflammation. Thyroid functioning will vary accordingly. Treatment of thyroiditis is focused on the underlying cause as well as regulating thyroid function based on symptoms.

Thyroiditis is of several types:

(i)   **Hashimoto's Thyroiditis** is the most common cause of hypothyroidism also known as **autoimmune lymphocytic thyroiditis**. It is caused by antithyroid antibodies by autoimmune or hereditary factors. The body's immune system attacks and damages one's own thyroid gland.

(ii)   **Silent or painless thyroiditis** is an autoimmune condition caused by antithyroid antibodies.

(iii)   **Postpartum Thyroiditis** occasionally occurs in approximately 5 - 10% of women, and it usually resolves on its own that is thyroid function returns to normal state within 12 to 18 months of the onset of the symptoms after childbirth.

(iv) **Radiation - induced thyroiditis** is a form of painful, acute thyroiditis resulting from radiation therapy to treat hyperthyroidism or from radiation to treat certain cancers like head and neck cancer or lymphoma or from radioactive iodine therapy.

(v) **Subacute thyroiditis or de Quervain's thyroiditis** is a painful condition thought to be the result of a viral infection. It is usually preceded by upper respiratory infection like sinus, throat, mumps, flu, common cold or a viral infection of the ear.

(vi) **Acute infectious thyroiditis** is a rare condition, usually seen in the elderly, chronically ill and immuno compromised patients. Generally, it is caused by an infectious organism or bacteria like Streptococcus, Mycobacteria, Pneumocystis and fungi.

(vii) **Drug - induced thyroiditis** is caused by the use of medications such as amiodarone, interferons, lithium and cytokines, occurring only in a small fraction of people.

(viii) **Riedel thyroiditis** is a rare disease caused by chronic inflammation and fibrosis (thickening or scarring of tissue) in the thyroid gland.

Thyroid Cancer – Thyroid cancer is a relatively less common cancer than oral, breast, lung, cervix, stomach and colon cancers in India. Its incidence is about 5 new cases of thyroid cancer per lakh population per year in India.

Thyroid cancer is primarily due to genetic factors with some environmental factors. There may be no symptoms, and it may be discovered incidentally as a lump in the neck or a thyroid nodule.

Warning signs of thyroid cancer – The physician while checking the patient in the clinic may feel a lump or growth in thyroid gland called a **thyroid nodule.** Most nodules are benign, only 3 out of 20 may be malignant or cancerous. Accompanying enlarged lymph nodes in the neck may be indicative of thyroid cancer.

Certain **symptoms** like difficulty in breathing or swallowing, hoarseness in voice, tiredness, loss of appetite, nausea and vomiting, unexpected weight loss are associated with a firm to hard thyroid enlargement.

Causes / risk factors for thyroid cancer include goiter, family history of thyroid cancer, thyroiditis, fluctuating thyroid hormone level during pregnancy or within the first year after childbirth, gene mutations like multiple endocrine neoplasia type 2A (MEN 2A) or type 2B (MEN 2B), low iodine intake, radiation therapy for head and neck cancer, especially during childhood, exposure to radioactive fallout from nuclear weapons or a power plant accident. Thyroid cancer can metastasize to other parts of the body like the liver, the lung, and the bones.

There are **four types** of thyroid cancer – some of which are less aggressive compared to others.

i) **Papillary thyroid cancer -** This is the most common, in about 80% of cases. It is a slow - growing differentiated thyroid cancer – i.e., the cancer cells are akin to normal thyroid cells. Papillary thyroid cancer spread to lymph nodes in the neck.

ii) **Follicular thyroid cancer** - This is the 2nd common thyroid cancer which is about 10 - 12% of all thyroid malignancies is. This develops from follicular cells which are cuboidal epithelial cells responsible for production of thyroid hormone. This is also a differentiated thyroid cancer. It can spread via blood stream to distant parts of the body and bones.

iii) **Medullary thyroid cancer (MTC) – this cancer accounts for** 2 - 3% of thyroid cancers, arises from C cells, which are special cells that make **calcitonin,** a hormone involved in calcium metabolism. This is a very aggressive cancer **with** a strong genetic predisposition. It can be part of a genetic syndrome called **multiple endocrine neoplasia type 2** (MEN2). It is poorly differentiated with very little, if any, similarity to normal thyroid tissue.

iv) **Anaplastic thyroid cancer (ATC)** accounts for 1% of thyroid cancers and can be very aggressive, poorly differentiated, fast growing and spreads quickly.

Treatment for both papillary and follicular thyroid cancer usually performed by complete removal of the thyroid gland – **total thyroidectomy**. MTC can sometimes be prevented by the technology of detecting proto - oncogene - *RET* (rearranged during transfection).

Meticulous surgical resection - total thyroidectomy and removal of lymph node from the neck may provide good survival to patients. Lifelong replacement of thyroid hormones is required after total thyroidectomy. ATC is usually nonoperable and does not respond to treatment. However, new therapy by immuno - oncologic methods with high throughput sequencing has paved the way to targeted therapies by revealing the molecular alterations of ATC. Like many other tissues, lymphoma, i.e., tumor of the lymphatic tissue, may develop in the thyroid gland from intrathyroidal **mucosa - associated lymphoid tissue** called MALT. These are generally treated by chemotherapy.

Thyroid Function Tests – Thyroid gland is examined by **palpation** if enlarged. An enlarged gland moves with swallowing and can be seen by a trained physician. Most of the time thyroid functions are tested and if these are normal, the patient is called **euthyroid**. The following table shows the normal values of the total and the free component of T3 and T4 hormones in blood. These values may vary between labs. Besides these certain antibodies are also tested in the blood. Serum levels of antibody against **thyroid peroxidase (TPO)** of 25 units/ mL and **anti - thyroglobulin** 1:100 titer is considered significant to diagnose autoimmune thyroiditis.

Diagnosis of Thyroid cancer is through various methods, similar to other types of cancer. These include **aspiration cytology** (fine - needle aspiration cytology or FNAC), sometimes done with ultrasound guidance, in which a needle is put into a thyroid nodule and thyroid cells sucked into a syringe for examination under the microscope. Biopsy is usually not done from thyroid gland. Ultrasound, X - rays, MRI scans and radioactive Iodine and Technetium scans are done to examine thyroid nodules, determine their size and assess their characteristics. Staging is done by screening the neck nodes and rest of the body by clinical examination, X - ray and PET CT scan.

Medications – The functional thyroid disorders are treated by replacement of thyroxine in case of hypo - functioning and anti - thyroid drugs in hyperthyroidism. Thyroid hormone is synthesized on a commercial basis.

Now synthetic thyroxine is available in plenty, and it is not very expensive. **Methimazole** and **propylthiouracil** are medications used to treat hyperthyroidism. **Beta - blocker drugs** may also be used to control symptoms of hyperthyroidism, such as a rapid heart rate.

Surgery – In cases of severe thyroid dysfunction - usually hyperthyroidism or thyroid cancer **thyroidectomy** (removal of the thyroid gland) may be performed. This surgery can be partial or total removal of thyroid gland, depending on the condition. The surgery of thyroid gland removal can be combined with lymph node dissection in the neck if so indicated.

It requires skillful surgery because the thyroid gland is closely associated with two vital nerves and para - thyroid glands which control body calcium levels. Nowadays thyroid gland can also be removed from inside the mouth or from axilla using laparoscope.

Radioactive Iodine Treatment – Radioactive iodine (radioiodine) therapy may be used to treat hyperthyroidism and thyroid cancer. This treatment requires lifelong replacement treatment with thyroxine.

In conclusion, the seemingly insignificant butterfly - shaped gland in front of the neck, nestled between the carotid artery and jugular vein, is the thyroid. Despite its small size, it acts as the master regulator of the body's metabolic activities. Hypothyroidism is its most common disorder, and it can also be affected by cancer. The absence of a functioning thyroid is incompatible with life, highlighting its critical role. It remains a focal point of medical discussions, underscored by the significant impact its dysfunction can have on overall health.

Chapter 38

Genetic and Hereditary Diseases

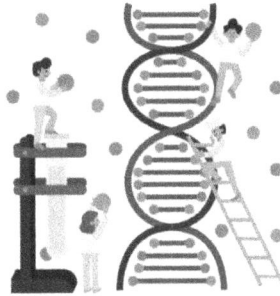

Learning Objectives:

- Genetic structure and functioning
- Difference between congenital, familial, hereditary and genetic diseases
- Chromosomal, monogenic and polygenic diseases
- Mendelian patterns of inheritance
- Investigation of genetic diseases

A gene is the fundamental unit responsible for determining physical and functional traits, which are passed down from parents to offspring. Congenital diseases or disorders, which are present from birth, may not necessarily be hereditary.

For instance, congenital rubella syndrome, caused by a mother contracting German measles during pregnancy, is congenital but not hereditary. Some congenital defects, such as heart defects or duodenal atresia, may not be evident at birth and require further investigation. The term **"hereditary"** typically refers to diseases with a known genetic cause. **Familial** disorders, on the other hand, are those that affect more family members than expected by chance and may have genetic and/or environmental causes.

Some genetic diseases are due to fresh **mutations** that arise in the affected individual (index patient). Modern medical science diagnoses such disorders through gene and chromosome testing and sequencing, offering a clearer distinction between these groups of diseases.

Genes are made up of **deoxyribonucleic acid or DNA**. The structure of DNA was elucidated in 1953 by two scientists – **James Watson** and **Francis Crick**. They described the DNA as a **double helix**. DNA and ribonucleic acid (RNA) are molecules essential for all living organisms. DNA consists of two long chains (double helix) made up of **nucleotides** (building blocks of DNA). Each nucleotide has **three parts**: **nitrogen base**, **phosphate** and **sugar** molecules.

There are 4 different nitrogen bases - **adenine (A), thymine (T), guanine (G) and cytosine (C)**. A always bonds with T, and G always bonds with C. The exact sequence of nucleotides determines the genetic code. There are about 3 billion base pairs, and 80,000 - 100,000 genes of varying lengths arranged on 23 chromosomes in the human genome. To **replicate** itself, the two chains from the double helical molecule separate, and then the complementary bases join to form a copy of the DNA. RNA is formed from DNA by a process known as **transcription**.

RNA is also made up of phosphate and sugar molecules bonded with nitrogen bases in sequence, but is single - stranded, the sugar is ribose, and the nitrogen bases are slightly different – **uracil** instead of thymine. RNA further forms protein by a process named **translation**. These proteins are often in the form of enzymes that take part in various vital biochemical reactions in the body. These biological processes of **replication, transcription and translation** which lead to incessant continuation of life from generation to generation are defined as **central dogma of genetics**.

The term **genotype** refers to the genetic makeup of an individual, or an allele, while **phenotype** refers to the effect of the genotype in terms of observable physical properties or function. DNA contains all the information needed for the functioning of the organism. Most of the DNA is in **chromosomes**, which are in the nucleus of the cell. Genes contain information about our inherited characteristics, such as color of hair or eyes, similarities in features of family members, etc.

Human beings have **23 pairs of chromosomes** (one of each pair from each parent), of which 22 are **autosomes** and the last pair are the **sex chromosomes** – X or Y. Males have X and Y sex chromosomes, while females have two X chromosomes. Every individual must have at least one X chromosome. Since the female is XX, each of her eggs has a single X chromosome. The male, being XY, can generate two types of sperms: half bearing the X chromosome and half the Y. If the egg receives another X chromosome from the sperm, the resulting individual is XX or female; if the egg receives a Y chromosome from the sperm, the individual is XY or male. The Y chromosome carries a gene that encodes a testis - determining factor which organizes the gonad into a testis, whereas XX chromosome organizes the gonad to produce ovaries in the fetus.

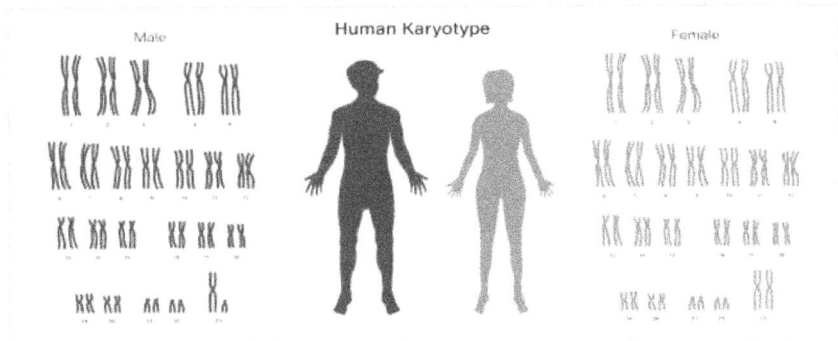

Human Karyotype

There are 2 types of **cell division** in all living organisms. **Mitotic** division occurs in all somatic cells (all cells except gametes – ovum, sperm). It does not involve the fusion of gametes (sperm from males and ovum from females), exchange of genetic material or change in the number of chromosomes. The other type of cell division is **meiosis**, which occurs only in the male and female gametes. In this process, "**crossing over**" of genetic material occurs between the strands of chromosomes. The cell divides to form a **haploid** cell with half the chromosome number. After fusion of male and female gametes each contributes their chromosomes to again form a **diploid** cell. In humans, this results in 23 pairs of chromosomes, for a total of 46 chromosomes. This union, known as **fertilization,** combines the genetic material from both parents and leads to the creation of an embryo and eventually a fetus.

Genes direct the production of proteins by the cell. Every living being and species has specific protein molecules that may have specific functions. There are about 80,000 - 100,000 genes in each human. Each person has two copies (**alleles**) of each gene, one of which is obtained from each parent. If both alleles are the same, the individual is **homozygous** for that allele. If the alleles differ from each other, the individual is **heterozygous** for that allele. The exact location of the allele on the chromosome is called the **locus**. Most genes are the same in each species. Only less than 1% of genes are different in different individuals, which play the role in defining different physical and mental characteristics and determining disease.

The **Human Genome Project** was a collaborative international scientific research endeavor with the aim of identifying, mapping and sequencing all of the genes of the human genome from a physical and functional standpoint. It started in 1990 and was completed in 2003.

Each gene has a different name, which are usually shown by English letters or groups of numbers. In this way, the name of the gene is written in a subtle way, such as cystic fibrosis gene is called CFTR. A permanent, disease - causing alteration in the DNA of a gene, is called **'mutation' or 'genetic variation'**. This mutation is usually on account of some fault during cell division. Mutations can be inherited from one or both parents or may occur *de novo*. If the mutation is present in the gametes, it affects all the cells in the body. Mutation may also occur in somatic cells during mitotic division due to chronic irritation, chemical substances or viral infections (contagion).Genes primarily have two functions – (1) to carry hereditary information and direct specific protein production (2) to enable gene reproduction, i.e. DNA replication.

Types of genetic disorders – Genetic disorders can be chromosomal, polygenic or monogenic (single gene disorders). These can vary from absence of a whole chromosome (as in **Turner syndrome** in which there is only one X and no Y chromosome) or presence of an extra chromosome (as in **Kleinfelter syndrome** which has XXY complement of sex chromosomes).

Trisomy – This is a chromosomal disorder in which there is an extra chromosome, usually due to **'non - disjunction'** during meiosis - trisomy. So, the person has 47 chromosomes instead of 46.

Down's syndrome, Edward syndrome and Patau syndrome are the most common trisomies. **Down's syndrome** or Mongolism is the most common chromosomal disorder and cause of intellectual disability. Apart from this, there are various other physical features – Mongoloid slant of the eyes, short stature, hypotonia (low muscle tone), flat occiput (back of the head), short broad hands, single palmar crease (or simian crease), clinodactyly (short curved little finger), increased distance between the first and second toes etc. Defects in internal organs include hypothyroidism, congenital heart defects, imperforate anus (blocked anal passage) and duodenal atresia (obstruction of first part of small intestine). Prevalence of Down's syndrome increases with maternal age.

Reciprocal Translocations – This involves the exchange of genetic material between two non - homologous chromosomes.

Robertsonian Translocation – involves the fusion of two acrocentric chromosomes (chromosomes with the centromere close to one end) where the entire genetic material of one chromosome is translocated to another chromosome. In Robertsonian translocation, the whole chromosome is joined end to end with another. This type of translocation involves chromosomes 13, 14, 15, 21 and 22 only because their short arms have similar repetitive DNA sequences that predispose to their fusion.

Apart from these, there are other **sub - microscopic** defects in chromosomes in which some parts may be either **deleted** or **duplicated**. These are called '**copy number variations (CNVs)**. They are often associated with intellectual disability with or without **dysmorphisms** (which are minor physical abnormalities, such as high arched palate, hypertelorism (increased distance between the eyes), simian crease etc.

Polygenic inheritance – Many traits are inherited through many alleles present in different loci, such as phenotypic characters present in plants and animals. Examples of such traits are hair color, height, skin pigmentation, tendency to lose hair in youth, etc. Multiple independent genes have an additive effect on a single quantitative trait.

Monogenic inheritance – Here mutation in a single gene is responsible for causation of disease. Single gene disorders follow the principles of **Mendelian inheritance**.

Gregor Mendel was an Austrian monk and biologist who in 1865 propounded the rules of inheritance through a series of tedious experiments on the pea plant. These rules apply even to human genetics to the present day. Mendel's laws are:

(i) Law of segregation

(ii) Law of independent assortment and

(iii) Law of dominance.

Autosomal Dominant disorders – Disorders in which only one defective copy of an autosomal gene is required to cause disease are called autosomal dominant. As a result, affected individuals have one normal and one mutated allele. Autosomal dominant disorders can therefore be inherited from one affected parent who also has one defective copy of the gene or can occur sporadically as a result of a new mutation in the patient with no family history.

Examples are Huntington's disease (mutation on chromosome # 4), **Marfan's syndrome** (mutation on chromosome #5) and **achondroplasia**. Fifty percent of offspring will get the disease from an affected parent and the remaining 50% will be free of the disease mutation. However, severity of the phenotype may be highly variable (**variable expression or penetrance**).

Autosomal Recessive disorders – Here, both the mother and father must have the mutated gene. Inheriting the mutated gene from one parent is not enough to produce the disease phenotype, which is why it is called 'recessive'. If parents have the recessive gene, then 25% of offspring will manifest the disease, 50% will be **carriers** of the trait (i.e. they could also pass on the disease to 25% of their offspring if their partner also had the trait), and the remaining 25% will be normal. The expression of these diseases is not necessary in every generation of the affected family, and complete generations may be 'skipped'.

Examples are **cystic fibrosis** (caused by mutations in the CFTR gene) which affects the lungs, pancreas, and other organs, **sickle cell anemia** (caused by mutations in the HBB gene) and many inborn errors of metabolism like **phenylketonuria**.

X - Linked Recessive disorders – These disorders occur when there are different forms of genes (antipodes) on the X chromosome. In females, there are two X chromosomes. The gene being recessive does not manifest in the heterozygous state as it is 'dominated' by the allele on the other X chromosome. In males, there is only one X chromosome, so the mutated gene remains unopposed and manifests the disease. Most patients are male. Fifty percent of male offspring develop the disease and 50% of female offspring are carriers. Examples are hemophilia (a bleeding disorder), Fabry Disease (accumulation of a specific lipid) and Duchenne's muscular dystrophy (a muscle disease).

X - Linked Dominant disorders – Here the gene mutation is on the X chromosome, but it is dominant. So, it manifests in 50% of both male and female offspring and there are no carriers. Examples are Rett syndrome and X linked hypophosphatemic rickets.

Trinucleotide Repeats – Trinucleotide repeat disorders are a group of human diseases primarily affecting the nervous system, that are caused by the expansion of trinucleotide repeats within a gene. There is repetition of a three - nucleotide sequence in the DNA. Examples of such disorders include **Huntington's disease** (neurodegenerative disorder that leads to motor dysfunction, cognitive decline, and psychiatric symptoms), **Fragile X syndrome** (intellectual disability, behavioral problems and social deficits)**, Friedreich's ataxia, myotonic dystrophy etc.** The number of repeats increases with each generation which causes a more severe disease with lower age at presentation.

Codominance – In genetics, codominance is the phenomenon wherein the two alleles of a gene are expressed to an equal degree. As a result, traits associated with each allele are simultaneously expressed in the phenotype.

The human ABO blood group system is an example of codominance. Persons with type AB blood have alleles for both A and B, *while* the O allele is recessive, and its expression is masked by the other alleles.

Mitochondrial Inheritance – Mitochondria are structures in each cell that convert glucose into energy that is easily used by our cells. They are the energy house of the cells.

Cells contain thousands of mitochondria located in the cytoplasm around the cell nucleus. Mitochondria also have some genetic material – DNA.

Mitochondrial disorders are **inherited from one's mother**. Defects related to mitochondria develop in the embryo while it is developing into a female egg. This type of disorder cannot be inherited from father to son. In each generation, due to mitochondrial variants, the altered form of DNA is expressed, resulting in some symptoms in offspring. Examples of mitochondrial DNA - related disorders include **Leigh syndrome, mitochondrial myopathy** and **MELAS syndrome**, among others.

Epigenetics is the study of how the environment can cause changes that affect the way genes work. Unlike genetic changes, epigenetic changes are reversible and do not changes DNA sequence, but they can change how the body reads a DNA sequence. Examples of epigenetic changes are :

(i)   DNA methylation i.e. addition of a methyl group, to a part of the DNA molecule, which prevents certain genes from being expressed and

(ii)   histone modification

Genomic Imprinting – This is a process whereby only one gene copy from one parent is expressed, and combined with mutations, may lead to disease. There is thus exclusive expression of specific genes from only one parent. Imprinted genes are more vulnerable to the negative effects of mutations. In addition, genes and mutations that are recessive can be expressed if the dominant allele is silenced due to imprinting.

This expression of genes is called uniparental (meaning originating from one parent). In this process, the DNA sequence remains unchanged, meaning that external agents or the environment do not alter the DNA gene sequence. Prader - Willi syndrome and Angelman syndrome are the first diseases discovered to be due to imprinting. Both conditions are caused by deletion of 15q11 - q13 region on chromosome 15. However, the parental origin of the defect is different. While Prader - Willi syndrome is caused by a deletion of paternally inherited genes on chromosome 15, Angelman syndrome is caused by the loss of a maternally inherited gene in the same region of chromosome 15.

Genome - Wide Association Studies (GWAS) – This is a research approach in which genomic variants are identified that are statistically associated with risk for a disease or a particular trait. This is a collaborative work in which the information is spread worldwide. Scientists are not only gaining knowledge about the origin of genetic disease but are also researching treatment for diseases caused by gene defects.

Genetic Disease Testing and Diagnosis

Karyotype – This test examines 23 pairs of chromosomes using G - banding and is observed under a microscope during metaphase. Gross defects in number and structure of chromosomes are elucidated.

Fluorescence In - Situ Hybridization (FISH) – This technique uses fluorescent probes to bind specific genes or regions of DNA. It is used when a specific defect is suspected.

MLPA (Multiplex Ligation - dependent Probe Amplification) – This approach detects DNA copy number variations - deletions and duplications through a multiplex PCR assay. It is commonly used for elucidating the cause of intellectual disability with a yield of about 10%. Specific suspected copy number variations are looked for and identified.

Chromosome Microarray – Sub - microscopic structure (sub - telomere) of the entire genome is studied by chromosomal microarray. Copy number variations in the whole genome are identified without looking for specific defects. Microarray has become the first line test for intellectual disability of unknown cause.

Next generation sequencing (NGS) is the most recent genomic technique of sequencing all the protein - coding regions (exons) of genes in a genome in a rapid and cost - effective manner. There are about 180,000 exons – about 1% of the human genome.

Whole Exome Sequencing (WES) – An exome is the sequence of all the protein - coding portions of a genome. In humans, the exome is about 1% to 1.5% of the genome. This type of genetic sequencing technique provides clues to genetic diagnosis. There are 2 steps in WES - the first step is to select the DNA that encodes proteins. The 2nd step is to sequence the exonic DNA using high - throughput DNA sequencing technology.

The idea of this approach is to find genetic variations that alter protein sequences in the exome, at a much lower cost than **whole - genome sequencing**.

WES is becoming more accessible and less expensive for use in modern genetic diagnosis but has many pitfalls as unexpected genetic variations may be identified, which opens the door to many **ethical dilemmas**. A discussion around such possibilities should be held with the family before going for the test.

Whole Genome Sequencing (WGS) – The sequencing of the entire genome is performed using Next - Generation Sequencing (NGS). Unexpected variations may be found, which are pathogenic, likely pathogenic or of uncertain significance. WGS has enormous scope in detecting variations in the entire genome, but at present it is mostly experimental and too expensive.

Genetic Counselling – This is a specialized process by which trained medical personnel help individuals and families who are affected by or are at risk for genetic disorders – this counselling helps patients/families to understand and adapt to the implications of genetic disease. The first step is usually to fully investigate and reach a final genetic diagnosis in the **index patient.**

The index patient is the first known case suffering from a genetically pre - determined cancer or mutation or genetically transmitted condition. The consequences of the disease in the index patient are explained. Chances of other family members and future offspring being affected are discussed. Finally, the options before the family are explained, allowing for an informed decision i.e. deciding the best choice suitable for them. In some cases, if the unborn child is also proven to be affected, the family may opt for abortion.

In conclusion, genetics, as a relatively new specialty in modern medicine, has advanced rapidly over the past 70 years. The understanding of DNA structure, the decoding of the genetic code, the elucidation of the central dogma, protein synthesis, and techniques such as whole genome sequencing have propelled genetic science into deeper exploration of human traits and diseases.

Genetics has illuminated medical science, enabling modern scientists to address some of the most complex challenges in clinical medicine. While certain genetic diseases are rare, their recognition and diagnosis are crucial, as they can impact future generations if left unchecked. Prenatal genetic diagnosis through fetal **chorionic villus biopsy** helps prevent the birth of genetically affected infants. Many genetic disorders are now considered treatable, offering new avenues for research and medical advancements. Genetic counseling is gaining prominence, highlighting the need for more skilled professionals in the field of genetics in our country.

Chapter 39

Ano - Rectal Problems – Constipation, Fissure, Piles, Fistula, Rectal Prolapse and Cancer

Learning Objectives:

- Understanding how Constipation may lead to anal fissure, piles and fistula

- Inadequate consumption of roughage and fibrous food reduces bowel motility and causes constipation

- Anal hygiene and proper ablution, *Yog* and exercise are the natural ways to abate anal problems

- Hemorrhoids, fissure and fistula-in-ano – types, grading and treatment

- Symptoms and treatment of rectal prolapse and anorectal cancer

Feeling hungry is a natural signal from our body to replenish energy and nutrients, and the daily cycle of eating and passing stools ensures the smooth functioning of our bodily systems. Food not only provides essential energy but also nutrients for growth and repair. Equally important, regular bowel movements and urination help detoxify the body. Maintaining regular and healthy bowel movements is crucial for overall well - being.

The anus, a small yet significant 4 cm long canal, follows the rectum and plays a critical role in controlling defecation. The complex structure of the anal sphincter, made of both longitudinal and circular muscle fibers, allows for precise control over stool release. The abundant mucus glands in the anus help lubricate the passage, ensuring smooth evacuation of feces.

The tightly sealed closure of the anus, with its richly supplied blood vessels and mucosal folds, ensures continence - allowing safe discharge of flatus (gas) without leakage or soiling.

The rectum, which is about 15 cm in length, acts as a storage site for feces until defecation occurs. After food passes through the small intestine, where the majority of nutrients are absorbed, it enters the large intestine. In the large intestine, water and remaining nutrients are absorbed, and the remaining waste is formed into stool. The process from the stomach to the large intestine typically takes about 6 - 8 hours. Gut bacteria in the large intestine play a key role in breaking down undigested food, turning it into stool for elimination. Understanding the importance of the digestive and excretory processes highlights the necessity of maintaining a healthy diet and regular bowel habits to support good health.

All this happens on account of ever continuing intestinal **gut motility**. At the end of the complete digestion the remaining food gets converted into well - formed fecal matter which is offloaded in the rectum. Rectum with its enormous capacity for receptive dilatation fills up with stool. With habitual morning hour 'prompting' or at an appropriate opportunity, the person goes to the toilet and evacuates. Normally, stool evacuation should take just a few minutes or 2 - 3 bouts of expulsion. However, in case of poor motility of bowel some people spend long hours and also strain in expelling stools. It is this habit of constant straining with the stools that leads to anal fissures, piles and perianal infections. Bowel movements can be regulated by various diet with lot of fiber, water, anal hygiene, exercise, *yog - pranayam*, meditation, mental equanimity etc. Various problems regarding anal diseases can thus be avoided.

Constipation - Fecal matter collects in the rectum and is expelled through the anus. Inability to completely clear the bowel within few minutes signifies constipation. Constipation is ubiquitous as most people suffer from it at some time or other. However, frequent, chronic or severe constipation is a cause of concern. Many have sequalae like fissure, hemorrhoids, abscess, fistula and pruritus.

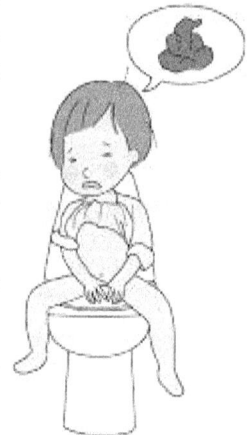

Medications for constipation are heavily advertised by celebrities at a high premium because constipation is a huge market for drug manufacturers. Constipation is a condition wherein the person remains uncomfortable in passing stool and his bowel movement is infrequent. Ideally, one should have bowel clearance once on each day, but it is said that three times a day to 3 times in a week may be considered normal bowel habit. However, a person is considered to be constipated when bowel movements result in passage of small amounts of hard, dry stool, usually fewer than three times a week. There may also be sense of incomplete evacuation, and the person may take more than few minutes on the toilet seat. How much time should one spend on the toilet seat is a matter of training from childhood. Careful parenting requires diet training with plenty of fiber and water. Stool training begins with spending only a few minutes in the toilet seat.

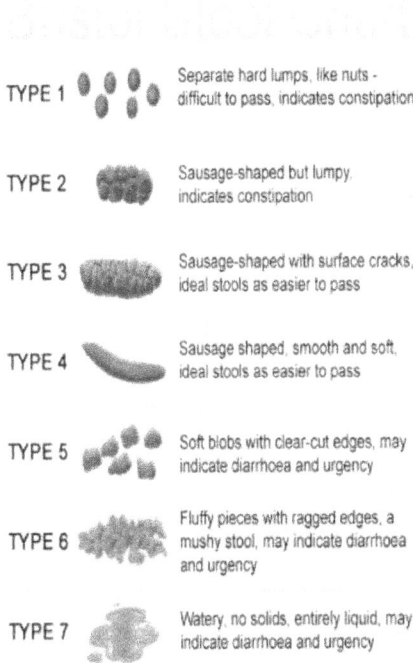

TYPE 1	Separate hard lumps, like nuts - difficult to pass, indicates constipation
TYPE 2	Sausage-shaped but lumpy, indicates constipation
TYPE 3	Sausage-shaped with surface cracks, ideal stools as easier to pass
TYPE 4	Sausage shaped, smooth and soft, ideal stools as easier to pass
TYPE 5	Soft blobs with clear-cut edges, may indicate diarrhoea and urgency
TYPE 6	Fluffy pieces with ragged edges, a mushy stool, may indicate diarrhoea and urgency
TYPE 7	Watery, no solids, entirely liquid, may indicate diarrhoea and urgency

Anal hygiene with proper ablution is inculcated from childhood and it develops as a habit. Constipation is best avoided by drinking 3 to 4 liters of water in a day, consuming lukewarm water and increasing the consumption of fibrous foods like salads, carrots, radishes, cucumbers and fruits. The intake of low residual diet consisting of *ghee*, oil, refined flour, white sugar and sweets, milk only diet, red meat, alcohol, etc. makes the stool solid hard (Type 1, 2, 3 in the image).

Traditional Indian medicines like *Triphala*, *Harad* (Terminalia chebula), *Amla* (Indian gooseberry), *Munakka*, *Chhuhara*, *Anjeer* and *Khajur*, are beneficial for constipation. Natural Remedies – seasonal fruits, *bel* (wood apple), *jamun* (Indian blackberry), *isabgol* (psyllium husk) and laxatives may fend off constipation. Jaggery and unrefined sugar are more beneficial than refined sugar. Excessive consumption of refined sugar leads to a decrease in friendly bacteria in the gut.

Similarly, harmful bacteria multiply with intake of processed, preserved and refined food. Changing one's diet, drinking plenty of water, yog, *manduk - asana* can alleviate the suffering borne out of constipation.

Types of Constipation – There are two types of constipation:

Functional constipation is occasional and without any specific cause. All internal functions remain normal or natural, but constipation occurs. No physical cause is traced even after thorough examination and investigations. Functional constipation occurs when people travel to another place; do not find a suitable toilet facility, diet change, altered water quality and oscillating duty rota. This is generally temporary and responds to home and traditional remedies. Functional constipation generally reverts after returning to normal domestic routine in food and wake–sleep pattern. Some people suffer functional constipation more frequently than others.

Chronic constipation: This refers to disturbance in propulsive movements (peristalsis) of the intestines. Feelings of blockage, lumps in the abdomen are described. Patients may resort to finger evacuation. Constipation can also be caused by factors such as depression or thyroid hormone imbalances. Pregnancy and old age both are associated with constipation, as are immobility and being bedridden.

Certain drug intake especially **opioids** can cause severe constipation. Young babies and children have troubling chronic constipation and pediatricians generally advise mothers to change their diet of children. Breast fed babies may not pass stools for several days because breast milk is very well absorbed. Stools remain soft, however. It is important to think of and exclude a severe motility disorder of the colon - **Hirschsprung's disease** which presents in infancy. In older people, cancer of the large bowel may present constipation.

When a person seeks medical advice for chronic or severe constipation, the physician may conduct a thorough examination of the anal region to check for signs like fissures, itching, redness, or other irritations. Assessing fecal leakage (incontinence), anal hygiene, and the tone of the anal sphincter is essential to determine the underlying cause of constipation. In many cases, physicians recommend a diet rich in fiber and encourage regular exercise to improve bowel movements.

However, if constipation persists, more detailed investigations such as **proctoscopy** (examining the anal canal and rectum), **colonoscopy** (viewing the entire colon), or **biopsy** (to analyze any abnormal tissue) may be necessary. These procedures, along with imaging studies, help to identify any underlying issues like **diverticula** (pouches in the colon), growths, or **motility disorders** affecting the rectum and anus.

Additionally, it is crucial to recognize that chronic constipation can increase the risk of developing **urinary tract infections (UTIs).** This is because prolonged straining and the buildup of stool can exert pressure on the urinary tract, potentially leading to infections. **Common conditions of anus, rectum and lower large intestine**

Anal Fissure or Crack at the anal opening – Anal fissure is a crack or tear (a linear ulcer) causing severe pain and some bleeding during defecation. It is usually caused by prolonged and excessive pressure on the anal canal by hard stools due to the forceful act of defecation. Anal fissure is a common problem that can occur at any age, often due to factors like poor dietary habits, lack of exercise or constipation. Once fissure develops and defecation becomes painful a vicious cycle sets in leading to more constipation. In **acute anal fissure** the anal sphincter can go into spasm leading to excruciating pain during and after defecation. Acute fissure is not a serious condition and can be treated with dietary changes, exercise, **sitz bath** (sitting with buttocks submerged in medicated warm water), lubrication and certain medications. Home remedies can also help in healing fissures within 8 - 10 weeks.

If a fissure persists for a long time, it is referred to as a **chronic or persistent fissure**. Chronic fissures can be associated with certain conditions such as **Crohn's disease, anal cancer, and anal tuberculosis**. The infected base of fissure harbors bacteria and leads to abscess in the anal area called **perianal abscess**. This abscess, when bursts, leads to a communicating infected track discharging pus which is also very painful. This is called anal or **perianal fistula**. Piles and fistulas may occur together.

Treatment of acute and chronic anal fissure involves avoiding constipation and prolonged straining during defection. All out efforts include dietary changes, exercises and identifying a secondary cause. Lubrication, home remedies and judicious use of modern medicines are suggested.

Attendant infection should be treated with appropriate antibiotic and anti - amoebic drugs. Oral and local cream of metronidazole is effective. Since fissure is a painful condition non - opioid pain - relieving agents orally and local anesthetic jellies are prescribed. The tight sphincter is relaxed by using smooth muscle relaxing agent like diltiazem, nitroglycerine and xylocaine anesthetic cream. Botox - injection in the internal sphincter may also do the trick. Hot bath fomentation is soothing and eases the passage of stool. Surgically acute and chronic anal fissures are treated with an excellent procedure called **lateral internal sphincterotomy** where a sharp cut at 3'O clock position is made in lower fibers of internal sphincter leading to almost instant easing of the passage of stool. Eminent relief of constipation is a must. Some pain - relieving medications and anal lubrication may also be prescribed. Not infrequently anal fissures have small or big skin tags hanging. This forms on account of constant straining and is fancifully called **'sentinel pile'** because it harbors and hides the fissure on its internal surface. Fecal particles collect underneath such skin tags. Fecal matter constantly rubs and infects the anal skin causing fissure. Thus, sentinel piles should also be removed to avoid recurrence of fissure.

Hemorrhoids – Also known as **piles**, hemorrhoids are a common condition worldwide. Hemorrhoids are a cluster swollen, distended and thickened blood vessels. Nearby supporting tissues, muscles and elastic fibers get amassed along with nerve endings. Thus, they torment us in the day - to - day activity. Hemorrhoids are known for familial predisposition and may occur in several members of the same family. It is said to be due to weakness in the vascular cushion (venous plexus) existing under the lining of anal mucosa. The blood vessels dilate and become tortuous, especially during constipation and straining during defecation. When managed properly, they can be cured, but if left untreated, they can become extremely **painful** and bleed. Hemorrhoids are of two types - **Internal and External Hemorrhoids.**

Grade I hemorrhoids are those that do not prolapse or come out when one sits to defecate. In case of strenuous and prolonged defecatory process these may bleed. Chronic bleeding from internal hemorrhoids for months and years can lead to severe **anemia**. A unique feature of this condition is its **intermittent character** – the symptoms of internal hemorrhoids exacerbate and abate.

Long duty hours, heavy diets, party and spicy foods, alcohol, smoking and tobacco, long and frequent travelling, neglecting proper anal ablution and lubrication lead to exacerbation in the symptoms of piles. **Grade II hemorrhoids** protrude outside during defecation and straining but go inside once relaxed. **Grade III hemorrhoids** are bigger and protrude so much that they have to be manipulated by fingers each time and pushed back inside anus after defecation. **Grade IV hemorrhoids** are those in which blood clots in these dilated veins (**thrombosed hemorrhoids**) become organized with fibrous tissue and cannot be pushed inside anus by fingers. Grade IV piles in substantively organized stage may develop a covering of skin - these are called external **hemorrhoids**.

Symptoms include pain and burning, itching, soiling with stools while bleeding may now become infrequent. There may be associated fissures which make it even more painful both during rest and defecation. Long standing hemorrhoids can be associated with idiosyncratic behavior, some **fecal incontinence**, constant pain, itching, a sense of incomplete evacuation and chronic anemia.

Treatments of hemorrhoids – In modern and traditional medicines hemorrhoid treatments are more or less similar in principle. Hemorrhoids in their initial stage (that is non prolapsed grade I hemorrhoids) can be treated by conservative therapy consisting of high fiber diet (25 - 35 gm per day), green leafy vegetables, fiber supplementation, increased water intake up to 2 - 3 liters, minimum defecation duration with thorough ablution, warm water sitz baths (anus dipped in water) with hot fomentation, pharmaceutical lubricants like oil, various piles alleviating ointments and stool softeners. In grade II hemorrhoids also, all - out efforts must be made to ease constipation. Similar measures are not so effective in grade III and IV piles. With the protrusion of hemorrhoids in grade III and grade IV, that is with the symptoms of heavy bleeding, strenuous, piercing and distressing pain one must also take **retreat from strenuous work** and heavy sports.

It is better to go 2 - 3 times to evacuate rather than sit in the toilet seat for long. Certain perineal exercises – **Kegel exercise or *Yog*** exercise *mula - bandha, uddiyana - bandha* may be helpful in which perineal muscles are repeatedly pulled up for strengthening. However, once the person returns to a hectic life and food the problem may return.

Surgical intervention is to ablate the tortuous and dilated venous plexus that form the protruded and bleeding pile masses. Several methods are available to achieve this. Ayurvedic treatments like ***Kshara Sootra*** or an **alkaline Seton** is used to tie the pile masses inside the anus. This leads to necrosis of distal pile mass which sheds away. One has to be careful not to tie the pile outside the anus where it becomes extremely painful and may cause an ulcer. An alkaline *kshara* liquid is also applied on the surface of protruding piles with lesser success. In modern medicine the same is achieved by putting a **rubber band** at the neck (pedicle) of the pile on the mucosal side. **Sclerotherapy** is used for internal piles like grade I, II and III and even actively bleeding piles. A sclerosant chemical is injected submucosally as high as possible. Three to five piles can be injected in a single sitting.

Infrared Rays (IR) or Radio Frequency Ablation (RFA) can also be used to fulgurate hemorrhoid tissue causing them to shrink and heal.

Similarly, Nd: YAG (neodymium - doped yttrium aluminum garnet) **laser** is also used to abrogate the protruding grade IV bleeding piles. Sclerotherapy, rubber band ligation of the pedicle or laser fulguration generally provide equivalent results in grades I – III piles and may have to be repeated a few times to treat remaining and new emerging piles.

Surgery for Hemorrhoids - In cases of Grade III and IV hemorrhoids with extensive internal and external masses, surgery that is **hemorrhoidectomy** may be performed. In this operation, both internal and external hemorrhoids, whether bleeding or not, are dissected from below upwards up to the neck or origin and tied or ligated with sutures.

The mucosa overlying the pile is repaired skillfully. Another procedure is called **hemorrhoidal artery ligation or HAL** Here an ultrasonic Doppler device or finger palpation is used to locate 3 or 4 hemorrhoidal arteries at the apex of the hemorrhoid mass which are tied off in a specific manner using a 5/8 curved needle and suture. This makes the hemorrhoids shrink back and fibrose. Another surgical method is by a gun like circular **stapling machine.** The hemorrhoidal masses are captured along with mucosal lining in the anvil of the stapling device and then they are cut. Steel staples approximate the upper and lower cut ends of mucosa removing the pile bearing mucosal donut.

The staples are removed *en - block* with all the pile masses in the entire circumference of the anorectum. Unfortunately for some people having hemorrhoids is not a one–time experience – these recur in 5 - 20% despite all kinds of treatment described above. Hemorrhoids recur on and off for various reasons like habit of sitting in toilet for long time and medical conditions like recurrent diarrhea or constipation. The recurrent piles are treated in the same way as above.

Fistula - in - Ano and Anal Abscess (Perianal Abscess) – An abscess or fistula can develop near the anus, commonly referred to as perianal abscess.

There are mucous glands in the anal canal which lubricate the anus and ease the passage of stools. Bacterial infection in the crevices of the mucous gland leads to the formation of an abscess adjacent to anal canal, causing severe pain. This abscess can burst inside the anus i.e. internally as well as around the anal opening (externally). In this manner, an outer opening connects to an internal cavity through a narrow passage called a **fistulous track**. The anal fistulae may be a single track, multiple tracks, straight - on with a short course and length, curvilinear or horseshoe shaped. The internal opening may be low down in the anus or may be high up in the rectum, traversing through the muscles of the ano - rectum - the internal and external sphincters. Several types of classifications are described for these fistulae.

There is a mild continuous seepage of fecal material from the internal opening and over time, it forms a chronic channel breeding several infections. This condition is known as **'chronic recurrent fistula - in - ano'**. The perianal skin is loose and the perianal area in the buttocks consists of fat and connective tissue where bacteria colonize easily. The infected anal crypt of the anal mucous gland becomes a continuous source of seepage of organic material where bacteria thrive.

Treatment of Anal Fistula - MRI or **magnetic resonance imaging** is done and also **blue dye test** is done to delineate the course and location of anal fistula. Maintaining proper anal hygiene, antibiotics for infections and all - out effort to treat constipation are cardinal to treatment of anal conditions. Warm compresses, antibiotics and anal ointments deliver soothing relief to patients with fistula.

Generally, antibiotics are given by family doctors but no amount of antibiotic or other medical treatment heals this condition. This is an ever painful, embarrassing, pus discharging problem next to anus and has been appropriately called a *nasoor* – surgical treatment though the ultimate answer also does not exclude frequent recurrences.

Simple fistula or sub - sphincteric fistula are treated simply by laying open the track, curettage and cleaning of its infected lining. This is performed at certain intervals to let the tissue heal speedily.

Treatment of deeper or higher fistulae is more challenging. Occasionally, there may be other types of fistulas as well like an inter - sphincteric fistula.

Surgery in Anal Fistula is usually performed in general, spinal, regional block or perianal anesthesia. Classical surgical treatment involves complete excision of the fistula track called **fistulectomy**. Although this gives good results in simple and superficial fistula, in deeper / higher fistulae fecal incontinence may result. Therefore, newer techniques like - **ligation of the inter - sphincteric fistula track (LIFT)** procedure is a treatment for fistulas that pass through the anal sphincter muscles, where a fistulectomy would carry a risk of fecal incontinence. The fistulous track is interrupted surgically by cutting and ligating to seal off the internal opening and the portion of the track below the anal sphincter muscle is excised. Another technique is **video assisted anal fistula treatment – VAAFT.** Here a long, thin tube with a small camera at the end is put into the fistula. An electrode is then passed through the endoscope and fistula fulgurated and sealed. Endoscopic ablation works well and there are no serious concerns about its safety. But the success rate may be low because frequently fistula tract is not a single linear track and has many out - pouching cavities, canaliculi and ramifications.

Laser fulguration of the fistulous track is done using a laser probe with success in about 65% patients. The failure mostly occurs in high or deeply situated curvilinear or horseshoe shaped trans - sphincteric or supra - sphincteric complicated anal fistulae. This encouraged the surgeons to adopt 5000 - years - old *Ayurvedic* technique of using **kshara soötra** a sleek, indigenously manufactured medicated Seton coated with highly alkaline plant juices and extracts. This is strung through the fistula track.

The high alkalinity of *kshara soötra* disrupts the pseudo - epithelium of the fistula and nurtures healing from crypt to surface. Continued regular work, toileting, defecation and bathing practices are advised. The Seton treatment is done on ambulatory basis and patients are sent home the same day. The Seton cuts through the track which gets shallow day - by - day. It is changed every 7 - 10 days. Treatment by Seton (*kshara soötra*) keeps draining the pus, its high alkalinity destroys the ramifications of the track, and the cut - thru track heals after withering in few days.

Rectal prolapse is a condition wherein the last part of the large intestine slips outside the anus. This happens because it loses its normal attachments inside the body, allowing it to telescope out through the anus, thereby turning "**inside out**." If only the inner lining comes out it is called mucosal prolapse. This is common in malnourished young children, in whom it subsides on its own when the nutrition improves. If the entire thickness of the rectum comes out during the act of defecation, it may be uncomfortable, bleed on expulsion and become non - reducible. It is an embarrassing illness with incontinence and soiling of undergarments. Overall, rectal prolapse is not as common as piles or fissures. Risk factors include multiple vaginal deliveries. Minor rectal prolapse (mucosal type) can be treated by **sclerotherapy** as described above by use of local injections of sclerosing agents. These are injected in the peri - rectal tissue to stabilize the rectum that prolapses outside. Patients are advised to treat constipation as above and not to strain on stools. Elderly subjects when they lose a lot of muscle power and become asthenic may also develop rectal prolapse and be treated by sclerotherapy. Rectal prolapse are usually circumferential and distinguished from grade III large piles all around the anus from a groove in the periphery once the prolapsing mucosal mass is pushed back. Definitive treatment of rectal prolapse requires surgery. Several types of operations have been described to treat rectal prolapse.

Rectal Cancer (Cancer of the ano - rectum) – Symptoms such as frequent bowel movements, continued urge to pass stool even after defecation – sense of incomplete evacuation – reported as constipation, fecal incontinence – soiling of undergarments, hard stool sticking in the anus, pain around anus, blood or fleshy pieces in stools, i.e. symptoms similar to fissures and hemorrhoids, can also occur in rectal cancer. Some individuals may experience urinary difficulties.

Congenital polyps in this area can transform into malignant ulcerated growth or cancer. Rectal cancer can occur in adolescence. Often, patients with rectal cancer get treatment for fissures, hemorrhoids, or fistulas and remain undiagnosed for cancer unless a digital finger examination of the ano - rectum is performed. Unfortunately, in anorectal symptoms patients carry on medicine without having undergone a digital rectal examination.

A watchful surgeon confirms the diagnosis by performing the rectal examination in the anal region. A biopsy is always done before starting treatment. A small piece of tissue is taken out from the lump or ulcer in the rectum for biopsy, which confirms the exact diagnosis of the disease. Depending on the type and stage of rectal cancer, treatment can involve chemotherapy, radiotherapy, novel forms of immunotherapy and surgery.

Lower down growth within 8 - 10 cms of the anal verge may involve removal of the lower anal canal in order to get clear margins for complete excision of the cancer. In such a case the anal sphincter gets disrupted, and a new diversion of the fecal passage is made in the lower abdomen which is called **colostomy**. Feces is collected in a disposable bag which is flushed out as and when needed. One should not be apprehensive of diversion colostomy but rather adapt to the new situation as function remains the same, only defecatory practice changes. Anorectal cancer though may feel painful and distressing, yet its efficacious treatment allows excellent prognosis that is survival with quality life years.

In conclusion, we have learned that anorectal health plays a pivotal role in maintaining overall human well - being. Abdominal issues and gastrointestinal disorders often stem from poor maintenance of gut flora, reinforcing the connection between gut health and anorectal wellness.

The body detoxifies itself daily through the expulsion of urine and stool, and regular bowel movements, particularly in the morning, are a sign of good health. In contrast, delayed or difficult bowel movements, as seen in constipation, can trigger a cascade of anorectal problems. Constipation is not just a discomfort but often a precursor to several common anorectal conditions, emphasizing the importance of digestive and bowel health in preserving overall wellness.

Chapter 40

Aching Legs and Feet – Leg Swelling, Prominent, Tortuous Leaking or Varicose Veins

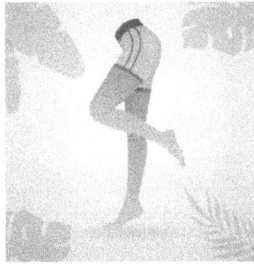

Learning Objectives:

- Reasons of persisting leg and feet pain

- Leg and feet pain continuing due to - peripheral artery disease (PAD), deep vein thrombosis, peripheral neuropathy, sciatica, arthritis, pulled muscles, sprains, restless leg syndrome, leg pain in growing children

- Examination and treatment of leg and feet pain

- Varicose veins i.e. prominent or tortuous veins in the legs, leaking veins or chronic venous insufficiency, skin changes, eczema, dark spots/mottling, swelling in feet in venous insufficiency

Our legs and feet are composed of a robust skeletal structure supported by muscles, making them essential components for movement. The lower limbs, including the thighs, legs, and feet, constitute roughly half of our body's length. These limbs play a crucial role not only in movement but also in circulation.

A significant proportion, approximately 25% to 35% of the heart's output, is directed toward the lower extremities, ensuring an adequate blood supply to sustain various activities. During more vigorous activities like brisk walking or running, the demand for blood in these regions increases, demonstrating their vital role in both mobility and cardiovascular health.

Leg & foot pain: Many people, usually between the ages of 40 - 50 years, experience fatigue and pain in one or both legs and feet while standing or walking. Usually, leg pain can have certain underlying causes like heavy physical activity, prolonged standing, injuries, sprains or strains, wear and tear, overuse, problems in joints, bones, muscles, nerves etc. However, leg pain in older people may also occur due to weakening of muscles, poor blood circulation in leg arteries and excessive use of the feet and knees. Diabetes, hypertension and tobacco consumption all contribute to **atherosclerotic** disease of **major** lower limb arteries, which may cause pain on walking. Excessive use of tobacco with nutritional deficiencies lead to leg pains. **Claudication** of **thrombo - angiitis obliterans** or **Buerger's disease –** peripheral artery disease occurs in young adults because of inflammation of arteries.

Valves in veins of the legs help in efficient return of blood from the feet and legs towards the heart. Incompetence of these valves venous leads to **varicose veins** or **chronic venous insufficiency** in the legs, which are a cause of swelling and pain in legs and feet. Deficiency of proteins and certain minerals like calcium can cause chronic and persistent leg and feet pain. Several immunological, vascular and inflammatory conditions can also lead to leg pains. Infections in feet and cracked heels also cause pain. Venous thrombosis leading to sluggish blood flow and clotting of blood in deep veins is described below and is a cause of severe pain in the calf. Stress related minor fractures in small bones of the foot in marching troops or exposure to frost in extreme cold weather are some other causes of leg pain. Filaria an illness caused by a worms transmitted by mosquito bite causes pain and swelling in lower limbs with lymph node enlargement in the groin. Later the swelling may become indurated and permanent leading to huge enlargement of the legs called **elephantiasis**. The purpose of this chapter is to apprise the reader of common disorders related to legs and feet in order to make him aware of taking adequate preventive measures and treatment.

Peripheral Artery Disease (PAD) – The arteries supplying the lower extremity arborise (branch repeatedly) and end in capillaries in the tissues. From there the blood collects in venules which in turn drain into veins and finally into the main vena cava draining into the right side of the heart. Large arteries are prone to the process of ageing - **atherosclerosis** and **plaque (atheroma) formation** which reduces blood flow, leading to weakness, numbness, coldness and cramps. **Claudication** is a type of muscle pain which occurs because of lack of oxygen. It is triggered by walking or running and relieved by rest, so the person is forced to stop walking. When blood circulation in the feet is severely restricted (critical limb ischemia) the skin of the feet becomes shiny and scaly, nails become lusterless and capillary refill in the nail bed slows down. The blood pressure in upper arm and ankle shows **ankle - brachial index** (an objective measure of poor blood circulation in the lower limbs) of less than 0.9. Foot pain caused by PAD is similar to angina in coronary artery disease. It is exacerbated in diabetes, hypertension and tobacco consumption. It is adversely affected in dyslipidaemia or when **low density lipo - protein (LDL)** is high. Prolonged uncontrolled diabetes causes neuropathy also which predisposes to skin infection, ultimately leading to **diabetic foot**. In this condition, the poor blood supply to feet, tendency to harbor skin infection and neuropathy produces a conundrum of foot ulcers, infection of foot bones and gangrene of toes and forefoot. **Angiography** and **color doppler** studies are used to diagnose this condition after thorough history and examination. Prevention and treatment of PAD involves maintaining excellent foot hygiene, exercise training, **'absolute no'** to tobacco consumption, eminent control of diabetes and hypertension, provision of high quality supportive and protective footwear and treatment of foot infection especially fungal infection. Treatment and dietary management to keep high density cholesterol (HDL) high and LDL low is also needed. Treatment of anemia, other nutritional deficiencies, suitable antibiotics for infection, wound debridement and dressings are required to treat PAD lower limbs. Surgical treatment involves careful assessment of angiography and arterial bypass surgery if indicated.

Buerger's disease or Thromboangitis - Obliterans – is a common cause of aching leg and feet in the smoking population of rural poor. The disease affects both the arteries and veins mostly in the lower legs and feet leading to severe handicap in walking and cycling.

It is a non - specific inflammation, spasm and blockage of **medium and small size arteries and veins**. Pain on walking gradually becomes more severe and allows less and less walking. Initially the patient can walk some distance without pain but starts feeling severe pain in the calf after covering a certain distance (**claudication distance**). This compels him to halt and take a rest and then starts to walk further. Day by day, increasing pain in the leg and feet of the patient, restricts him from covering that distance which he did previously. Eventually, **pain occurs on rest** and a person is unable to walk. This state progresses to **paresthesia** (feeling of numbness and tingling) due to poor blood supply to nerves in the leg. **Gangrene** may develop in toes and forefoot leading to need for **amputation**. **Treatment** involves complete abstinence from tobacco, full attention to treatment of anemia and nutrition, foot hygiene, comfortable and protective footwear, exercise training and surgery by sympathetic nerve ablation to improve blood supply.

Deep vein thrombosis (DVT) – The blood from the lower limbs – feet, legs and thigh, returns to the heart through veins. The veins located under the skin that we can see are superficial veins and those located under muscles closer to bones are deep veins. Whenever there is indolence, dehydration, hypercoagulability states, cancer or injury in the lower limb, blood clots may form in the deep veins. This can lead to deep vein thrombosis (DVT). Mild DVT may simply pass off with some pain and swelling in legs and feet without being diagnosed. More severe DVT causes induration, swelling and tenderness in calf muscles and foot pain. This condition is serious because blood clots can loosen, travel to the heart and lodge in the lungs leading to severe breathlessness and even death due to **pulmonary embolism**. Conditions or risk factors which predispose to DVT are old age, dehydration, recumbency after a major illness such as surgery, especially cancer surgery etc.

Preventive measures include blood thinning agents (anti - platelet) like **aspirin** and **clopidogrel. Heparin and its analogues** are used as injectables for short durations. Continuous or frequent wriggling of toes when standing, sitting or lying is advised. **Crepe bandage or compression stockings** on legs and feet are advised. In case of long - term bedridden patients **bubble mattress** are advised. Blood clots may be surgically removed from the deep vein using endo - venous procedures.

Peripheral Neuropathy – The brain and spinal cord makes up the central nervous system. The nerves are the wires that transmit signals to and from the brain and peripheral organs like the hand, feet, eyes, tongue, etc. and are called peripheral nervous system.

Our body has three types of nerves;

(i)   **Sensory nerves** which transmit sensations like touch, pain, pin prick, pressure, weight, hot and cold, taste from the tongue etc. to the brain.

(ii) **Motor nerves** follow the instruction and intention from the brain and move the appropriate muscle or a group of muscles to do any voluntary action like lifting a cup of tea, playing tennis, walking, running etc.

(iii) **Autonomic nerves** function automatically and are responsible for functioning of internal organs like bowel movement, urination etc.

In **neuropathy**, the body's nerves become unable to transmit information to and from the brain. Several diseases affect our peripheral nerves which may present as altered sensation, tingling, numbness, loss of sensation, loss of pain sensation, inability to distinguish between hot and cold sensations, severe and sharp pain and burning (neuralgia), muscle paralysis, sexual dysfunction or impotence, digestive problems, fecal and urinary incontinence etc. Peripheral neuropathy can be caused by **deficiencies of vitamins** E, B1 and B6., and B12. External pressure on nerves as in **carpal tunnel syndrome** (pressure on the median nerve in the wrist), nerve impingement in bone fractures, pressure at the nerve roots as they pass out of the vertebral column are common causes of neuralgic pain.

Nerve and nerve sheath tumors like neuromas also cause symptoms of peripheral neuropathy. **Diabetes** and **chronic kidney disease** frequently affect the peripheral nerves. Certain drugs, exposure to volatile substances like pesticides may lead to neuropathy. Certain cancer chemotherapeutic agents cause mild to severe, short term to permanent peripheral neuropathy. Chronic infection like **leprosy** due to *Mycobacterium leprae* may affect peripheral nerves causing anesthetic patches in skin.

Some viral infections like *Herpes* virus and autoimmune diseases (in which immune system attacks its own cells) such as rheumatoid arthritis and lupus erythematosus may also affect the nerves.

Diagnosis – Neuropathy is diagnosed by electrophysiological studies – the **nerve conduction velocity**.

Treatment – Peripheral neuropathy associated with diabetes, Buerger's disease, leprosy and those associated with deformity of leg and feet require close attention with physical medicine and rehabilitation experts. Attending foot hygiene and providing comfortable, protective footwear are basic requirements. Correction of the primary causes like diabetes or deformity of the foot is important. Protection of the foot from further injury, adequate supportive aids, skin care and foot appliances are given. **Pregabalin** and **gabapentin** are drugs used for neurologic pain. Surgical release of nerve compression is done in fractures and carpel tunnel syndrome. Replacement of vitamin B_{12} and other nutritional deficiencies may be required. Peripheral arterial disease of diabetes with superadded peripheral neuropathy causing diabetic foot is a complex condition to treat. In autoimmune peripheral neuropathy **plasmapheresis** is carried on removing auto antibodies.

Dehydration and lack of vitamins and minerals – may lead to aches in legs and feet. Dehydration caused by diarrhea, excessive sweating etc. may be associated with electrolyte imbalance. Replenishing the body with adequate water intake, salts or glucose and mineral enriched drinks after heavy exercises or sports in hot and sultry weather give relief. Usually, people indulging in these activities are able to fix their problem by adequate intake of fluid and electrolytes. Cancer chemotherapy and heavy urination after diuretics can also cause leg pains.

Nerve Root Compression/Slipped Disc/Spondylolisthesis – our spine or **vertebral column** has several bones that are stacked above each other with intervening disks of fibrous tissue which keep them in place. Over the years twisting and bending the spine and continuous working in wrong posture may cause muscular spasm. Disruption or prolapse of the inter - vertebral disk (slip disc) may cause pressure on the nerve roots. Spinal cord may also be compressed due to bone fractures, spinal degeneration, hematoma, tumor etc.

Compression of the spinal cord may occur with cervical or lumber stenosis, symptoms of which are almost absent in the initial stage. This may lead to back, neck, shoulder, hip, thighs and leg pain. Slip disc may occur at a young age or manifest in adulthood, especially in obese subjects. Lower back is the most common site. Slip disc **grade I** is less than 25 percent displaced, **grade II** is 26–50%, **grade III** 51–75%, **grade IV** is 76–100% and **grade V** is over 100% displaced and is referred to as **spondyloptosis**. Bed rest, muscle relaxants and several muscle strengthening exercises are advised.

In severe cases offending disc or discs causing neurological symptoms are removed by surgery and adjacent vertebral bodies are fixed to each other using metal plates and screws. More recently micro - discectomy using endoscopic surgery to remove the offending disc is undertaken without inter - fixing the vertebral body. This is a minimally invasive surgical procedure for this condition.

Sciatica or sciatic pain is characterized by continuous shooting pain in the outer part of thighs radiating to lower thigh and knee while standing or sitting. It is caused by compression of nerves in the lower part of the spine. The problem of displaced or herniated discs (vertebrae) and spinal stenosis (narrowing of the spine) also exacerbates the condition. Diagnosis is made through X - rays and MRI imaging. Treatment includes pain killers and muscle relaxants followed by physiotherapy. If this does not provide relief, surgery has to be resorted to. If only one disc is affected micro - discectomy may be advised as described above.

Arthritis of various joints such as the hips, knees, and ankles cause pain along with swelling and stiffness, making it difficult to walk, stand, sit or run etc. Various types of arthritis are described in Chapter 34. Arthritis requires comprehensive treatment according to the cause. Losing weight, doing *yog* and appropriate joint and muscle exercises can be beneficial in addition to specific treatment.

Muscle Pull / Sprain occurs when a person suddenly performs a heavy muscular activity, when certain fibers or tendons of the muscle snap all of a sudden and thus get partially injured. This can happen with sudden weightlifting, climbing, engaging in sports or ankle twisting.

Sprain occurs especially when foot turns inwards and causes injury to the outer lateral ligament of the ankle. This can cause immediate or sudden pain in legs and feet. It is prudent to rule out stress bony fractures due to avulsion. This can be done by good clinical examination of point bony tenderness and focused ultrasound and x - ray. Treatment consists of resting the snapped muscle, hot and cold compresses, pain relievers, muscle relaxants, compression bandaging and limb support by temporary plaster cast. Pulled muscles are generally treated by the technique called **RICE** (rest, ice on the injured portion, compression, elevation).

Muscle Cramp can occur in leg and foot muscles, causing intense shooting pain when walking, standing, sitting and in bed etc. Muscle cramps happen more frequently in women, during winter or with air - conditioner exposure. The exact cause is not known but there may be a familial or a genetic tendency to this symptom. Weak muscles, unaccustomed exercise, electrolyte disturbance etc. are implicated. Thyroid, kidney functions, sodium, potassium and calcium levels should be tested. Reassurance, muscle relaxants, hot compressions, warming up the bed, correction of dehydration and electrolytes, use of muscle protein called L - carnitine and Vitamin E are prescribed with some success.

Stress Fracture in feet occurs when there is a crack (fracture) in the small bones of the foot called **metatarsals.** These are due to repetitive stress and strain without adequate rest. These fractures are often seen in athletes, marching troops or individuals who engage in rigorous physical activities without proper rest. Diagnosis can be made through X - rays or MRI imaging. Treatment involves resting with bandage or plaster for 6 to 8 weeks followed by exercise and physiotherapy.

Tendonitis (Inflammation of tendon) – Tendons are tissues that connect muscles to bones. Inflammation of a tendon, known as tendonitis, can cause pain in the feet, buttocks, knees and ankles. Tendons that attach to the heel bone (Achilles tendon) and control ankle movement are very powerful ligaments. Tendons have a sheath covering with a thin layer of lubricant jelly fluid so that tendons can slide on each other and manipulate movements of joints. Un - noticed injuries can cause inflammation in these tendons and their sheath. It can result in difficulty in foot movement and pain.

Treatment is usually done through rest in a relaxed position, medication and physiotherapy – i.e. treatment through RICE technique.

Restless - leg syndrome – is a nervous system disorder that causes an overpowering urge to move legs. It has been considered as a sleep disorder if patients fail to fall asleep. Pain in legs can be described variously as itching, aching, throbbing and paresthesia (pins and needles sensation) etc.

Some possible reasons for this discomfort during rest include the accumulation of fluid in the legs, excessive caffeine or alcohol consumption, irregular sleep patterns, stress or anxiety, kidney disease, diabetes, anemia and a sedentary lifestyle. X - rays, MRI and ultrasound can be conducted. Relief can be achieved through exercise and massage. Treatment includes supplements of iron, folic acid, vitamin B_{12} and vitamin C and D supplementation and lifestyle changes like regular exercise, maintaining proper sleep patterns and reducing stress. In some cases, medication like benzodiazepines may be used.

Growing Pains or **leg pain in growing children** – Children often complain of leg pain for weeks, months or even years during their growing age, which is called "growing pains." The reason for such pain is considered to be excessive running and playing during the day. Pain occurs in their legs, often behind their thighs, calves, and knees, especially in the evenings or while lying in bed at night. This pain usually goes away on its own by morning. Treatment for growing pains includes leg massage, hot fomentation and mild pain relievers. Children may also experience pain in their legs due to flat feet or the inappropriate feet arches from birth or the use of ill - fitting shoes or sandals.

Varicose Veins – These are abnormally tortuous and prominent superficial veins affecting the lower limbs. The blood from the lower limbs – feet, legs and thigh return through veins. The veins running under the skin are superficial veins and veins running underneath the muscles are deep veins.

There are **valves** in the walls of the leg veins which direct the flow of blood upward towards the heart. If these valves become weak, blood in the legs cannot continuously and efficiently flow back to the heart, and it pools in the legs. This usually affects superficial veins and is also called **venous hypertension** or **venous insufficiency**.

Symptoms include swelling and pain in legs and feet. It is a common condition affecting 5 to 10 per 1000 people. The dilated and tortuous superficial veins are visible under the skin. Prominent tiny veins – called spider naevi (**telangiectasia**) develop near ankles and elsewhere in the lower extremity. Because of venous hypertension small venules disrupt and blood leaks in small quantities into the skin. The iron content in hemoglobin causes pigmentation, mottling of skin, itchy eczema like rash (**venous dermatitis**) and skin ulcerations (**venous ulcer**). The texture of the skin of the legs changes due to seepage and accumulation of blood protein (**patchy dermo - sclerosis**).

The skin of the leg in long standing cases becomes heavily pigmented and parchment - like. The underlying muscles also take the brunt of the leaking blood from incompetent veins leading to reduced muscle tone. Various stages of this condition have been described as C0, C1, C2, C3, C4, C5, C6, etc.

No visible symptoms and a healthy leg in the presence of disease is C0, only prominent veins and spider veins is C1, tortuous visible veins are C2, swelling in ankles due to oedema is C3, pigmentation and eczema is C4, venous ulcer is C5 and gross skin changes with non - healing painful ulcer is C6. Skin loses its elasticity and becomes eczematous, with nonhealing ulcers altogether called **lipodermatosclerosis**. Risk factors for developing this condition are familial pre - disposition, obesity, long standing hours, pregnancy, lack of leg movements, hormonal changes and superficial venous infection called thrombophlebitis.

Treatment involves keeping the legs elevated, using specially designed elastic stockings, crepe bandages, deep breathing and exercise for relief.

Medications are not very effective in this disease. Traditionally this condition when severe was treated by surgery. Most of the treatment nowadays concentrates on obliterating the leaking veins. The offending veins on the outer and the inner aspect of the leg and thigh where they join the deep vein in the groin are ligated and the rest of the vein is stripped out and removed. The blood returns to the vena cava through remaining and deep veins. Several treatments are in current practice which include **laser** and **radiofrequency endo - venous ablation** under ultrasound guidance.

A thin tube is inserted into the faulty veins, and when the tube is properly positioned, laser beams or radiofrequency waves are used to fluctuate the veins and destroy the lumen. This causes the veins to collapse, and leakage stops. **Sclerotherapy (chemical closure)** is the most popular and least expensive technique. **Glue, foam and other sclerosing agents** are injected in the varicose and leaking veins under ultrasound guidance. Treatment is usually successful in the first phase, with up to 85% success. Several veins can be targeted in one treatment session.

In conclusion, our legs and feet are fundamental locomotory organs, enabling us to move, travel, and maintain mobility. In Hindu culture, feet symbolize energy, agility and strength. The prayer, "O God, when you call me to your abode, let me travel on my feet," underscores the cultural and spiritual importance of maintaining strong, healthy feet throughout life. Regular care, nourishment, and massage are customary practices to ensure foot health, especially in old age, to avoid reliance on aids like sticks, walkers, or wheelchairs. To emphasize the importance of lower extremity health, National Foot Health Awareness is observed every April, highlighting the need for continued attention to foot and leg care.

Chapter 41

Urinary Tract Problems – Infections, Urinary Stones, Prostate and Cancer

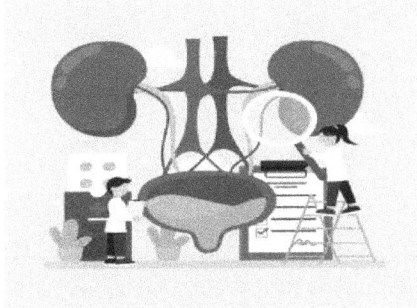

Learning Objectives:

- Urine formation and its excretion from kidneys

- Common diseases of the urinary tract – urinary tract infection (UTI), Lower Urinary Tract Symptoms (LUTS), urinary retention

- Kidney malfunctioning due to raised blood pressure, uncontrolled diabetes and other causes

- Kidney failure and dialysis

- Stones in the urinary tract – diagnosis and new treatment modalities of shock wave lithotripsy and minimally invasive endoscopic treatment of urinary stones

- Enlarged prostate, prostate cancer, urinary bladder cancer

The kidneys play a crucial role in maintaining the body's health by filtering out unwanted waste products and toxins, ensuring **homeostasis** is achieved. These beans - shaped organs, located in the lumbar region of the abdomen, function through about one million microscopic units called **nephrons**, which filter blood and form urine.

Urine flows from the kidney through the ureters into the bladder and is expelled from the body through the urethra. In children, urination occurs reflexively when the bladder is full, whereas in adults, it is controlled until a convenient time and place. On average, a healthy adult produces 2 - 3 liters of urine daily, urinating 4 - 6 times. The volume of urine produced depends on fluid intake and body functions. If urine output falls below 30 ml/kg/24 hours in children or less than 1 ml/kg body weight per hour in adults, it could signal dehydration or kidney malfunction. Urinary control is regulated by a combination of voluntary and involuntary muscles, allowing normal control over the urinary stream. The urinary tract consists of the kidneys and ureters (upper urinary tract), and the bladder and urethra (lower urinary tract). Malformations such as polycystic kidney disease, posterior urethral valves, or vesico - ureteral reflux may be present from birth and often manifests in childhood. Symptoms indicating potential issues with the kidneys or urinary tract include frequent urination, burning sensations while urinating, poor urinary flow, incontinence, urgency, hesitancy, blood in the urine (hematuria), pain in the kidney area, high blood pressure, or the passage of stones, blood, or tissue in the urine. Early detection and treatment of these symptoms are essential for preserving kidney and urinary health. Common conditions of kidneys, ureter, urinary bladder, urethra and prostate gland are briefly described below. Sexual problems are not discussed in this chapter.

Kidney – The kidneys are major excretory organs that detoxify the body by continuously removing unwanted metabolic waste products. For example, nitrogenous product **urea** from proteins and **creatinine** from muscles and some acids from our body are removed in the urine. Kidneys maintain the intricate electrolyte balance of sodium and potassium in our body. Kidneys are a site for **vitamin D** and calcium metabolism through production of **calcitriol**. It also produces a hormone **erythropoietin** which is important for the formation of red blood cells. Another function performed by the kidneys is the control of blood pressure and fluid balance by **Renin - angiotensin system.** Kidney or **renal failure** means inability to maintain kidney functions as per the needs of the body. It can be acute or chronic. **Acute renal failure (ARF)** occurs when there is **sudden decrease in renal function** with **low urine output**. It can result firstly from certain conditions affecting the body (systemic conditions) like state of **shock** and low blood pressure and **septicemia.**

Poisoning and wrong blood transfusion adversely affect kidney. Secondly, there are **primary diseases** of the kidney like auto - immune diseases (**acute glomerulonephritis**), hemolytic uremic syndrome, kidney stones and infections of the kidney (**nephritis or pyelonephritis**). Mostly ARF is associated with **sudden decrease is urine output**, with increase in blood urea and creatinine (**azotemia**). Although the patient may be critically ill, ARF is usually self - limiting and reversible with treatment of shock and septicemia. A temporary mechanical procedure called **dialysis** may be required for acute renal failure.

Chronic kidney disease (CKD), also called **chronic renal failure**, is characterized by a gradual loss of kidney function. **The glomerular filtration rate** reduces progressively. Advanced CKD may be associated with toxic levels of waste substances like urea and creatinine and deranged levels of acid, fluid and electrolytes in the body. The causes of CKD like **uncontrolled diabetes** and **hypertension** must be treated. Other causes of CKD include glomerulonephritis (autoimmune inflammation of glomerulus or filtering apparatus), polycystic kidney disease, and recurrent kidney infection causing scarring. Any obstruction in the urinary tract – either congenital or acquired can cause dilatation of the urine collecting receptacles called calyx and pelvis due to back pressure. This condition is called **hydronephrosis** and can cause renal failure. **Kidney infection** or **pyelonephritis** can occur if bacteria enter kidneys usually traveling upwards from lower urinary tract. This is especially common if there is stone or any urinary tract obstruction or reflux. **Polycystic kidney disease** (PKD) is characterized by congenital cysts in the kidneys and may lead to high blood pressure and kidney failure. **End stage renal disease** (**ESRD) is** a terminal illness when **glomerular filtration rate** is less than 15 ml/min. Treatment for CKD aims to slow down the progression of kidney damage to ESRD, which is fatal without artificial filtering (dialysis) or **kidney transplant**. Kidney transplant for ESRD has become common now-a-days. Appropriate brain dead (cadaver) persons after due matching are deployed as donors for kidney transplantation.

Urinary Tract Infection (UTI) are common infections caused by bacteria, often from the skin, vagina or rectum, which enter the urethra, and infect the urinary tract. The most common bacteria of UTI are **E coli or Escherichia coli.** The infection can affect several parts of the urinary tract, but the most common type is a bladder infection (**cystitis**) and kidney infection **(pyelonephritis)**. Common symptoms are burning, itching, frequent urination with urgency, pain while urinating, blood in the urine and / or redness of the genitalia and urethral orifice.

Infections in the urinary tract are more common in women. Any congenital abnormality in the urinary tract or obstruction in the flow of urine predisposes to UTI. In men prostate gland enlargement especially in old age or infection in prostate (prostatitis) give rise to severe UTI. Uncontrolled diabetes is associated with troublesome recurrent UTI. Other pre - disposing factors are stricture in urethra. Inability to completely evacuate the bladder with each act of urination leads to residual urine which attracts bacteria to thrive leading to chronic UTI. Many a times a pre - disposing cause may not be found. Urine samples are taken for microscopic examination, culture and bacterial sensitivity. Intake of plenty of water is advised to all patients. Urine generally is acidic in nature. Alkalinizing agents may be prescribed to check bacterial growth in acidic medium. Antibiotic use can initially be empirical but more precise antibiotics can be used after bacterial sensitivity laboratory report is available. Recurrent UTIs especially in women may warrant a prolonged course of antibiotics.

Urinary Tract Stones or calculi may develop in the kidneys and then pass through the ureter to the lower urinary tract. Stone formation in urinary tract affects 1 - 13% of the global population. Kidney stones are usually composed of calcium oxalate and phosphate or uric acid. Defects of calcium metabolism and disorders of para - thyroid gland should be checked for in patients with recurrent kidney stones. Urinary stones, if they get trapped or block the urine flow, cause UTI. The stones may be small crystals (**crystalluria**), sand like particles or sometimes large single (**stag horn**) or multiple stones. They form by precipitation of salts from urinary contents and gradually enlarge over months and years. Some people and some geographical areas are more prone to urinary stone disease. The patients may have no symptoms, and the stone may be discovered on an incidental ultrasound or X - ray. Both severe, acute pain (renal colic) or low - grade renal pain may also be an indication of renal stones. Patients are advised to drink plenty of fluids while avoiding calcium and oxalate or uric acid rich diet (in uric acid stones). There are several remedies prevalent in alternative medical systems to get rid of stones in the urinary tract.

These are *Berberis vulgaris* in homeopathy, *Kulthi* (horse gram) and sugarcane juice in *Ayurveda*, *Sharbat Bazoori Motadil and Badyan arq* (fennel seed) in Unani medicine etc. Small stones, typically 2 - 5 mm in size, can often pass through the urinary tract spontaneously with urine but many people do take some or the other medicine which may be credited with stone expulsion. Passage of urinary stone and process of expulsion through the urethra can be excruciatingly painful. There are several endoscopic, open surgical and mechanical methods to remove kidney stones. Large and irregular stones or multiple stones in the kidney, ureter and bladder may require **surgical** intervention by making an incision in the abdomen and opening the kidney or its pelvis, ureter or bladder to remove the stone under vision. Nonsurgical technique of breaking stone by focusing targeted shock waves to the stone by **Extra - corporeal Shock Wave Lithotripsy (ESWL)** is deployed. Approximately 1 to 3 cm stones can be broken into pieces and removed through the urinary route by cystoscopy. This may be followed by placing a **stent** in the ureter to keep its mouth open so that the fragments and sand of the stone keep coming out.

The stent is removed after a few days. There are also now several **minimally invasive surgical methods** to tackle stones in kidney and urinary tract. With the technique of **nephroscope** direct puncture into the kidney is done from the back with the patient under anesthesia and X - ray screening machine (C - arm). The stone is visualized and broken by the targeted energy source, sucked out and removed. The procedure of removing stone through nephroscope is called **Per - Cutaneous Nephro - Lithotomy or PCNL**. A **laparoscope** insertion by making a small hole in the abdomen is used to remove kidney and ureteric stones. Stones may become impacted in the uterer, for which equipment called **ureteroscope** is inserted in the ureter from below through the urethra and bladder. These scopes are manipulated to directly inspect the impacted stone. A camera is fitted at the surgeon's end of the scope and the image is seen on a television or video screen. These scopes have an operating channel through which various devices to break stones can be negotiated. Depending on where the stone is lodged in the kidney and urinary tract, the surgeon chooses the most appropriate route and equipment to remove the stone or let small pieces and sand pass through the urinary tract. Stones trapped in the kidney and urinary tract are removed successfully without making a major incision, achieving a success rate up to 90 percent.

Minimally invasive endoscopy techniques have revolutionized several surgical procedures and thus have built up confidence in patients and surgeons to go through highly successful and least painful experiences, especially in the field of urinary stones.

Urinary Retention occurs when someone is unable to pass urine despite several efforts. The urinary bladder being filled with urine feels acutely painful. Advanced pregnancy, spinal cord injury, severe urinary tract infection, blood clot obstruction from bleeding from a bladder tumor, injury in the pelvic bone and urethra, stricture of the urethra and prostatic enlargement are common causes of urinary retention. History, examination and tests are conducted which usually reveal the cause of urinary retention. A catheter or tube is inserted through the urethra to remove urine from the bladder. A commonly used latex catheter is called **Foley's catheter**. This tube is retained in the bladder by inflating a bulb or a balloon and connecting the catheter into a urine collecting bag. People who experience urinary leakage and lose control over it may need to have a catheter inserted for an extended period. At times or when there is stricture and injury to urethra, it may not be possible to negotiate a catheter from below and urine is drained out by putting a catheter directly into the bladder through the lower abdominal wall. This is called **supra - pubic catheterization** or urinary diversion. After giving temporary relief thorough examination and assessment is done to treat the underlying cause.

Prostate Enlargement and Prostate Cancer – The prostate is a walnut - sized gland in men only and it is an accessory part of the reproductive system. Prostatic secretion is necessary for semen and sperms. It is situated just below the bladder surrounding the urethra. Prostate gland is often enlarged as men age, more so after the age of 40 or 50 under the influence of testosterone hormone. This is called **Benign Prostatic Hyperplasia (BPH)** – an extremely common condition with prevalence of around 50% in men above 60 years. This is a result of disproportion of estrogen and testosterone, with higher concentration of estrogen within the prostate causing prostatic enlargement. Enlarged prostate at the outlet of the urinary bladder where it surrounds the urethra can cause pressure and impede the outflow of urine. **Symptoms** of prostate enlargement include shortening and thinning of urinary stream, increased frequency, urgency, hesitancy, bifid urinary stream, intermittent stream, dribbling, post micturition dribbling, double micturition (going to pass urine successively 2 times), application of force to micturate, painful micturition (dysuria) and symptoms of UTI like burning, hematuria etc. Nodular, hard and rapidly enlarging prostate in older age may be due to **Carcinoma** of the Prostate.

Prostate gland when enlarged, secretes a protein in the blood called **Prostate - Specific Antigen (PSA)**. Various views and values of PSA have been described in the literature. PSA above a certain level is indicative of prostate cancer. Thus, PSA is a **tumor marker**. PSA levels of 4.0 ng/mL and lower were considered normal. and PSA levels higher than 10 ng/mL usually indicate prostate cancer.

Doctors examine the prostate gland by a finger in the rectum or ultrasound by putting a probe in the rectum (transrectal ultrasound). When suspicious, a biopsy is performed through rectum. The latest technique is MRI - US fusion and grid **guided perineal biopsy** for precise sampling of suspicious nodule in the prostate gland.

The evaluation of the urinary stream is done by observing the flow of urine during urination and using a **uroflowmeter**. In the case of urinary retention due to prostate enlargement catheterization as described above may be necessary. There are several ways of treating benign and malignant prostatic enlargements. BPH in majority can be managed by a drug called alpha blockers which are pharmaceutically known as **Terazosin, Doxazosin, Tamsulosin, Alfuzosin** and **Slodosin. Dutastride** a 5 - alpha reductase enzyme blocking agent is added to stop the further growth of prostate.

Benign enlarged prostate is removed piece - meal through the urethra using a diathermy cutting device under flowing current of liquid. This process is known as **Trans Urethral Resection of Prostate (TURP)**. **Holmium Laser or Robotic Prostatectomy** is performed for very large benign prostatic enlargement.

Cancer of the prostate is now the 2nd commonest cancer in men worldwide and the 3rd commonest cancer in men in India after oral cancer and lung cancer. It is often an androgen hormone dependent cancer. There are many advancements in its treatment also - removing both the testes (**orchidectomy**), several **anti - androgen drugs, chemotherapy, targeted therapy, hormonal treatments,** etc.

Surgically it can be treated with TURP, open laparoscopic or **robotic radical prostatectomy**.

Bladder Tumor (Bladder Cancer) - Urinary bladder cancers are relatively uncommon. Constant irritation by carcinogens and chemicals excreted in urine cause cancer of the urinary bladder. Its main symptom is **painless hematuria** (blood in urine). Small pieces of tumor tissue may be passed out in urine also. **Ultrasound** of a full bladder or endoscopic examination of bladder (**cystoscopy**) may clinch the diagnosis by seeing a coral like abnormal growth at single or multiple places in the bladder.

Cystoscopic biopsy is obtained by cutting and pinching a piece of frond like tumor. An important parameter is how deeply the tumor is rooted in the bladder wall. The primary treatment for bladder cancer is surgery, where the bladder tumor is resected through a procedure called **Transurethral Resection of Bladder Tumor (TURBT)**.

Accordingly, using a cystoscope, the tumor tissue is removed, and the depth and grading of the tumor are determined. Further treatment options are medications, surgery, chemotherapy and radiotherapy. Instillation of agents like BCG, Bleomycin and others in the bladder may be advised.

Surgery for advanced bladder tumor may require partial or complete removal of urinary bladder and diversion of urine into a neo - tubing created by small intestine which discharges urine in a bag.

Cancer of the kidney: The most common renal cancer in adults is **renal cell cancer**. This is an adenocarcinoma arising from cells lining the renal tubules. It presents painless hematuria, a mass in the abdomen or back pain. Other symptoms are fever, fatigue and weight loss.

Metastatic spread is to the lungs or brain. Renal cancer is treated either by removing the affected portion of the kidney (**partial nephrectomy**) or removing whole kidney **(total nephrectomy)**. New drugs are now available to treat renal cell cancer.

Another renal tumor which occurs in childhood is the **Wilm's tumor**. This also presents hematuria and mass in the abdomen.

In conclusion, life without functioning kidneys becomes incompatible with survival, as kidneys serve as the body's essential drainage system.

Much like a home or city without proper drainage, the absence of this vital organ would lead to the accumulation of toxins, making life unsustainable.

The Almighty has intricately designed the human body with an efficient system of filtration and excretion through the kidneys, which, like the heart, lungs, and intestines, work tirelessly day and night without pause. Kidneys maintain homeostasis - ensuring a balance of fluids, electrolytes, and other vital components within the body. This state of equilibrium is crucial for the survival of all living beings.

Modern medical advancements have greatly improved the treatment of urinary conditions, particularly kidney stones. Innovative oral medications now effectively manage symptoms of prostate enlargement, reducing the need for surgery significantly. Likewise, new techniques have revolutionized the management of prostate cancer.

World Kidney Day, observed on the second Thursday of March every year, serves to raise awareness of kidney health and diseases. In 2024, the theme is "**Kidney Health for All**," emphasizing the importance of kidney care and health for people across the globe.

Chapter 42

Mental Disorders and Indian Mental Health Act – 2017

Different Mental Disorders

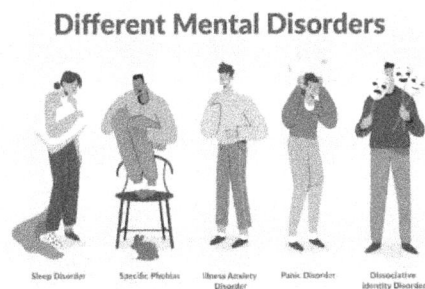

Sleep Disorder Specific Phobias Illness Anxiety Disorder Panic Disorder Dissociative Identity Disorder

---

Learning Objectives:

- Difference between mental and neurological illness
- Various mental diseases – depression, neurosis, psychosis and hypochondriasis
- Understand the difference between neuroses and psychoses
- Understand importance of suicide and its prevention
- Indian Mental Health Act 2018 explains how to manage patients empathetically and help them to rehabilitate

---

The fast pace of modern life often brings stress, tension, and conflict, leading to mental strain and negatively impacting well - being. Prolonged stress can upset mental equilibrium, resulting in the widespread occurrence of mental disorders. It is important to distinguish between **'mental'** and **'neurological'** disorders. Neurological disorders are typically linked to identifiable pathological processes in the **central nervous system (CNS),** making them organic in nature. In contrast, mental disorders, as defined by the **World Health Organization (WHO),** are characterized by **"clinically significant disturbances in an individual's cognition,**

emotional regulation, or behavior," often leading to distress or impairment in daily functioning. Unlike neurological conditions, mental disorders usually lack an identifiable organic cause and are primarily diagnosed based on behavioral and psychological symptoms. These disorders are treated by both **psychiatrists** and **psychologists**. Psychiatrists, being medical doctors, can prescribe medications to manage symptoms, whereas psychologists provide therapeutic support through counselling and psychotherapy. Both play critical roles in mental health care, offering different but complementary approaches to treatment.

Two broad categories of mental disorders are **neurosis** and **psychosis**. In the former, the patient remains in touch with reality while in the latter the touch with reality is lost.

Neurosis is a state wherein recreating and molding the personality in consonance with the needs of society becomes difficult or unattainable.

Neurosis originated from the Greek root word Neuron + Latin word 'Osis' denoting neurosis as the abnormal condition of neuron or nerves.

Neurotic patients establish the relationship with the external real world but are unable to mold their personality as per the needs of the external real world. Patients suffering from neurosis build and maintain their relationships and acceptability in society. Symptoms of neurosis have been detailed in the **Theory of Psychoanalysis by Sigmund Freud.**

Anxiety disorder – This is a common mental disorder characterized by getting perturbed over minor issues. Associated symptoms include digestion problems, sweating, headache, palpitation, restlessness, sleeplessness etc. This makes them unable to solve small problems occurring in day - to - day life. These are petty mental disorders which augment sorrow, displeasure, despondency, indifference and tiredness.

Obsessive Compulsive Disorder or OCD – This is a lasting disorder wherein the person experiences recurring, unwanted and uncontrollable thoughts (obsessions) or engages in repetitive behaviors (compulsions) or both, causing significant distress and interfering with daily life. Examples of such obsessions and actions are fear of contamination or dirt, fear of leaving home unlocked, needing things to be symmetrical and orderly etc.

The patient feels compelled to commit actions such as washing hands again and again, checking the door lock frequently, arranging items in the home repeatedly, to the point of causing distress to self and family members.

Somatoform Disorder (SD) – The term 'soma' is Greek for 'body'. Somatoform disorders are a set of neurotic conditions where a person complains of and experiences symptoms suggesting a physical disorder. Symptoms can range in severity from mild and infrequent to chronic and severe and are out of the individual's conscious control. However, there is **no demonstrable organic finding** and instead there exists a **strong link to psychological factors** or conflicts. Many people who have SD will also have an anxiety disorder. Regardless, they cause excessive and disproportionate levels of distress often long term. The symptoms can involve one or more different organs and body systems, such as neurologic, gastrointestinal and pain. People with SD are not faking their symptoms. The distress they experience from pain and other problems they experience are real. For example, stress can cause some people to develop headaches, chest pain, back pain, nausea or fatigue. Somatoform disorders include somatization disorder, pain disorder, hypochondriasis, functional or conversion disorder, body dysmorphic disorder and undifferentiated somatoform disorder – NOS (not otherwise specified) i.e. where specific diagnosis is not possible.

Somatization is a milder, brief form of somatoform disorder in which mental stress causes physical symptoms.

Functional disorder, earlier called **conversion disorder** – Here the patient believes he/she has physical symptoms, but these cannot be explained by a physical disease or other medical condition. Onset is usually abrupt. Symptoms may be those of convulsion, coma, paralysis, asthma etc. Like other somatoform disorders, the symptoms are not intentional or under conscious control of the patient, but the patient does not appear to be so distressed or worried about their symptoms. Characteristically, symptoms are maximum when there are other people around to witness them.

Body dysmorphic disorder - a mental health condition in which patients perceive defects or flaws in their appearance and cannot stop thinking about them, making them ashamed and embarrassed to the extent that they avoid social occasions. These flaws appear minor and unnoticed by others.

Pain Disorder – Somatoform pain disorder refers to recurring pain without a known cause, in any part of the body. The pain cannot be accounted for by any known organic illness.

Hypochondriasis – Here the person is obsessed with fear of having a serious illness or becoming sick. Mostly such conditions develop in adulthood. For example, elderly persons feeling insecure due lack of support from children, losing a life partner, dearth of finances etc. may get obsessed with different symptoms at different times like nervousness, palpitations, bowel disorder, chronic respiratory or cardiac diseases etc.

Hypochondriasis is also described as a type of obsession which agonizes the patient but equally affects their family members because of frequent complaints by the hypochondriac person. The person may remain consulting doctors very frequently and they change the types of doctors also. A lot of tests are done to rule out several diseases whose symptoms the person may be complaining about. Diagnosis of hypochondriasis is made by intelligent physicians mostly on history and listening to the patients and his emotions. Sympathetic listening, counselling and short - term medication may help the concerned person.

Treatment of Neuroses– All the above forms of neurosis are treated by the norms described in the Theory of **Psychoanalysis,** which propounds the norms of treatment as following – neurosis is a disorder caused due to emotions and aspirations **suppressed in the subconscious mind** of the subject. Neurotic patients require the assistance and personal involvement of the therapists.

The suppressed impulses, emotions and memories of the patient are revived in order to enable them to relive the past and revisit such memories. This process is necessary to emancipate the patients from their past complexes and terrifying experiences. The emotions of the patients are **desensitized** so that their past feelings may be reconditioned and reformed according to the present situation.

Thus, their phobia of the past is treated, and they are rehabilitated to live a good social life. Pharmacological treatment is done by **anti - anxiety and anti - psychotic** drugs. Patients suffering from acute disorders may need to be given **electroconvulsive shock.**

Depression is a mood disorder which penetrates deep into the mind. Gloominess causes persistent emotional unrest along with the feeling of restlessness. Depression is identified in 2 dimensions viz; **unipolar** and **bipolar** disorder. Here we are describing unipolar depression which consists of experiencing depressive episodes only. Bipolar depression occurs when a person experiences both manic and depressive episodes and it has been described later.

Characteristic symptoms of depression are feelings of **dejection, despondency, melancholy, gloominess, lack of self - worth** etc. It may be accompanied by **restlessness, difficulty in falling asleep or insomnia, lack of concentration and poor decision - making capacity.** Depression affects the patient in many ways like losing activity and dynamism. Absent mindedness and vacuum reigns supreme in depression, usually patients do not remain aware of time span, thus their bonds of inseparable relations are often worn away. Usually, patients in depression are submerged into emptiness, aloofness, indifference, thus are induced to derive the pleasure from drug abuse, get detached from their marital life, very often they are overpowered with the feeling of worthlessness.

Depression is a type of inner unhappiness or downheartedness persisting in the human psyche in various shades and hues. It is a feeling of something lost or something missed or bygone. It is a state of sorrow which transforms the mind time and again. **Sadness** is momentary sorrow caused due to some squabbles or difference of opinion, but **depression** is a mental state continuing and sustaining for a long time. Depression is a deep - down feeling in the heart and mind of the person concerned. Depression is inadvertently expressed in various modes of personality deviation or personality impairment. Depression is a common disorder affecting up to 3 - 4% people worldwide i.e. 1/25th of 8 billion population of the world.

Approximately 250 - 300 million people are victimized by some symptoms of this mental disorder. Women are affected more commonly than men. About 50% of severe depression is **familial.**

Causes and triggering factors for depression may be:

Depression is known to run in families. Therefore, hereditary or familial factors are important predisposing factors for depression.

Precipitating factors for depression are strained social relations, mental shock, natural disasters, bereavement from death of a close relative, physical injuries, new employment, broken marriage, losing employment, financial loss, etc. Delinking of family bonds, acute illnesses viz; heart attack, paralysis, cancer and after childbirth (postpartum depression) Drug abuse like alcohol, cannabis, heroin, smack

Treatment of depression proceeds in following ways – **cognitive behavioral therapy** (**CBT**), inter - personal **psychotherapy** and **certain medicines** are proving effective in depression and a number of psycho - somatic disorders. Deviated thoughts and lifestyle can be controlled by reforming responses and behavioral pattern of the concerned person during behavioral therapy and psychotherapy sessions.

The patient should be counselled not to ponder deeply over negligible issues. Use of medicines for unipolar depression should be minimal and for short term, strictly under supervision of an expert. Drugs like benzodiazepines, agomelatine, amitriptyline, citalopram, duloxetine, escitalopram, imipramine, mirtazapine, paroxetine, sertraline, monoamine oxidase inhibitors, selective serotonin reuptake inhibitors and tricyclics are commonly used to treat depression.

Suicide - A major tragedy caused by depression is **suicide**. According to World Health Organization, more than 700,000 people commit suicide globally every year and it is the 4th leading cause of death among 15 - to 29 - year - olds. For every suicide death, there are many attempted suicides. In fact, a prior attempted suicide is an important 'risk factor' for suicide. The most common methods of suicide are ingestion of pesticides, hanging and use of firearms. Suicide is not only a problem of developed nations, and about 77% of suicides globally occur in low - and middle - income countries. Suicide is a major public health problem in India where suicide rates are on the increase. In 2022, 1.71 lakh suicides were recorded which is an increase of 4.2% over 2021 and 27% compared to 2018.

Who is at risk? - A definite link exists between mental disorders (especially **depression and alcoholism**) and suicide. However, many suicides occur impulsively during moments of crisis and stress – financial problems, broken relationships, feeling of isolation and chronic pain.

Prevention of suicide: Suicides are preventable. Effective evidence - based methods are

i)   limiting access to means which the individual may use – such as pesticides and guns

ii)   fostering life skills in adolescents to make them more resilient

iii)   improving awareness of symptoms and treatment options for patients with mental health issues

iv)   improving access to mental health specialists. In patients with depression, the psychiatrist tries to identify **suicidal thoughts**. If present, proper treatment is an emergency.

Psychosis is a paranormal mental state. Usually in psychosis the person concerned starts relying too much on such sensory experiences as are completely superficial. This dichotomy of real and superficial and the unresolved mental conditions is a state of psychosis. Symptoms of psychosis usher in with trusting the virtual experience as real and true, false notions and beliefs overpower the individual with a veil from where returning becomes almost impossible. The couplet of Urdu - Shayri elucidates the symptom of psychosis as follows –

दूरियां जब बढ़ी तो गलतफहमियां भी बढ़ गईं, फिर उसने वो सुना जो मैंने कहा ही नही .. !!

Explanation –

Ever increasing distance, reached mistrust to pinnacle, what they heard, never did I whisper…

In psychosis, the patient is found unable to make the distinction between the real and the virtual – his experiences have no locus standi of reality. The fundamental difference between neuroses and psychotic disorders is that the psychotic patients isolate themselves from the external real world and lose their acceptability in society. **Psychosis** is an extrasensory mental state which ultimately culminates into occultism and mimics clairvoyance. The patient believes and lives only in virtual experiences.

For example, without actually hearing any noise or music listens to sounds and similarly objects or colors not visible to others are visible to the patient.

They smell odors without the presence of any smell in the atmosphere. Thus, the symptoms of psychosis are manifested in two ways; viz: **Hallucinations** and **Delusions. In Hallucination**, the patient perceives **false sensory stimuli** through the sensory organs. No stimulus is presented to the patient, but their sensory organs feel a variety of false experiences – visual, auditory and olfactory.

In the initial stages, false or hallucinatory experiences emerge and remit automatically, but hallucinatory experiences may transform into **delusion**. **Delusion** is a **false belief** despite incontrovertible evidence to the contrary, that is persistently held. Hallucinations and delusions may lead to a state when the patient feels that others are conspiring against him (**paranoid state**).

Very often patients of psychosis have a fear of being followed or being conspired against by others. Delusions having their genesis in hallucination get consolidated and reinforced as trustworthy in the eyes of those engrossed in their own notional processes.

Thus, in delusion whatever were false experiences transformed into settled and trustworthy belief. The vicious cycle of hallucination and delusion continues as long as the patient is not treated and cared for empathetically.

Hallucination and delusion, though different, occur simultaneously, augmenting each other time and again. Apart from hallucination and delusions, other mild to severe symptoms also occur, such as depression, attention deficit hyperactivity disorder (ADHD), sleeping late at night, insomnia, anxiety, dubiousness, too much suspicion, isolation from the society, incoherent speech, and unkempt living, negligence of physical cleanliness, etc.

Causes of psychosis – There is no single cause of psychosis, which appears to result from a combination of genetic risk, differences in brain development and exposure to stressors or trauma.

Psychosis may be **triggered** by a number of factors such as physical injury or illness, high fever, head injury, or lead or mercury poisoning, recreational drugs, smoking, alcohol, and prescribed medication.

Important types of psychoses include:

- Brief psychotic disorder

- Schizophrenia.

- Bipolar disorder

- Schizoaffective disorder

- Delusional disorder

Brief Psychotic Disorder – Psychosis may occur for a short period of time, such as a few days or a few weeks, after the sudden death of a beloved relative or a divorce, but such brief psychotic disorders may vanish away or dissipate on their own. Sudden drug or alcohol withdrawal in subjects addicted to these may result in hallucinations - auditory, tactile etc.

Schizophrenia, the acute, delirium or frenzied stage of psychosis wherein hallucination and delusion reaches the peak is identified as schizophrenia. This is a chronic, debilitating illness. Combination of genetics, environment and altered brain chemistry and structure are believed to play their role in causation. Schizophrenia has a strong genetic component and may run in families. The course may have exacerbations and remissions.

The illness often first appears in men in late teens or early twenties, while onset in women is typically in 3rd or 4th decade of life. Patients with schizophrenia cannot distinguish as to when they are shackled tersely by their hallucinatory or delusional experiences or by both and thus they remain far away from reality. Schizophrenia can be effectively treated with drugs but there may be poor compliance with treatment. Its treatment is generally lifelong involving medicines, psychotherapy and coordinated specialty care services.

Bipolar Disorder – In this disorder, the individual experiences extreme mood swings that include emotional highs (mania or hypomania) and lows (depression). These periods of mood swings may occur multiple times a year. When depressed, he/she may feel hopeless, sad and lose pleasure or interest in most activities. When the mood shifts to mania or hypomania (less extreme than mania), there may be a feeling of euphoria, increased self

- esteem, being full of energy or unusual irritability, racing thoughts and distractions. These mood swings can affect sleep, behavior, judgment and the ability to think clearly. Between episodes, most patients will have some emotional symptoms. Bipolar disorder is a lifelong condition but can be managed by medications and counselling.

Schizoaffective disorder is different from schizophrenia in that there is no decline in role functioning and mood disorder is prominent.

Delusional disorder is usually manifested as the inconsistency and antagonism between the real and the imagined. It is commonly exhibited in three ways, viz, persecutory, jealous, and grandiose types. Sometimes, the state of psychosis is transformed into a paranoid state in which dependence on grand and grandiose thoughts torment the patient acutely and adversely. The onset of this mental state typically is in middle age. Delusions are present but with less impact on daily life.

Diagnosis of psychosis is made by experienced psychiatrists on the basis of patient's history and by asking certain questions ascertaining feelings, emotions and deep - rooted reasons due to which deviation has crept into patients' personality. **Tests** are done to rule out certain metabolic diseases of calcium, parathyroid hormone, chronic liver disease etc.

Treatment of psychosis in acute situations is by tranquilizers to the patients behaving in anomalous manner like doing violence. Hallucinations and delusions in psychotic patients are treated by antipsychotic drugs. The mental health of the patient is reconstructed by **cognitive behavioral therapy** (CBT) and counselling. Rehabilitation is done in residential homes and asylums so as to bring them back into mainstream. Mental hospital in Agra and Bareilly established by British Government around 150 years back are called mental asylum by the people. These are actually Institutes of Mental Health and Hospitals wherein empirical research is going on. Mental patients are treated with intense care in conducive surroundings so that they are rehabilitated to become useful members of society. The expenditure incurred on their treatment is borne by the Government. In the past family members used to leave and forget their beloved, near and dear in these hospitals. The patients even after being rehabilitated were not accepted by their society and had to live a life of loneliness till long.

Therefore, the best and humanistic rehabilitation of patients with psychoses is in their own home and efforts are made to capacity build the family for domiciliary care.

Nowadays, due to multidimensional advancement in research on mental diseases, skilled and specialist psychiatrists are treating psychotic patients in favorable environments.

Indian Mental Health Act

One in 30 - 40 adults is agonized with some or the other mental disease, though this scenario is not very transparent in society. Mentally ill patients have been usually ill - treated and tormented in every society.

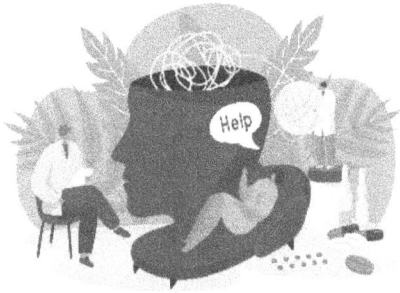

Objectives of the Act 2017– The existing Mental Health Act of 1987 was reformed drastically and ratified in the year 2018 in order to safeguard human rights of mentally ill patients. Thus, the act of 2018 superseded the previous existing act of 1987.

1. **Right to Mental Healthcare:** Every citizen is guaranteed the right to mental healthcare, including treatment, care, and rehabilitation.

2. Every district must have accessible and affordable mental health services.

3. Every person with mental illness has the right to information, confidentiality, and personal contacts.

4. **Decriminalization of Suicidal Behavior:** The Act recognizes suicidal behavior as a symptom of mental illness rather than a crime.

5. The role of nominated **representatives** such as parents/ guardians is outlined in decision - making for mental healthcare of minors.

6. Infants and toddlers must not be separated from mothers receiving treatment for mental illness unless there is a risk to the child.

7. **Prohibition of Unmodified electroconvulsive therapy (ECT):** The Act restricts the use of ECT except in emergency. Even in emergency situations, it cannot be used without anesthesia and muscle relaxants. ECT is prohibited for minors. The **Mental Health Review Board (MHRB)** must review and approve the use of ECT, especially when a patient lacks capacity or in emergencies. Patients can refuse ECT with a valid **advance directive (AD)**, and the medical officer would need to approach the MHRB to review the AD.

8. The act provides that mental illness will not be stigmatized in the society.

9. Inhuman treatment of the mentally ill patients will be illegal.

10. A concerned in charge officer of any police station may take any mentally ill patient into their custody to provide reasonable and required protection.

In conclusion, urbanization, pollution, the rise of nuclear families, and the quest for worldly pleasures fuel mental anguish. Movements like Romanticism, with their poetic and lyrical expressions, call us to seek peace in the natural world, emphasizing that our disconnection from nature is at the root of much of our mental suffering. Philosophers, poets, and thinkers have long argued that humanity's estrangement from the natural environment has played a significant role in the rise of mental illnesses. To regain balance, a return to nature, simplicity, and mindfulness may offer a path toward mental well - being and fulfillment.

Chapter 43

Neurological Disorders & Diseases

Learning Objectives:

- Structure and function of Central Nervous System (CNS) Brain and spinal cord
- Common disorders of CNS – seizures & epilepsy, headache
- Infections in CNS
- Stroke leading to weakness in body and paralysis
- Demyelinating disorders of CNS, Parkinsonism
- Brain and spinal cord tumors
- Coma & Brain death
- Spinal cord disorders
- Neuro-muscular disorders
- Neuropathy, myasthenia

The brain is the central organ that governs and interprets sensations received from all sense organs - eyes, ears, tongue, skin, etc. It controls vital involuntary actions like breathing, heartbeat, intestinal movements, temperature regulation, and blood pressure. In addition, the brain also manages voluntary movements such as walking, running, and maintaining balance.

Beyond these basic functions, the brain oversees complex cognitive activities such as learning, memory, reasoning, emotions, and decision - making. It is responsible for higher functions like analyzing information, comparing, forming judgments, and creative thinking.

What sets the human brain apart is its size and complexity relative to body size compared to other species. In absolute terms, the human brain is larger than that of most mammals. This is one of the primary reasons humans are considered the most evolved species.

The brain's capacity for intelligence allows us to plan, innovate, cooperate, and share knowledge, making human society and development far more advanced than that of other animals.

The brain has a soft, gelatinous consistency, similar to that of soft cheese. To protect this delicate organ, it is encased in a hard, bony structure called the **cranium** or skull. This protective casing shields the brain from injury and external forces, serving as a vital safeguard for such a complex and sensitive organ.

Inside the cranium there are 3 layers of covering called **meninges** (layers of membranes), which hold the brain in place and have a cushioning effect. There are 3 main parts of the brain –

i) The forebrain or bilobed **cerebrum** fills up most of the cranium. It is the cerebrum which controls senses, vision, memory, hearing, cognition, analyzing, making judgement etc. The left side of the cerebrum controls the right half of the body and vice versa. It is involved in remembering, problem solving, thinking and feeling;

ii) The bilobed **cerebellum** at the back and lower part of the head, under the cerebrum is responsible for coordination and balance; and

iii) The **brain stem** sits beneath the cerebrum and in front of cerebellum. The brain stem helps regulate some vital body functions - breathing and heart rate, consciousness, blood pressure and sleep. It is the relay station between the brain and rest of the body and also controls balance, coordination and reflexes. The brain stem is the site of origin of the cranial nerves (nerves to the head region). It has 3 parts – the **midbrain, pons and medulla oblongata.** The brain stem continues downward through the spine as **spinal cord.**

The brain along with spinal cord extends to form the **central nervous system or CNS.** The nervous system links thoughts to actions by sending electrical impulses from the brain cells (**neurons**) to all other parts of the body.

Apart from neurons, the brain also contains **glial cells** which support the neurons. The CNS has **grey and white matter**. The grey matter contains mainly cell bodies and white matter consists of **axons** or long fibers continuing from the cell bodies. Most of the grey matter is found in the **cortex** or **folded outer layer** of brain, while the deep, inner part is mostly made up of white matter.

Besides the CNS has **cerebrospinal fluid** (CSF) circulating through the inner most parts of the brain (ventricles) and spinal cord (spinal canal).

Apart from the CNS, there is the peripheral nervous system which includes the **peripheral nerves**. These nerves carry electrical impulses travelling from brain stem and spinal cord to muscles and from sensory organs to the spinal cord and brain. Any movement in and through the body depends upon communication between the brain and the muscles. A component of the peripheral nervous system is the **autonomic nervous system.** It is responsible for regulating involuntary physiologic processes like respiration, heart rate, blood pressure, digestion and sexual arousal.

Diseases of CNS

Seizures & Epilepsy – The brain functions through electrical signals. A seizure is a single event characterized by sudden uncontrolled body movements, sensations or change in behavior due to abnormal electrical activity in the cerebral cortex. Symptoms include loss of muscle control, awareness and shaking.

The term **epilepsy** refers to a tendency to recurrent seizures. There are many types as well as causes of seizures and epilepsy – both acquired and genetic. In most cases imaging of the brain and electro - encephalogram (EEG) are done, which may shed light on the cause and type of epilepsy.

Acute seizures are a medical emergency, especially if there is loss of consciousness. Usually, a seizure would last less than 2 - 3 minutes. The patient should be made to lie on one side with face downward and nothing should be put in the mouth until full consciousness is regained. If the seizure continues beyond 5 minutes, medical help in the form of intravenous injection or intranasal dose of antiseizure medication is required.

Status epilepticus is a prolonged seizure lasting for more than 5 minutes or recurrent seizures without regaining consciousness. It should be treated in hospital according to protocol.

For epilepsy, the patient is put on long term (2 years or more) regular antiepileptic drugs. In addition, driving is prohibited and so is unsupervised swimming, cycling or crossing the road.

Headache – Pain in the head or face is a very common symptom which most people experience during their lives. Headache often occurs as recurrent episodes. Causes of headache can be primary or secondary. The main primary headaches include migraine, tension headache and cluster headaches. Tension headache is the most common cause.

Migraine is a common type of headache which runs in families. Often it is throbbing in character, on one side of the head and associated with nausea. It is worsened by physical activity, bright lights and noise. Primary headaches are generally not dangerous but can disrupt daily life. Secondary headaches are those associated with underlying medical conditions i.e. headache is the symptom which draws attention to an underlying brain lesion. Sudden onset of new and severe episodes of headache or any of those following head injury, associated with fever, neck stiffness or neurological signs or any new type of headache after age 55 should be investigated to exclude any brain mass or tumor, bleed or infection.

Cerebrovascular Disease & Stroke – Here, the arteries of the brain are affected. Blood flow to the brain is obstructed or retarded mainly due to atherosclerosis. Arteries supplying oxygen and nutrition to the brain are ruptured, narrowed or blocked. Brain **stroke** occurs which means permanent damage to part of the brain supplied by the artery, leading to permanent paralysis of limbs (usually on one side of the body) and disability, or the patient may even die. Strokes are usually sudden in onset and are of 2 main types - ischemic and hemorrhagic.

Transient Ischemic Attack is a precursor or warning of a stroke. Transient paralysis occurs but later recovers. High blood pressure, diabetes and frequent tobacco consumption must be controlled for preventing actual stroke.

Ischemic Stroke – This is the commoner type (80%) of stroke caused by atherosclerosis in which blood clots obstruct blood flow in the cerebral arteries, causing paralysis. This attack is similar to a heart attack.

Again, there are 2 types of ischemic strokes –

i) **Embolic** – when a blood clot or debris (embolus) formed in one part of the body or heart travels to and lodges in a narrower brain artery, blocking the blood flow to the brain. Onset is most sudden with embolic stroke

ii) **Thrombotic Stroke** – this type of stroke occurs when a thrombus (blood clot) develops in an artery supplying blood to the brain. It is not as sudden as embolic stroke and may have a 'stuttering' onset.

Hemorrhagic Stroke – this type of stroke occurs due to rupture of blood vessels causing bleeding into the brain. Increased pressure in the brain causes severe headaches and irritation of meninges. Uncontrolled high blood pressure is another reason due to which hemorrhagic brain stroke may occur at any time. Hemorrhagic stroke can also occur due to bleeding disorders or some intrinsic abnormality of the artery such as **aneurysm or arteriovenous malformations**.

Aneurysm – This is another type of arterial disease. A part of the arterial wall is weak and ballooned out. Often these are present from birth but may go undetected until they rupture – often with devastating effects. Rupture of brain aneurysms lead to hemorrhagic stroke. Sometimes this stroke may be fatal causing untimely death of the patient.

Arteriovenous malformation (AVM) – Multiple, irregular and abnormal connection (tangle of blood vessels) between arteries and veins may occur anywhere in the body but such malformations most commonly occur in brain or spine. AVM is usually present at birth (congenital). Rupture of AVM in the brain causes hemorrhagic stroke.

Peripheral Arterial Disease – Narrowing or blockage of the arteries of legs occurs. It is primarily caused by the buildup of atherosclerotic or fatty plaque in the arteries of the legs, similar to atherosclerosis in the coronary (heart) arteries.

Pain in the legs may occur during exercise – this is known as (intermittent **claudication**) and later may recur at rest.

Infections of CNS – A wide variety of infectious agents – viruses, bacteria, protozoa, fungi etc. can invade the brain and may cause **meningoencephalitis** (inflammation of brain meninges and brain parenchyma). The usual symptoms are fever, headache, vomiting, seizures, coma and paralysis of body parts. Brain infections are usually serious with risk of mortality and disabling sequelae and must be diagnosed and treated urgently. Brain infections can be mimicked by non - infectious conditions if fever is present due to another cause. Investigation of brain infection often involves examination of cerebrospinal fluid (by lumbar puncture) for cell count, protein and sugar levels and culture of the organism.

Specific antibodies to infectious agents are tested for. Neuroimaging in the form of **Magnetic resonance imaging** (MRI) or **computed tomographic** (CT) scan may give a specific picture. Apart from meningoencephalitides, other forms of CNS infection are **brain abscess, granulomas** and **spinal arachnoiditis** (inflammation of meningeal covering of spinal cord).

Demyelinating disorders are a group of autoimmune disorders in which antibodies are formed which attack the myelin sheath of nerve cells. Due to this, the impulses between neurons cannot travel as fast as usual. The common symptoms of demyelinating disorders are muscle weakness or paralysis, muscle stiffness, vision loss, symptoms related to urinary bladder and bowel and sensory changes (tingling, numbness). The cause of these disorders is not well understood. There may be a genetic predisposition coupled with an environmental trigger (such as virus infection). The most common of the demyelinating disorders is **multiple sclerosis**. This is a chronic disease with a remitting and relapsing course.

Other demyelinating disorders are **acute disseminated encephalomyelitis (ADEM), transverse myelitis, Guillain Barre syndrome, neuromyelitis optica, etc.** Investigations include MRI scan and tests for specific antibodies. Treatment is usually in the form of immunosuppressive agents and physiotherapy.

Parkinson's disease – This is a chronic progressive disorder that is caused by degeneration of nerve cells in a part of the brain called the substantia nigra, which controls movement. Onset is usually after age 55 years. These neurons then lose the ability to produce an important chemical (**neurotransmitter**) called **dopamine**.

Without enough dopamine, the delicate balance between various neurotransmitters is disrupted, resulting in movement disorder in the form of **bradykinesia** (slowness of movement) **rigidity** (stiffness of the limbs); **tremor** (trembling in the hands, arms, legs and jaw) and **impaired coordination**. **Dementia** and **depression** may cause further difficulties.

The cause of Parkinson's disease is not fully understood but genetic coupled with environmental factors are believed to play a role. Diagnosis is based on clinical features and exclusion of other causes of such symptoms.

Treatment is in the form of medications – **levodopa, anticholinergic drugs and dopamine agonists**. Surgery and **deep brain stimulation** (DBS) are other options.

Brain Tumors – A brain tumor is an abnormal growth of cells in the brain. They can originate in brain tissue or other structures like nerves, glands, glial cells and membranes covering the brain surface. They can be benign or cancerous (malignant). Malignant brain tumors may be primary (arising within the brain) or secondary i.e. metastasis of a primary tumor elsewhere in the body. Brain tumors are common in childhood in which they are the 2nd most common malignancy after leukemia. Any growth in the brain would lead to pressure effects on surrounding tissue and impair its function causing seizures, paralysis, problems with balance and coordination, memory, personality and behavior changes etc. So, symptoms depend on the location of the tumor. Ultimately, because the brain is encased in a bony structure there is no space to expand and pressure within the cranium increases (**raised intracranial tension**) causing headache, vomiting, blurred vision, double vision etc. Growth within the cranium can also lead to obstruction in the flow of CSF and accumulation of CSF (**hydrocephalus**). Types of brain tumors include astrocytoma (arising from glial cells – astrocytes), medulloblastoma, acoustic neuroma (arising from nerve), germ cell tumors, pinealomas, pituitary tumors, meningiomas, choroid plexus tumors etc. Diagnosis can usually be made on neuroimaging (CT scan or MRI) but **stereotactic needle biopsy** may be required for delineating type and grade.

Treatment options might include surgery, radiation therapy, radiosurgery, chemotherapy and targeted therapy. Brain surgery has to be performed very carefully so as not to injure vital parts of the brain. For this reason, surgery may have to be subtotal and followed up with radiosurgery.

Coma – This refers to a state of **prolonged** loss of consciousness. There are two main types of comas – structural and functional. In structural coma the cause is within the brain that is structural abnormality in the brain itself like traumatic head injury, brain infection, stroke, tumor, injury due to low oxygen etc. Functional coma occurs due to some general illnesses (like diabetes, uremia, abnormalities in electrolytes etc.), poisoning, drug or toxin affecting both the cerebral hemispheres. It is important to find the cause of the coma and treat it. The severity or depth of coma is assessed by various scales – the **Glasgow Coma Scale and AVPU scale** (Alert - response to Verbal commands, response to Pain – Unresponsive). A quick assessment of the need for resuscitation needs to be made. Airway, breathing and circulation need to be assessed and supported if necessary.

A detailed physical and neurological examination should follow. Supportive care includes medicines to bring down fever (if febrile), medicines to prevent seizures (if present) and measures to bring down raised intracranial pressure as needed. Nursing care is very important. The patient should be made to lie on one side with face downward (recovery position) and frequent changes from side to side are made to prevent bed sores. Care of the eyes is important to prevent corneal ulcers. Chest physiotherapy is done to prevent pneumonia of the dependent part of lung.

Persistent vegetative state refers to a state of recovery from coma when the patient returns to a wakeful state but without awareness.

Brain Death – Refers to complete permanent cessation of all brain function including the brain stem. The heart muscle can go on beating even indefinitely if respiration, oxygen level and blood pressure are maintained. However, once the patient is brain dead, the individual is dead for all practical purposes and can never return to a functional state. Diagnosis of brain death is important because in this state the organs can be removed for **organ donation**. Different countries have their own laws and criteria for diagnosis of brain death. For E.g. the proximate cause of death should be known and should be irreversible, and all brain stem reflexes should be lost.

Spinal Disorders – The spinal cord is a long, fragile structure extending downward from the base of the brain. It is protected by the vertebral column, which is made up of vertebrae separated from each other by discs made of cartilage. The spinal cord is the main pathway through which the brain communicates with the rest of the body. The **anterior horn cells** in the spinal cord project from the grey matter of spinal cord directly to muscle fibers.

The spine is divided into four sections – cervical, thoracic, lumbar and sacral. The spinal cord may be compressed by mechanisms **external** to the cord, such as vertebral fractures, herniated disc, collapse of vertebrae due to tumor or disease, abscess or spinal canal narrowing (stenosis). Causes inside the spinal cord are fluid - filled cavity, (syrinx), blockage of the blood supply, inflammation (as occurs in acute transverse myelitis), tumors, bleeding, vitamin B_{12} deficiency, infections, multiple sclerosis and radiation therapy. Damage to the cord often produces specific patterns of symptoms according to where the damage occurred.

These symptoms include back pain, muscle weakness or paralysis involving both lower limbs (paraplegia) or all 4 limbs (quadriplegia), loss of sensation or abnormal sensations, change in reflexes, loss of bladder and bowel control, decreased sweating and erectile dysfunction. Diagnosis is made by neurological examination, X - rays of the spine and MRIs and occasionally myelogram.

Neuromuscular disorders – A **motor unit** consists of an anterior horn cell and all the muscle fibers innervated by it. Neuromuscular disorders are those affecting the motor unit at any level – anterior horn cell, peripheral nerve, neuromuscular junction and muscles. Specific damage to anterior horn cells is caused by **polio** and some chronic progressive diseases – **spinal muscular atrophy (in infants and children)** and **motor neurone disease** in adults. Peripheral nerve damage occurs in diabetes, vitamin deficiencies, leprosy, some genetic conditions and **Guillain barre syndrome**. The latter is an autoimmune disorder characterized by generalized neuropathy. The prototype of neuromuscular junction disorder is **myasthenia gravis** – which again is autoimmune in nature.

Finally, there are many types of primary muscle diseases – such as **myopathies, muscular dystrophies, polymyositis** etc.

Diagnosis of neuromuscular disorders is made by examination in which there is weakness and diminution in deep tendon reflexes. **Nerve conduction** and **electromyography** studies are done. **Antibody levels** and **exome sequencing** studies may also be done.

In conclusion, the brain is integral to all life processes. It enables us to hear, smell, feel, and perceive everything presented before it, making it the epicenter of existence. If the brain ceases to function, all life processes come to a halt, underscoring its critical role. Research has revealed that all living beings possess some form of consciousness, allowing them to continue their existence. While lower beings function with a more limited form of awareness, higher beings, such as humans, operate with an enriched and developed consciousness that enables complex thought, sensation, and interaction with the world. This higher level of consciousness sets humans apart, guiding not only individual life processes but also the continuity and progress of human evolution.

Chapter 44

Accidents and Injury – Prevention, Minimization, First Aid, and Basic Life Support

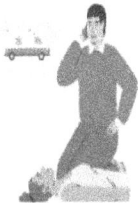 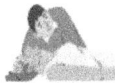 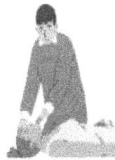 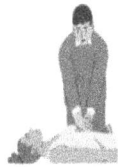

CALL EMERGENCY NUMBER   CHECK BREATHING   LIFT CHIN CHECK BREATHING   GIVE RESCUE BREATHS   PERFORM CPR

Learning Objectives:

- Physical injuries and damage due to various accidents
- Occurrence and causes of accidents – traffic, violence, drug abuse, drowning, burning, dog bite, snake bite, poisoning, bleeding, seizure
- Utility of Basic Life Support (BLS) training and drill
- Accidents due to radiation, radioactive carcinogens, volatile inhalants etc.
- Implementing rules and measures to avoid accidents

Accidents occur in various settings - on roads, in factories, homes, sports fields, and workplaces - despite constant warnings and awareness campaigns. Whether minor or major, accidents often have serious consequences, including injury, loss of life, and psychological trauma. Globally, road traffic accidents alone account for approximately one million deaths annually, with millions more suffering serious injuries. When accidents impact multiple people, they are classified as disasters, requiring specialized management efforts from government and rescue teams.

In India, disaster management protocols are robustly established by central and state governments, ensuring prompt responses to large - scale emergencies. Disasters such as landslides, floods, earthquakes, fires, bridge collapses, gas leaks, and terrorist attacks demand highly trained personnel. Teams, consisting of fire workers, divers, helicopters, and advanced machinery, collaborate to rescue individuals and mitigate damage.

Local populations often act as first responders, playing an important role in providing immediate aid. Paramedical professionals and emergency response units administer **basic life support** and **cardiopulmonary resuscitation (CPR)** to stabilize victims. The injured are then transported to hospitals for advanced medical care.

Each type of accident, whether it occurs in a natural setting or as a result of human activity, presents unique challenges. Preparedness, vigilance, and an effective response system are crucial in minimizing the damage caused by these unfortunate events. Discussions regarding various types of accidents are detailed below.

Road Traffic Accidents wherein **three causative factors** that emerge may be indicated as follows.

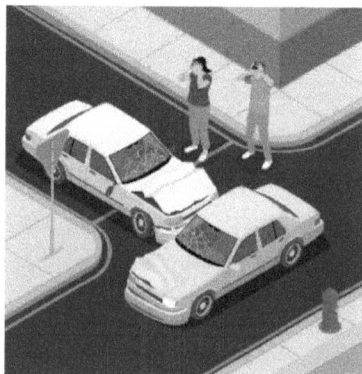

The **first factor** is the **host,** that is the person injured who can save themselves from accidents. Non - adherence to traffic rules may cause an accident resulting in serious injuries or trauma. Fastening the vehicle seat belt, putting on helmet, having children use child seat, promptness at road crossing, driving in proper lane, being vigilant for cleanliness of vehicle glasses, care as regards vehicle and crossing light, driving the vehicle with cautious view through the mirrors, avoiding alcohol while driving, observing speed limits, not driving the vehicle while sleepy or affected by diseases like epilepsy, hypoglycemia, night blindness, etc. can save and protect us against sudden traffic accidents on the road. Sleep usually overpowers during 2 - 5 AM resulting in serious traffic accidents. Certain rules must be adhered to while walking in the pedestrian lane.

The vehicle owner should have the right attitude of investing on safety measures like getting the seat belt fitted, purchasing a helmet, buying car fitted with air bags, efficient brake system, changing worn out tire, etc. are behaviors which save precious lives. Parents, social organizations, schools and elders must teach their children road traffic rules.

The **second factor** is the **agent -** that is the vehicle involved. The various 'built in' modern safety technology in the vehicle include brake system, seat belt, **self - inflating balloons**, collapsible steering, side - view and back - view mirrors without blind spot, auto brake in case of impediment etc. prevent accidents. Expressway accidents may occur due to over - heating up and **bursting of tires**. To prevent this, good tires with less air pressure filled with nitrogen gas are used.

The **third factor** is the **environment**, as for example – road, railway line, air space, sea, river, weather, heavy rain, visibility etc. Animals suddenly coming in front of vehicles, ditch on roadside, inadequate light, potholes in the road, vehicle standing in the way, vehicle running on another lane taking a sudden turn, etc. sometimes are a significant reason in causing serious accident. The host, being prompt and vigilant, may be able to avert a serious accident. Providing safe roads, pedestrian lanes, making the traffic rules, safety signages etc. are obligations of the government.

Avoiding a road journey when weather is bad, visibility poor, and driver sleepy speaks of wisdom of the man. Not allowing children to drive, not using mobile phones while driving, not going near unguarded ditches or water bodies etc. are pragmatic measures to avoid accidents. Special care has to be exercised while removing the helmet in an accident involving a 2 - wheeler.

Two rescuers are required. The first immobilizes the head with hands on each side of helmet and fingers on patient's mandible (jaw bone). The assistant cuts or loosens the strap and places hands either side of the head to **support the neck**. The rescuer at the head end then gently removes the helmet and glasses. Support the head, neck and spine in a **neutral position** at all times to prevent twisting or bending movements or apply a **cervical collar**, if trained to do so, to minimize neck movement.

Drowning is caused due to **immersion, or submersion** in water. In **immersion** the body is surrounded by cold water but the airway is above the water level, while in submersion the airway is below the water surface and inability to breathe is obvious.

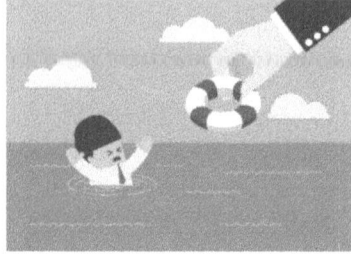

Sometimes drowning may also mean suffocation caused by submersion of the nose and mouth in a liquid. Ninety percent of drowning occurs in fresh water (river, lake, pond or pool) and 10% of drowning in sea water. Drowning in various liquids may occur in industrial accidents.

Different types of drowning are detailed as below –

Near drowning – means that the person survived after reaching to the brink of drowning. About a third of such people would experience complications in the form of **acute respiratory distress syndrome (ARDS) or acute lung injury (ALI).**

Drowning This can be considered in four stages:

In the first stage, as water enters the respiratory passage in a conscious person, there is **spasm of the larynx** which prevents water from further entering the airways. The laryngeal spasm persists till **the buildup of carbon dioxide** becomes overwhelming. If most of the water goes into the stomach and not into the lungs still choking may be felt - is called dry drowning.

In the 2nd stage, **fluid is aspirated** into the airways and lungs and also **swallowed** into stomach and intestines.

In the 3rd stage, the presence of fluid impedes **gas exchange** in the lungs. This leads to low oxygen levels in the blood. A low oxygen level in the brain causes loss of consciousness and stops breathing.

Brain injury due to low oxygen becomes **irreversible**.

Fresh water drowning – Ninety percent of drowning takes place in fresh water.

Swallowed fresh water from pools, lakes, ponds etc. has low **osmotic pressure** and quickly gets absorbed into blood. After complete drowning and swallowing fresh water, it percolates into the lungs and enters the blood stream causing **hemodilution.** The pH value of blood is reduced, and death occurs in this **secondary drowning**.

In hemodilution blood volume is increased as a result of which blood cells swell up and rupture (**hemolysis**). Intensive and critical emergency treatment of hemodilution saves life.

Saltwater drowning – Here the lungs get filled with salt water. The salt water being **hypertonic** (higher osmotic pressure) pulls water from the bloodstream into the lungs. This liquid build - up in the air sacs stops air exchange in the lungs. Oxygen then does not reach the blood stream. Sea water drowning is rare because of high buoyance due to the presence of 3.5% salt in it. Drowning in sea water results in death because high viscosity of saltwater which makes the blood highly viscous, thus retarding heart beat.

First aid for drowning includes:

(i)   calling for help

(ii) pulling the victim out of water

(iii) turning the victim onto the belly and thumping the back for letting the water come out from the lungs

(iv) lying the victim on the back for providing cardio - pulmonary resuscitation.

(v)   starting cardio - pulmonary resuscitation (CPR). This means giving **rescue breaths** *and* **cardiac massage.**

Burns – These are injuries to skin or other body parts caused by heat, radiation, radioactivity, electricity, friction or contact with chemicals. In day - to - day fire accidents, usually the surface skin and sometimes the tissue under the skin is burnt. Thermal (heat) burns occur when some or all the layers of skin or other tissues are destroyed.

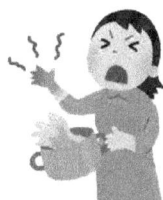

Burning caused on account of boiling water or steam, hot tea, hot oil, sugar - syrup etc. is called **scalding**. Similarly, burning caused due to contact with hot solids is contact burn and burning with flames is flame burn.

Burns are a public health problem, accounting for an estimated 180,000 deaths globally every year. The majority of these occur in low - and middle - income countries. In India, over 1 million people are moderately or severely burnt every year. Burns are also a leading cause of morbidity, prolonged hospitalization, disfigurement, disability, stigma and rejection.

Burning with flames in *saree, dupatta* etc. in kitchen and burning because of friction i.e. abrasion in muscles or tissues due to traffic accidents are common.

In India most of the casualties viz; 90% burn cases happen on account of accidents in the kitchen mostly in women, 5% burn occur due to fire out - breaks and industrial accidents, 3% due to suicides and 2% due to homicides.

Burn Assessment is done by the burnt body area and the depth of burn as given below. The flat hand of the person is approximately equivalent to 1% body surface area. More than 10% body surface burn is considered serious, and patients are admitted to a hospital or burn unit. The depth of burn is documented below:

First - degree burns are superficial, mild, involving only the top layer of skin (epidermis), which turns red, is painful but doesn't blister. If somehow blisters erupt, these are punctured to let the fluid ooze out; dressing is applied with the burnt skin itself, new skin grows shortly.

Second - degree burns affect skin's top and lower layers (dermis). The upper portion of the skin gets inflamed, swollen and thickened. There may be pain, redness, swelling and blistering. **Blisters** filled with water fulminate over the skin - surface which if torn heal in 8 - 10 weeks after dressing etc.

Third - degree burns affect all three skin layers: epidermis, dermis and fat. Full thickness skin is burnt and hair follicles and sweat glands are also destroyed. The burnt portion is thickened and becomes stiff.

Because third - degree burns damage nerve endings, **pain is not felt** in the burn area itself, rather adjacent to it. Burnt skin may be black, white or red with a leathery appearance. Such burnt cases do not heal automatically - they need skin grafting otherwise contractures develop.

Fourth degree burns – it is severe burn in which torrid and oppressive heat and flames infiltrate through all the layers of skin and damages the underlying muscles, tendons or bones. All the wounds turn black, and the burnt portion of the body is severely damaged.

First aid for burns – The burnt area should be kept under cool (not cold) running water for 10 minutes.

For facial burns a cool, wet cloth should be placed over the burnt area till the pain eases. For a mouth burn from hot food or drink, a piece of ice should be kept in the mouth for a few minutes. Rings or other tight jewelry or clothing items should be removed from the burnt area.

First and second - degree burns are treated by **pain killers and soothing anesthetic ointments**. Usually, these burns do not lead to scarring.

Third - and fourth - degree burns need emergency medical care at **burn treatment centers.** The patient is stabilized, and measures are taken to prevent infection. There may be loss of proteins, fluids and electrolytes through the burnt area. The wounds of third - and fourth - degree burns are washed and cleaned by saline water and dressed in antiseptic ointment or may be kept open. The amount of body surface area and degree of depth of burn indicates severity. Treatment for third - degree burns may include early cleaning and debriding (removing dead skin and tissue from the burnt area) every day till it heals. Plastic surgery with **skin grafting** is planned.

Partial thickness of the healthy skin from another portion of the body is taken out and grafted on the wounds for quick healing – this grafting is called **autologous**. Nowadays research are going on for resurfacing the burnt area with stem cells that generate skin. Even after best treatment of acute, deep burns stiffness, numbness, scarring and white skin may remain.

Sometimes the interiors of the lungs of the industrial workers are burnt due to the excessive heat of smoke. Inhaled poisonous gas like carbon monoxide may cause acute interstitial lung diseases.

Dog Bite

Instances of dog bites are a common occurrence. Some dogs are dangerous for biting habitually while others seldom bite. Dog bite is a common problem in India. There was a dip in dog bites in India since 2018, but since 2022, dog bite cases are again on the rise – rising from 21.8 lakh in 2022 to 27.5 lakhs in 2023, with 18,000 - 20,000 deaths due to dog bite, according to data tabled by the Ministry of Health and Family Welfare in parliament. Under the **Bharatiya Nyaya Sanhita (BNS),** if a pet animal attacks a human, the owner can be fined up to Rs 5,000 with imprisonment of up to six months.

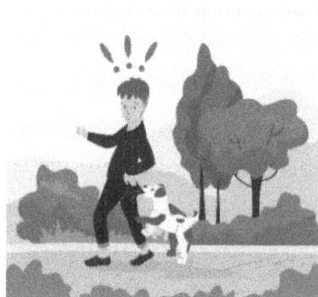

The most dreaded consequence of dog bites is rabies. **Rabies** is caused by a viral infection of the brain – the rabies virus travels along with nerves to the spinal cord and then to the brain where it multiplies. From there it travels to salivary glands and into the saliva. Rabies is endemic in 150 countries, including India, which accounts for 36% of global rabies deaths. The true burden of rabies in India is not fully known and is probably understated.

Dogs are the cause of the vast majority of human rabies deaths, contributing up to 96% of all rabies transmissions to humans. Infection of rabies occurs due to biting by **rabid dogs** (rabies infected dogs or mad dogs) or rabies infected animals. Apart from dogs, other **mammals** - cats, mongooses, jackals, foxes, wolves, horses, donkeys, monkeys, bats and rats can spread rabies. Rabies is spread through saliva of the infected animal. Symptoms start typically after 20 to 90 days, although incubation periods as short as 4 days and longer than 6 years have been documented. The first symptom may be tingling or itching at the wound site. Rabies infected humans also fear water which is referred to as **hydrophobia**.

As the disease progresses, high fever, over excitement, memory loss, offensiveness, delirium, abnormal behavior, paralysis, hydrophobia (fear of water) and insomnia ensue, ultimately resulting in death. Once symptoms start, rabies is almost uniformly fatal and only supportive treatment is given.

Prevention of rabies – Social security rules in all countries provide for anti - rabies vaccination of pet dogs, other pets and stray dogs to deter rabies infection. Nonadherence to these rules entails strict actions by Governments – though these rules are generally poorly implemented in India. If a bite by a stray animal occurs, it is helpful to keep an eye on the animal.

Immediate **first aid** in animal bites is **thorough washing** of the wound in running or flowing tap water. Never rub the wound lest the saliva should be inoculated. Use soap and antiseptics only if readily available or else wash under running water for 10 minutes, which should remove most of the saliva from the surface. The wound may be covered with a clean lint and bandaged only if bleeding. A medical practitioner should be consulted as soon as possible. Bite through clothing like trousers retains most of infectious saliva in the cloth and may be of less severity. Infected clothing should be removed with care.

Bites on the head and neck area and on upper limbs are more dangerous. Depending on severity of bite, **anti - rabies immunoglobulin** is administered. Rabies can be prevented by regular vaccination of pet dogs, possibly stray dogs, animal handlers and **post exposure prophylaxis (PEP)**, which means timely administration of anti - rabies vaccines as per schedule. Either intramuscular or intradermal vaccine can be used, with the latter using smaller volume in shorter schedule. **Tetanus** also needs to be prevented after bites by appropriate measures.

Snake Bite occurs mostly in villages, fields, forests, construction sites etc. Snakes usually bite if scared of human movement or being trapped. Fangs of snake penetrating into the body is called snake bite. Different species of snakes exist in this world - some of which are venomous while others are non - venomous – thus every snake bite is not similar in toxicity. Even among venomous snakes, different species carry different types of venom. Venomous snakes are **kraits, cobra, mambas, viper, sea snake** etc. Remaining cautious of snake bite is important because venomous snakes are found all over the world. Venom enters the victim's body through the fangs. The fang marks leave an impression on the skin.

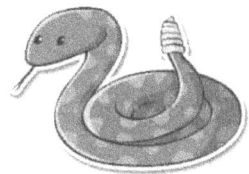

Snake bite fang marks are identified from which the genre of the snake is also deciphered. Usually, 2 fang marks indicate a poisonous snake.

There are at least **four major classes of venoms**, namely

i) **neurotoxins**, which affect nervous systems causes paralysis;

ii) **cytotoxins**, which kill cells leading to local area redness and swelling;

iii) **mycotoxins**, which damage muscles; and

iv) **hemotoxins**, which disrupt blood clotting leading to bleeding points.

Symptoms and signs after snake bite include

(i) puncture or fang marks at the site

(ii) redness, swelling, bruising, bleeding or blistering around the bite within one hour of bite

(iii) severe pain at the site of the bite and

(iv) nausea, vomiting, diarrhea and other systemic symptoms.

Symptoms of **neurotoxin envenomation** (as in cobra bite) include blurred vision, drooping eyelids, tremors of hands and feet, weakness, drowsiness, sweating, slow heart rate, and paralysis. Viper venom contains **hemotoxin** which may result in severe hemorrhage and kidney failure. Sometimes, faintness and vertigo may also occur due to hypotension.

First aid for snake bite – Immediate first aid measures if snake bite is suspected include

(i) removing any tight clothing or jewelry from around the bitten part (e.g.: rings, anklets, bracelets) as these can cause harm if swelling occurs

(ii) victim is made to lie or sit in a neutral position of comfort

(iii)   washing the site with soap and a gush of water

(iv)   Covering the bite with a clean, dry dressing

(v)   immobilizing the limb by splint

(vi)   providing analgesia. Tourniquet and sucking the venom, tearing or splitting the wound with a knife may cause harm to victim and are not recommended.

The victim should be hastily transported to a medical Center where **anti - snake venom (ASV)** is available - ASV is the mainstay of treatment.

Anti Venom is an anti - body or antiserum immunoglobulin used to neutralize the effect of snake venom. Developing anti venom of snakes of different species is exorbitantly expensive and time taking. Inaccurate or erroneous anti - venom may inflict more harm to the victim by causing **anaphylaxis (acute allergy)** etc. In the year 1950, the first anti - venom was developed by the USA from coral snake. Different countries develop antivenom according to their own local / regional snake species.

Now a day's **polyvalent ASV** vaccine is being developed from the commonly prevalent snakes. In India, polyvalent ASV effective against all the four common species - Russell's viper, common cobra, common Krait and saw - scaled viper is used. Monovalent anti snake venom (ASV) sera are not available in India because preparation of each type of snake venom will involve huge resources. Treatment of snake bites may require intensive care.

Bee sting - Stings by a bee can cause

(i)   mild temporary pain and discomfort

(ii)   significant swelling or

(iii)   severe allergic reaction.

First aid for bee stings

• Gently slide or scrape your fingernail across the sting to remove it. It should not be pulled out.

- Wash the area, and then apply a cold pack (this will reduce swelling).

- In case of significant pain and swelling, pain relief with paracetamol or an antihistamine may give relief.

- If the person is allergic to bee stings, **anaphylaxis** can occur. They need to be taken to hospital and may need an injection of **adrenaline.**

- If the person is stung in the mouth or stung multiple times in a single incident (adults more than 10 times or children more than 5 times) they also need to be taken to hospital.

Poisoning – This refers to exposure of the body to harmful or toxic substances – **accidental or intentional.** According to the WHO (2012), poisoning caused approximately 200,000 deaths worldwide of which 84% occurred in low - and middle - income countries. Poisons may be inhaled, ingested, injected or absorbed through skin. Effects of poison may be immediate or delayed.

Poison may be due to chemicals used in households (bleach, kerosene, phenol, pesticides, rat poison, acids or alkali ingestion etc.), industrial substances (methanol, ethylene glycol, cyanide, arsenic, lead etc.), gases such as carbon monoxide, overdose of drugs (iron, aspirin, paracetamol, barbiturates, antidepressants etc.) plant poisons (poisonous mushrooms etc.) etc. If a possibility of poisoning exists, immediate steps to be taken are – get the victim into fresh air (if inhaled poison), take off any contaminated clothing and rinse skin with running water for 15 to 20 minutes if absorbed through skin. Identification of the poison is done by history, laboratory tests or by toxicology screen. If possible, the ingested material should be saved for testing. Immediate medical help should be sought. Intensive care may be required. Measures to remove poison before absorption into blood include **induced vomiting, activated charcoal and gastric lavage.** Measures to enhance elimination of the poison are done by **dialysis**. Specific antidotes if available should be administered.

Exposure to Radiation and Lethal Substances refers to exposure to radioactive substances like uranium, thorium and other carcinogens in industrial zones.

Chemical reactions and vaporization of toxic gases in toxicological and health laboratories can cause irreparable loss and fatal diseases to humans. Specific precautions, preventive measures and highly specific treatments are undertaken.

Food poisoning – food poisoning may occur due to eating preserved or stale food, such as salad and fruit peeled and cut hours before dinner. It is caused by bacterial infection in consumed food. Food poisoning may cause acute vomiting, diarrhea, abdominal cramps and fever etc. Deficiency of water and electrolyte may be caused.

Consumption of country liquor like methyl alcohol or hooch (inferior or illicit alcohol) or poisonous liquor may have serious consequences. Victims should be rushed to the hospital for immediate treatment.

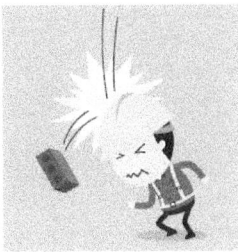

Workplace and Industrial Accidents – Examples of workplace accidents are injuries like falling in the workplace while lifting, carrying or unloading heavy loads, due to derangement in body balance. Similarly, injuries from heavy machines, apparatus handling, electrocution from high - voltage - electricity, amputation of fingers, toes, thumbs of limbs in various machines, sparks from welding causing burns in the eyes, ears or other organs, mud - sliding in mines, quarries, ditches, fire accidents are sometimes precursors of disasters.

Stern industrial rules and regulations exist for preventing industrial accidents. Machine designs are constantly evolving to prevent industrial accidents. Adherence to **good working, construction and manufacturing practices** are important.

Workplace fatigue reduction and shift duty have been recognized as important determinants towards restraining accidents. Safety gadgets like helmets, thick shoes, gum boots, gloves, barring loose clothes, wearing fluorescent clothes are effective measures to prevent accidents in workplaces or industrial places.

Rules regarding maintenance of apparatus, equipment and their time bound expiry utility should be audited and scrutinized at specific intervals.

As exposure to **radioactive substances - uranium, thorium,** carcinogens and other toxic gases are detrimental to health of workers, entry of common people to industrial places is prohibited. Health - assessment laboratories remain dynamic and vigilant in monitoring radioactive exposure and harmful effects of substances like uranium, thorium, toxic liquids and gases and other chemical substances for safeguarding the environment.

Major industrial disasters include the **Bhopal Gas Tragedy** which occurred on 2nd December 1984 due to leakage of the highly toxic gas methyl isocyanate (MIC) in the pesticide plant of Union Carbide India Limited (UCIL). As per the affidavit of Government of India this leak caused more than 5 lakh injuries leading to permanent disability and death. Distress like breathlessness, circulatory collapse, pulmonary edema, cerebral edema etc. were caused to the people living in the surrounding vicinity.

Long term health hazards like corneal opacities, early cataracts, obstructive and restrictive respiratory disease, aggravation of tuberculosis, etc. are still taking place. The **Chernobyl Meltdown, in erstwhile USSR (now Ukraine)** which occurred on 26th April 1986 is an example of a nuclear disaster. In spite of various restorative efforts 5 lakh people were affected by acute diseases and many people died. Another such accident is the **Fukushima - Daiichi Meltdown, Japan** which occurred on 11th March 2011. This was ascribed to a violation of safety rules. Due to this nuclear disaster around 600 people died soon after and another one lakh were displaced. Presently Fukushima has converted into the ghost town, homes situated around the radius of 30 kms were declared hazardous and thus vacated. Helicopter rain is still going on to cool down the heat caused due to radiation. The effects of all these calamities are still seen till the present day in various manifestations.

Injuries due to fall – People fall in many ways. Children fall from bed, sofa, stairs, roof etc. Laborers fall from terrace, stairs etc. Often, people during construction of houses and buildings remain inattentive or neglect measures to prevent falls from height. Similarly, not constructing walls or railings around the terrace or staircases lead to children falling. Multiple fractures, injuries to chest and abdomen and serious head injuries occur. Elderly people fall while walking on the ground due to loss of balance, especially on uneven or slippery floors.

This is known as falling on the surface in which their weakening bones are fractured easily. A fracture of the femur (thigh bone) can lead to prolonged immobility in elderly people. This in turn often leads to a chain of events culminating in death. Elderly people often fall while wearing trousers – they are advised to put on pants and pajamas in a sitting position. Toilets should be illuminated, and floor should not be slippery and there should be no hindrance or obstruction on the way from bed to toilet. Sturdy handles and railings should be fixed up for getting up in the toilet.

Household Bleeding – A deep cut can cause severe bleeding and frighten the onlookers. Many times, it is observed that people start rubbing the wound, which only increases the bleeding. The best thing to do is to **press the wound tightly and continuously** for a few minutes. This should stop the bleeding and after that the wound can be attended to. Bleeding from the nose (**epistaxis**) is a common occurrence. Here again, the patient should be upright so that blood flows out rather than being swallowed. The nose should be pinched tightly just below the nasal bridge and continuously for about 5 minutes.

Faint – Faint is a state when loss of consciousness occurs for a brief period of time due to inadequate supply of blood to the brain or sudden drop in the blood pressure. It is usually preceded by a period of feeling lightheaded. If anybody feels faint, he/she should lie down or sit down with head between the knees and not try to get up quickly. **First aid for faint** – Usually fainting occurs when the person is standing upright. The onlooker should help the person lie down on the back or turn to the left side.

Check for **pulse and breathing**. All adult citizens should know how to check their pulse and breathing. This can be learnt by practicing on one's own wrist on the side of the thumb or feeling on the side of windpipe in the neck (**carotid pulse**).

Breathing is checked by '**look, listen and feel**'. This means that one looks for rise and fall of the chest wall, placing your ear near the chest to listen for sound of breathing and to feel the air coming out of the nostril. If pulse and respiration are present, the **feet and legs of the patient should be raised by about 12 inches,** which increases blood flow to the heart and brain.

The **face of the patient should be turned to one side** so as to prevent the tongue from falling back and obstructing the airway. Usually, the patient will regain consciousness within a few minutes.

Seizure – A seizure or a **'fit'** is a common medical emergency in both adults and children. It occurs due to abnormal electrical activity in the brain. A **convulsion** is a seizure with movement abnormality. **Epilepsy** is a tendency for repeated seizures. Seizures are usually **paroxysmal** i.e. they start and stop suddenly. The patient may be unconscious. They are more sudden than faints and often associated with rolling or turning of eyes to one direction, frothing at the mouth, tightness of stiffening of the body and rhythmic (clonic) movements of the limbs. Occasionally there may be tongue bites and involuntary passage of urine or stool (**incontinence**).

First aid for seizures – It may be quite frightening for a lay person to witness a seizure, so the first thing is to be **calm and reassuring**. The patient should be **made to lie down on one side with** their face turned toward the floor or bed. Nothing should be put in the mouth as the patient is unconscious. Most seizures last less than 3 minutes, so this is all that needs to be done. The patient will gradually regain consciousness or go to sleep. However, if the seizure does not stop within 3 - 5 minutes they are treated as '**status epilepticus**' and should be taken to the hospital or a doctor called. If a patient has had seizures before, **Midazolam nasal spray** may have been advised to be given during seizures, which usually stops the seizure within about a minute.

Basic Life Support (BLS) – This is medical care given by **'first responders'** to suddenly collapsed patients usually outside of hospital to 'revive' or **resuscitate** them until they can be given full medical care by **advanced life support** providers. Earlier the term **cardiopulmonary resuscitation** (CPR) was used instead. BLS can be provided by trained medical personnel (paramedics, nurses, physicians) or lay people. It is needed in **cardiac (heart) or respiratory arrest, choking and drowning.** Various countries have standardized and introduced **BLS training courses** for paramedics, ambulance drivers, medical students and interested citizens, who are then **certified** to administer BLS. Properly performed BLS can save lives.

The **following link** can be used to obtain training in BLS in India.

https://certify.savealife.com/grants - bls
certification/?utm_source=google_grants&utm_medium=cpc&utm_campa
ign=india&utm_content=acls|bls|pals|cpr|bbp&gad_source=1&gclid=Cj
wKCAjwnqK1BhBvEiwAi7o0X61s4NjZd1JylvH7aXorxewjiuA2f6KzkUJT
GBIkCKfpevMkTKN0oRoCA9MQAvD_BwE

The elements and steps of BLS are:

(i) **scene safety** – this may mean moving the victim to a safe place (such as away from the middle of the road) Having the patient laid down supine (on the back) on a firm surface with chest exposed is advantageous.

(ii) giving a **firm tap on the shoulder** of the patient and asking if he/she is all right. If there is no response, it means that consciousness is lost and BLS should start right away.

(iii) Before starting the BLS drill, ask or **send for help** so that others are alerted.

(iv) Look, listen and feel for **breathing.**

(v) **Feel for carotid pulse** in the neck just to one side of the windpipe (trachea). If carotid pulse is not felt, immediately start **chest compression** at 30 compressions a minute. The palms of both hands are kept one on top of the other with elbows straight and the lower part of the chest is compressed by 2 inches with each compression. After 30 compressions, breathing is rechecked. In absence of breathing, **rescue breathing** (mouth - to - mouth ventilation) is done twice then chest compressions are continued.

(vi) **Automatic External defibrillators (AEDs)** are now available in public places in western countries. Personnel providing BLS should be trained so as to use AEDs skillfully.

BLS should be continued till the patient regains pulse, respiration and consciousness or help arrives.

In **conclusion**, accidents have caused irreparable loss to humankind in various ways and means. With fast - track urbanization, deforestation and industrialization, competition for nuclear proliferation among nations, threat of chemical and biological war is increasing, greenhouse gas effect is intensifying, and **global warming** is escalating day by day, decade over decade and century after century. Many injuries can be prevented by simple common - sense measures. Natural disasters are increasingly occurring. **New injuries will afflict mankind**. The acclaimed poet *Ramdhari Singh Dinkar ji*, expresses such disasters with the poetic rhythm:

हमने खुद को यूं बसा लिया, वैज्ञानिकता की बाहों में, अवरोध खड़े कर दिए बड़े, हर एक दूजे की राहों में।
धरती माता का दोहन तो कर लिया, गगन की बारी है, ये बिना शस्त्र का युद्ध है, जो महाभारत से भी भारी है!

Science Oh' science! Technology Oh' technology!
Developed thee to procure comforts, Created barriers over the way through / Extracted earth resources, now unravelling the sky this war in disguise; though without ammunition / Is far reaching colossus, vanquishing and bashing Mahabharat

Einstein made the forecast that "I do not know the consequences of the 3rd World war but if there will be 4th world war man will fight with stones", thus the continuity and existence of this global culture will come to an end if there happens any event like world war – once again injuries will be the major burden.

Chapter 45

Necessary Medical Equipment, Gadgets and Medicines to be kept at Home

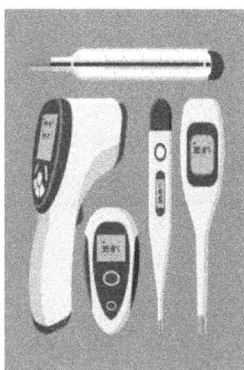

Learning Objectives:

- Utility of maintaining **medical gadgets** in homes – which help in the measurement of fever, blood pressure, diabetes, body weight, tissue oxygenation

- Treatment of disorders occurring in day-to-day life as fever, diarrhea, dysentery, constipation, cough-cold, allergy, productive cough, sneezing, stomach-pain, small injuries, indigestion etc. with over-the-counter medicines

---

We all encounter minor health issues such as headaches, colds, stomach upsets, or minor injuries that can be managed at home with simple remedies. In some cases, a phone consultation with a trusted doctor can provide quick relief or guidance. Keeping basic medicines, first - aid supplies, and equipment like thermometers or blood pressure monitors at home or during travel can obviate the need for an immediate visit to a hospital, doctor, or pharmacy.

Medications purchased without a prescription from a pharmacy are known as "**over - the - counter**" **(OTC)** medicines. These include pain relievers, cold medications, antacids, and other remedies for minor ailments. In India, many medicines can be bought directly from a chemist without a prescription, but regulations may vary between different countries. Having a well - stocked home first - aid kit ensures that minor ailments are handled promptly, offering convenience and reducing the need for urgent medical visits. However, it is important to use OTC medicines responsibly, read labels carefully, and seek professional advice when necessary. Medical instruments or equipment useful in our home are:

Thermometer – This is a common instrument for measuring body temperature. Earlier, mercury thermometers were in vogue but with the advent of technology mercury containing instruments are being phased out and digital thermometers are sweeping into the market. The latest thermometers use infrared rays without touching the body and the gun - like instrument is kept at nearby range to the forehead or the hands. This method of measuring fever in masses and airports became popular during Covid pandemic. A thermometer provides objective measurement informing the doctor or family regarding the normalcy or raised body temperature. The doctor may instruct the patient or family to maintain a **temperature chart.**

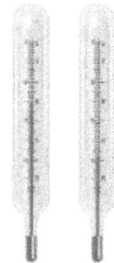

The temperature of the body is measured in degree Fahrenheit (°F) or degree Celsius (°C). Normally, body temperature is measured by keeping the bulb of the thermometer for one minute under the tongue, in the armpit or groin. No hot or cold solids/liquids should be taken just before putting thermometer sensor in the mouth. Usually, the temperature of the armpit is 10 F below the **core body** temperature, which is the temperature of the internal organs, such as liver. The normal core temperature is maintained within a very narrow range of 36.5 - 38.5 **°C**, 97 - 99 °F but accepted normal temperature is 98.4 °F at which the various metabolic processes occur optimally.

Blood Pressure (BP) Instrument – The BP machine is also known as **sphygmomanometer.** Now **aneroid** BP machines not containing mercury are popular. In both the techniques only trained personnel can measure BP.

First the cuff is tied over the upper arm, the tube is connected, then the bulb is pumped to insufflate the cuff beyond the systolic blood pressure (usually till 170 - 180 mm). The cuff is then deflated slowly while the person measuring holds the stethoscope diaphragm over the brachial artery. As the cuff deflates and reaches the **systolic** blood pressure, 'Korotkoff sounds' are heard. As the cuff reaches the lower or **diastolic** blood pressure, the sounds become faint and disappear. The most recent BP machine is **digital** without stethoscope requirement by which the patient can measure their BP easily. BP is generally measured in the right arm with patient lying flat on the back (supine position) and the instrument kept at the level of the heart. Normal adult blood pressure is 120 mm of Hg (mercury) systolic and 80 mm of Hg diastolic expressed as 120/80 mm Hg. It should be noted that BP varies with size of cuff, age, sex, height and emotional state etc. One measurement is not enough to label a person as having high blood pressure or hypertension.

Glucometer – Maturity onset Diabetes is extremely common in India so much so that India is called the diabetes capital of the world. A glucometer is a small hand - held device for measuring blood glucose and monitoring diabetes. The machine is easily available in the market and costs Rs 1500/ only but the strip which measures blood sugar costs Rs 15 - 20/strip. Those who are suffering from severe diabetes are often advised to measure blood sugar either once or many times daily, so that the patient may practice living and eat as per medical advice and take the medicines at scheduled time. After making the glucose meter ready, finger - pulp is pricked by lancet so that blood oozes out. The blood - drop is touched to the strip, the strip is inserted into the device after which reading is displayed on the monitor. A recent innovation is the **continuous glucose measuring (CGM) device**. This uses a small disc stuck to the upper arm of the patient. The disc with a sensor piercing the skin continuously samples the blood and a chip which measures the sugar level transmits it to a mobile phone through blue tooth technology, the blood glucose graph retrieved is proportionate to food intake and activity.

Pulse Oximeter – This instrument has become part of the armamentarium kept in many homes since the COVID pandemic. It measures the **oxygen saturation** of the blood. It is considered the **5th vital sign** (after pulse/heart rate, blood pressure, respiratory rate and temperature).

It is an easy, non - invasive and painless measure of how well oxygen is being carried to peripheral parts of the body such as the arms and legs. Normal oxygen saturation varies from 95 - 100%. Pulse Oximeter, a small portable device, is now readily available at a low cost. It can be clipped on to a finger, toe or ear lobe. The instrument uses light to measure the level of oxygen in the blood thereby helping the healthcare provider to decide if a person needs extra oxygen. It estimates the functional level of respiratory and circulatory systems. The oxygen saturation readings are accurate up to 2% of the arterial oxygen saturation from arterial blood gas analysis.

Medicines to be kept at home – Certain medicines required for particular disorders should be kept in the home to provide instantaneous or quick relief. Wise people maintain a *kit* of routine medicines like paracetamol and aspirin for pain and fever. The kit contains cotton gauze, vicks, *amrutanjan, amritdhara, pudinhara*, liniments for sprain, medicines for itching, antiseptic solutions like Dettol, Savlon, Povidon iodine for cleansing wounds and abrasions. A person suffering from watery **diarrhoea** is sometimes **dehydrated**. Children are more prone to such a disorder. Packets of oral rehydration salts may be kept at home to treat dehydration.

They are prepared as instructed on the packet. Otherwise, lime juice with a pinch of salt and 1 - 2 teaspoons of dissolved sugar in a glass of water could be used to prevent or treat dehydration.

Excessive dryness of the eyes may be relieved by **artificial tears** eyedrops like **refresh** for lubricating the eyes. A sudden feeling of some irritation in the eye may be due to some foreign body like straw or blade of grass. Washing your eyes with clean water may remove the foreign body. If unrelieved, do not try to remove it yourself, simply pad the eye and go to a specialist. Redness, stickiness or excessive discharge from the eye is a sign of **conjunctivitis**. Antibiotic eye drops are used for this. Splints to support suspected bone fractures can be made from wooden scales and flat wooden/steel planks. Crepe bandages are useful for spraining ankles and wrists common during hill expeditions.

The following table gives some medicines to be kept in the house.

S. No	Category	Name
1.	Cardiovascular System	Sorbitrate or Nitroglycerine (5 mg), Aspirin, (300 mg) Clopidogrel (300 mg) and Atorvastatin (40 mg). **These 4 drugs can be kept as a kit for chest pain and can be taken before seeing a doctor.**
2.	Non - steroidal Anti - inflammatory Drug (NSAIDs)	Paracetamol, Diclofenac, Aspirin (check its sensitivity)
3.	Antibiotics or Antimicrobial	Ciprofloxacin, Azithromycin, Ornidazole, Cefixime, Amoxycillin + Clavulanic acid
4.	Gastrointestinal Tract (for vomiting and acidity)	Ondansetron, Omeprazole, Pantoprazole, Domperidone, Antacids, Digestive enzymes
5.	Cough Remedies	Bromhexine, Dextromethorphan, Guaifenesin
6.	Anti Allergic	Levocetirizine, Montelukast, Betamethasone
7.	Central Nervous System – sedatives	Lorazepam, Alprazolam
8	Eye Drops	Moxifloxacin eye drops, gentamycin eye drops
9.	Urogenital	Flavoxate, Alkalizer, Fluconazole (for fungal infections), Norfloxacin & Ampicillin (for UTI)

In conclusion, being a "**half doctor**" at home or while traveling means being prepared with a well - stocked first - aid kit to assist family members and fellow travelers during emergencies. Whether it's cleaning and dressing cuts and bruises, bandaging sprains, splinting fractures, managing chest pain with essential medications, or administering common over - the - counter remedies for headaches, fever, dehydration, and digestive issues, such preparedness can make a significant difference. While offering immediate care, it's also crucial to call an ambulance or consult a doctor when the situation demands professional attention.

Chapter 46

Triage – Treatment Priority

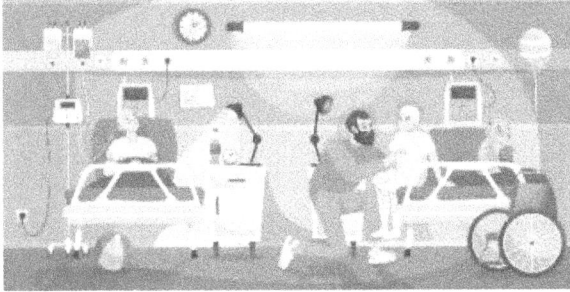

Learning Objectives:

- Sorting out patients into those needing immediate medical care, those serious but less emergent and those who can wait
- Imparting justice by prioritizing the severely ill

Triage is the process of sorting and classifying patients based on the urgency of their medical needs. It originated during the Napoleonic Wars, where limited resources had to be allocated efficiently to maximize survival among soldiers. This prioritization system was established to ensure that the most critical cases received prompt attention, while less urgent cases waited for care.

In modern healthcare, particularly in emergency departments and disaster situations, triage remains vital. It focuses on providing care to patients based on the severity of their illness or injury, prognosis, and the availability of medical resources. The approach is grounded in utilitarian principles, aiming to maximize the well - being of as many people as possible. This ethical framework prioritizes treatment to achieve the greatest good, sometimes even applying the "last come, first serve" principle when resources are scarce, emphasizing the human values of fairness and compassion in critical times.

Triage provides permission to doctors to impart services and to take care of the seriously injured or ill patients on priority, as follows –

1. Which patients need immediate attention and treatment?

2. Which patients are emergent but not critical?

3. Which patients can wait in the queue?

4. Which patients require treatment using the available resources?

In triage patients are given a **tag** on the basis of priority of treatment. Triage usually involves a **quick assessment** by a doctor or nurse, who then sorts out patients into 3 categories and allocates them the **tag** or **category** like **Red, Yellow or Green**. The Red category, being the most serious and critical, are wheeled into the red area of the emergency ward where life - saving equipment is available. With treatment or relief and with the passage of time, the categories may change from red to yellow or vice versa. But in situations when several people are affected of same calamity as war, construction site, bus accidents, land slide etc. triage is done as according to traditional method and patients are sorted out into 5 categories viz: **Black, Red, Yellow, Green and White**.

Various triage systems have been developed and are in use:

The Emergency Severity Index, Manchester; the Canadian, Australian Triage systems and WHO Emergency Triage and Treatment (ETAT). Some of these use the above red, yellow, green or 3 - category system while others use 5 category system detailed below:

Traditional 5 Category System

1. **Black Tag** – seriously wounded patients counting the last breaths of their life, where all the resources to save their life have been exhausted, are given "*black tag*". As for example cardiac arrest, multi - organ failure, bomb blast in the abdomen in war field or natural disaster. In such catastrophic conditions pain killer and **palliative** medicines like morphine injections are administered, they are provided with **life support** systems like oxygen and wound bandage. Medico - legal - aid documents are given to fulfil their last desire.

2. **Red Tag** – persons with acute life - threatening conditions are given the 'red tag'. These are those who suddenly became **unconscious**, subconscious or lose consciousness due to **severe heart attack**, stroke, active and **severe bleeding**, **shock** (falling blood pressure) **acute respiratory obstruction** etc. Thus, patients in dire emergency are provided with **intensive care** like emergency medicines, life saving procedures and sometimes surgical intervention. In severe respiratory failure oxygen is given with the tube inserted in the trachea – **endotracheal intubation**. **Ventilatory support** may be given. The procedure of **cardioversion** is performed during acute conditions of cardiac arrest. Intravenous fluids are also administered for volume restoration. Secondary survey is done for other needs.

3. **Yellow Tag** – such persons are put up with "**yellow tag**" who inspite of doing activities like walking, talking, speaking etc. scream aloud. As for example patients due to acute pain in abdomen or the chest, as of bone fracture in the hips or waist, high fever, snake bite, injury, poisoning, bleeding are sorted out in triage again and again for appropriate treatment.

4. **Green Tag** – only those persons are given "**green tag**" who though appear troubled due to trivial problems like headache, abdomen or chest pain, fever, vomiting, bone fracture, sprain or small injury etc. but can wait in the queue and get the treatment. Such patients are given some emergency and supportive treatments and relieved to go to their home within 24 hours otherwise their triage is done again.

5. **White Tag** – only those persons are given "**white tag**" who can wait in the queue. Such patients are provided primary medical care and are told to return to their home. Such patients are advised to consult OPD.

The above 5 tag system has evolved into 5 levels of priority

Level 1 – Immediate: Life threatening. Waiting time 0 - 10 minutes.

Level 2 – Emergency: Could become life threatening. Waiting time 60 minutes.

Level 3 – Urgent: not life threatening. Waiting time 120 - 240 minutes.

Level 4 – Semi - urgent: not life threatening.

Level 5 – Non - urgent: needs treatment as and when time permits.

Triage systems have gradually developed in scientific temper. Various research performances, validating experiments and literature throw ample light on the testimony as to how modern medical science is dedicated to human service.

Providing wellness and good health to all the members of society or nation is the pivot of medical care – listen to those first who are sorrow stricken. Not all can be attended as and when they come. The popular maxim of **first come - first serve** is not applicable in emergency departments. Triage systems developed in different societies in different forms and sorting serious patients to give them treatment according to their priority is the aim of all types of medical care.

Societal and Organizational Triage - - Providing treatment to high social profiles, kith and kins, friends and relatives in preference to the general population is often an obligation. Now most of the government hospitals and clinics are organizing societal triage. The hierarchy like politicians, bureaucrats, owners, employers, personal relationships and family members expect doctors to attend to them immediately on priority. The value system interwoven with triage philosophy provides sanction to organizational or societal triage and accordingly has provided fast track service corridor for fulfilling such demanding obligations without disturbing the triage in red tag zone. There are specific hospital protocols for handling the medical emergency of statesmen and laureates. Another type of organizational triage noticeable is when a single clinic is multi - tasking.

They perform flagging and chaperoning on assembled patients for various tasks like dressing change, catheter removal, stitch removal, internal examination, endoscopy, blood sampling, sending for ultrasound/X - ray, dietary consultation, detailed clinical history and examination of a first - time visitor etc. A patient might be requiring several facilities on the same visit and all his needs are fulfilled by watchful organizational triage. **Triage on request** for reasons like having a train to catch, getting children from school, attending to sick at home may also need to be accommodated.

In **conclusion**, we have understood the significance of triage in hospitals and clinics. Triage is a procedure which has stood the test of time. Following the standards and principles of triage, health institutions are contributing to saving the lives of thousands who might otherwise have succumbed. Triage procedure is a type of medical service which is carried out by the medical professionals on the principles of **distributive justice**.

The severely ill patient may be last in the queue, but they have the right to obtain priority in their treatment and it is incumbent on medical professionals to provide the best treatment on priority to the seriously ill patient.

Chapter 47

Quest for Excellence

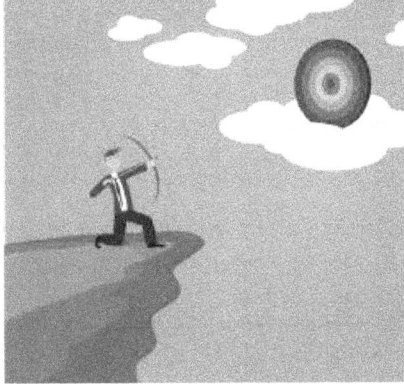

Learning Objectives:

- Various types of plastic surgery performed for functional improvement, structural and aesthetic showcasing
- Trying to improve height, maximizing strength & energy by sportsperson through hormone therapy
- Removing wrinkles, warts from face or neck, transplanting hair, removing excessive skin and fat from abdomen by abdominoplasty
- Side effects of unnecessary medical interventions to modify natural beauty

---

Fly along like birds is a quest for excellence resonating in the folk song

पंख होते तो मैं उड़ जाती रे !

Bestowed with wings, I would take flight far off…

Man's desire to fly led to the invention of airplanes. The quest to imitate birds and fly with wings has challenged human ingenuity for centuries.

Similarly, the desire to look more beautiful, fairer, taller, and attain perfection has motivated mankind to achieve excellence.

Modern medical science has developed treatments such as hormones and steroids that can temporarily enhance strength and virility. Various surgical procedures now restore or enhance body functions, while cosmetic surgeries improve appearance and contour. Some of these procedures are essential for correcting birth deformities, repairing tissues after surgery, or restoring functionality to amputated limbs. Others, such as hair transplantation for male pattern baldness, are elective and pursued based on individual preferences.

This chapter aims to introduce readers to essential medical procedures that serve a functional purpose, as well as those driven by the desire for beauty and enhanced strength - often the result of boundless ambition or a quest for excellence.

Typically, human height ranges from 5 to 6 feet, and those outside this range often draw attention. A person's complexion may be dark, or their nose may be crooked. High heels can disguise height, makeup can conceal a dark complexion, and rhinoplasty can surgically correct a crooked nose. These temporary measures, like visiting beauty parlors or going to the gym to build strength and muscle, are popular. However, only a few people choose to consult a doctor or plastic surgeon for therapy or surgery. These pursuits may be justified in specific circumstances. Let us discuss how modern medical science has evolved in this area.

Hormonal Treatments - Hormones are substances secreted form glands to maintain several functions of our body. For example, pituitary hormones, adrenal gland hormones, insulin, thyroid hormones and ovaries and testes secreting sex hormones do one or the other metabolic function. Medical treatment with natural or synthetic hormones is done to treat common deficiencies of thyroid hormones in hypothyroidism and insulin in diabetes.

Hormonal treatment is commonly done in women to conserve pregnancy and treat menstrual disturbances. Contraceptive pills are generally small doses of hormones estrogen and progesterone.

These hormones can also be utilized for enhancing or upgrading certain body functions for example growth hormone to increase height, cortico - steroids to improve temporary performance in sports, sex hormones to improve sexual drive or virility. Hormones used indiscriminately without pros and cons, can be harmful to the body. Use of sex hormones and steroids is strictly prohibited in sports. Use of growth hormone for routine request for increasing height of adolescent children is generally denied by pediatricians.

Plastic Surgery is performed in different areas:

Restoration of body organs, for example if a hand is severed in an accident and the cut hand is brought to the hospital in good condition, the micro - vascular plastic surgeons undertake re - implantation of this hand through arduous time - consuming surgery. Such surgery may take 8 to 10 hours where nerves, arteries and veins are joined together under a microscope which is called microvascular surgery. Many children are born with cleft lip and palate or deformed genitalia.

Corrective and restorative plastic surgical procedures are undertaken for such congenital deformities – the objective of restorative plastic surgery is to impart functional utility to the dysfunctional organ. Such surgeries are regularly performed by respective specialists.

Reconstruction and reformation of body organs, for example making breast from nearby tissue or silicone implants after breast removal or mastectomy. Cheek, jaw and face are reconstructed after major surgery in oral cancer using skin, muscle and bone along with the composite pedicle or free vascular flap. The objective of reconstructive plastic surgery is to revive maximum utility to such organs which are surgically removed in injury or cancer. Cosmetic surgery serves dual purposes: restoring lost shape or function and enhancing appearance when desired. For instance, after severe burns, contractures may develop on the skin, leading to deformities on the face, hands, and other areas. Cosmetic surgical procedures aim to release these contractures, remove fibrosed skin, perform skin grafting, and correct functional issues of the face, eyelids, and hands. As people age, wrinkles and loose skin folds often appear, and cosmetic procedures such as facelifts or wrinkle removal are performed primarily to enhance beauty and appearance.

However, the excessive use of these therapies, surgeries, and technologies can sometimes lead individuals to conceal their natural features in the pursuit of a more charming, beautiful, or glamorous look, or to develop greater strength. While the desire to improve natural traits can be valid, such procedures often come with risks and side effects that must be considered.

Additionally, motivations such as lack of self - esteem, societal pressures, or an overwhelming desire to upgrade appearance or performance can push some people toward unnecessary or harmful treatments. In such cases, it is important for medical professionals to recognize these motivations and discreetly decline treatments that could harm the patient's health. Often, such clients may remain unsatisfied with the results, reflecting a deeper dissatisfaction driven by an unrealistic quest for perfection.

Increasing Height – A stranger visits the clinic of my medico - friend along with his 14 - year - old son, saying, "Dr. Sahib, my son's height is just 5 feet…" My friend gives a faint smile and asks, "What are you expecting?" The man responds, "Sir, I've heard of certain hormones, maybe some hormonal therapy… Can we help him grow to 5 feet 6 inches?" The medico - friend replies calmly, "Your son may naturally gain a few more inches, up to 3 - 6 inches, as the body continues to grow until about 20 years of age. Hormone injections are not advisable in such cases. Let's run some tests just to rule out any underlying conditions."

He hands them a prescription, adding, "If the thyroid is malfunctioning, we'll treat that. But it's unlikely that your son has a thyroid disorder.

Administering growth hormone is not suitable here, and such therapies can have unpredictable side effects that may interfere with healthy growth factors." He continues, "We'll ensure that your son is not dealing with conditions like dwarfism, achondroplasia, or other genetic disorders leading to short stature. But if both parents are short, the child will naturally be a bit short as well. Hormone treatment in such cases isn't justified. There is no scientific method in modern medicine to increase height other than ensuring a healthy, protein - rich diet from childhood."

Physical Strength Enhancement – with the objective of proving excellent performance, winning awards and medals sportspersons attempt to boost and intensify physical strength by taking hormone injections.

As for example male - hormone - traits viz; testosterone may be enhanced by anabolic steroid, androstenedione, human growth hormone may be enhanced, erythropoietin for raising hemoglobin, fluid buildup may be reduced by diuretics, stimulant hormones like carnitine and various dietary supplements help in being victorious in sports and competitions.

Such therapies leading to short lived utility may help in winning the competition but not prepare the contender for all time to come. Hormone therapy create several problems to all males, females or sport - persons during old age viz: baldness in women, irregular menstruation, early prostate hyperplasia, liver cirrhosis, high level bad cholesterol (LDL, low level good cholesterol (HDL), high BP, cardiac diseases, hepatitis, arthritis, diabetes, vision - diseases, nervous system diseases, anxiety, sleep - disorder, depression and weight - loss. Hormone therapy is completely banned for sportspersons. Sports clubs, organizations and institutions have made provisions regarding hormonal therapy prohibitions – if the dope and other tests of the samples of urine sweat, saliva, blood, hair, nails report the presence of such drugs and stimulants the concerned sportsperson is disqualified from the competition.

Hair Transplantation is usually sought by youth living in big cities with the objective of hiding baldness. After due counselling **dense hair locales** are selected as the site from where hair is taken out – **donor sites**. From the donor site, hair follicle is taken out and each hair is skillfully sowed at the **bald site**. **Hair transplantation** and **skin grafting** are two different techniques performed in different methods. In hair transplantation **epidermis** and **dermis** are taken out together along with **hair follicle** from **donor site** but in skin grafting **full strip of the skin** is taken out from the donor site. **Side effects** – donor sites and transplantation sites may be infected with virus and bacteria frequently due to which vellus (रोंआ) grow out. These symptoms bring forth baldness time and again.

Face - Lift– with growing old age wrinkles start appearing over the face and neck and muscles of the neck, face and cheeks become loose. Removing wrinkles and sagging skin folds by **cosmetic surgery** is called **face - lifting**. Similar to this surgery, skin folds spread around the neck are removed. This surgery is known by the name **neck - lifting** or **platysmaplasty**.

Fine creases and wrinkles especially on the forehead and face below the eyes associated with ageing and some illness can be treated surgically by 'face lift' surgery as many actresses undergo. Subcutaneous or under the skin injections of Botox or platelet rich plasma (PRP) are administered by cosmetologists, dermatologist and plastic surgeons.

In face lifting, moles, old scars and marks on the face are eliminated. **Side effects** – in these surgery sensations in the nerves may be lost, and wounds may be infected. F**acial hematoma** may occur due to blood clotting on the wounds. The wrinkles spreading on the face may be prevented by a healthy diet and massage on the face. Surgical interventions are best avoided.

Abdominoplasty – similar to above cosmetic surgeries, **abdominoplasty** is a cosmetic surgery in which the fat on the abdomen is removed by surgical process – this surgery is also known as tummy **tuck**. In this surgery excess skin and fat are removed from the middle and lower abdomen. After removing the fat and skin around abdomen, the muscle and fascia of the abdominal wall are tucked up tightly.

Sometimes, there may be an associated abdominal hernia with a large hanging abdominal 'apron'. Surgery of hernia and **dermo lipectomy** (removal of redundant skin and fat over abdomen) are done together which is both correction of a troubling defect and cosmesis at the same time.

Vaginoplasty is a surgical procedure to construct, repair or rejuvenate the vagina with local tissue. Some female children are born with normal ovaries and normal female hormone levels and normal breast development; however, the vagina and uterus are vestigial and underdeveloped. Vagina may become loose or large and sagging due to repeated vaginal delivery or uterine prolapse. Vaginoplasty is undertaken surgically to reshape and tighten it up by **colporrhaphy**.

Thus, slack and asymmetric vagina are corrected. Complications are infection, inflammation, pain, bleeding, and blood clotting. Rarely, the vesico - vaginal fistula (abnormal connection between bladder and vagina) after vaginoplasty may result if careful dissection in the correct plane is not done.

Breast Augmentation and **Reduction mammoplasty** or one side breast size and shape adjustment may be requested for cosmetic reasons. Many young ladies consult doctors for breast augmentation medicines and surgery. Breast size generally increases after marriage, childbirth and weight gain, so they should be adequately counselled regarding the side effects of augmentation and reduction mammoplasty.

Silicone breast prostheses are implanted on both sides for augmentation through retro - mammary or behind the breast approach, under the pectoralis muscle. Breast reconstruction after mastectomy for cancer (oncoplastic breast surgery) creates a soft mound at the breast site, but the mound does not perform functions like lactation. At best it mimics breasts.

Breast reconstruction is also done by using skin and muscle flaps from neighboring areas of the body. Nipple and areola may also be reconstructed by transferring and sharing a part of it from the breast of the opposite side. Sometimes, breasts being too large and pendulous, become painful too, thus backache may also occur. A reduction mammoplasty by plastic surgical method is undertaken. Adjustments between 2 sides of unequal breasts may be done by augmentation or reduction. Complications include fat necrosis, calcification and sclerotic nodules.

Fat - graft and Lipo - suction are commonly performed by plastic surgeons. Fat grafting involves that fat and adipose tissue or fat stem cell is trans - positioned from one place to another in the body. This is done for filling up dimples, augmenting tissues, contouring and shaping the body as and where desired. Conversely, in obese subjects, double chin (excess fat under the chin), fat in the arms and thighs, abdomen and breast area in men (gynecomastia) is removed by liquefaction and suction of the fat. This surgical procedure is called **liposuction**.

Skin Procedures and piercings - Removing small warty growths, pox marks, little dents in skin or other ugly or offending lesion on the body surface is done at request of the patient.

In conclusion, attributes like beauty and strength can be either God - gifted from birth, genetic, or gained through hard work, lifestyle changes, diet, exercise, and practice.

Pursuing artificial or medical methods to enhance beauty or strength, often driven by the desire to win a tournament, medal, or to satisfy personal ego, is often described as the "Quest for Excellence."

In certain cases, such as an abdominoplasty (tummy tuck) during an abdominal hernia surgery or vaginoplasty during a uterine prolapse surgery, these procedures are considered nominal surgical interventions that yield both functional and cosmetic benefits. Providing a prosthetic limb after an amputation, like an artificial hand or foot, falls outside the scope of cosmetic surgery, as it addresses a functional necessity.

Similarly, correcting birth defects like a cleft lip or genital abnormalities is a natural and essential requirement. The discussion of these procedures, especially those performed by plastic surgeons, highlights the distinction between essential medical interventions and those undertaken for cosmetic enhancement. Ultimately, it is up to the reader to take a pragmatic view and carefully judge whether a procedure is genuinely necessary.

Chapter 48

Preparation For Old Age – Healthy Old Age, How to Live Long and Quality of Life (QALY)

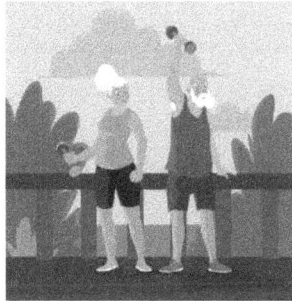

Learning Objectives:

- Life expectancy

- Physiological changes in ageing

- Factors associated with longevity

- Common problems which people face when ageing

- Developing lifestyle in preparation for healthy old age

- Philosophy of life as one ages

- Understanding the concept of Quality of Life

Growing older is a natural, continuous process that occurs from birth, advancing with time until one reaches old age. Despite knowing this, few people actively prepare for the challenges and changes that come with aging. Wise individuals, however, take steps to ensure a healthy old age before physical decline sets in. As health improves across populations, **life expectancy** has progressively increased - a global trend. Over the last century, this rise in life expectancy is largely due to reductions in infant mortality, improved hygiene, better living standards, healthier lifestyles, and access to quality education and healthcare advancements. In India, for instance, life expectancy at birth has risen dramatically from 33.21 years in 1950 to 70.62 years in 2023. The rate of increase has slowed over time, from 1.51 - 1.68% annually in the 1950s to 0.33% per year in the 2020s, reflecting more gradual improvements in recent years.

As life expectancy has increased, the definition of old age has also changed. The World Health Organization now defines **young old age as 65 - 75 years** (transition from working life to retirement); **75 - 85 years as advanced old age** – a period when functional changes start being observed and above **85 years as very advanced old age** – a period when special care and support are required.

With the increase in longevity, there are demographic changes expected. In the European region for instance, it is estimated that by 2024, the population of individuals aged over 65 years will outnumber those under the age of 15. Therefore, more focus needs to be given to 'healthy aging'. In fact, the decade of 2021 - 2030 is targeted by the United Nations as the **'Decade of Healthy Ageing'** to improve the lives of older people, their families and communities.

Biology of Ageing: Aging is believed to occur because of degenerative processes leading to dysfunction and death at cellular and tissue level. The most widely held theory about ageing is the **mitochondrial free radical theory of aging,** according to which, aging occurs due to accumulation of **free radicals** or **reactive oxygen species.** The latter are unwanted toxic byproducts of aerobic metabolism formed in the mitochondria – the tiny organelles within the cell – also called the powerhouse of the cell. Free radicals are atoms or molecules whose outer shell have a single unpaired electron, making them unstable. The free radicals induce oxidative damage to various cellular macromolecules. Oxidative damage is limited by **antioxidants** which are actually **reducing agents,** Antioxidants neutralize free radicals from the cells to prevent damage caused by oxidation. The most well - known antioxidants are **vitamin C, Vitamin E and beta - carotene.**

Determinants of longevity – Research have shown that the following factors are related to longevity. Many of these factors are inter - related.

1. **Gender** – At all ages, women have lower mortality rates than men. This has been attributed to higher risk - taking behavior in men and also because men are predisposed to certain diseases. The current overall life expectancy after achieving the age of 65 in USA is 82.9 years for men and 85.5 years for women.

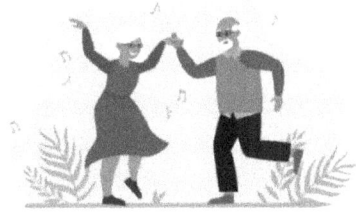

2. **Genetics** – Again, this is partly explained by occurrence of many diseases which have a genetic basis and may cause early death. Research studies on identical twins have shown that about 20 - 30% of an individual's lifespan is related to genetic factors, and the rest to modifiable environmental factors and lifestyle choices.

3. **Prenatal and early childhood conditions** – Prenatal and intrauterine growth retardation are associated with higher mortality even in advanced age.

4. **Education** – Higher education levels are associated to improved longevity, According to Centre for Disease Control, USA, 25 - year - old men with a bachelor's or higher degree have a life expectancy 9.3 years more than those without a high school diploma. Higher education levels were also associated to lower levels of obesity and tobacco use, which again correlate to greater longevity.

5. **Socio - economic status** – This is closely related to education. It is believed that the higher the socio - economic status is, higher the longevity will be. This is not a hard and fast rule as inner strength of austerity may endows longevity. Even the poor and uneducated may reach the pinnacle of longevity by their talent and diligence.

6. **Hygiene** –Although not so applicable to affluent societies today, poor hygiene had a great influence on occurrence of infection leading to early death especially in low - income countries.

7. **Diet and nutrition**: A balanced diet, rich in fiber and low in refined sugars and flour is conducive to healthy old age.

Nowadays, a **'vegan' or plant - based diet** is believed to be strongly protective against coronary artery disease – a major killer in middle or young old age. **Obesity** is strongly associated with premature death. People living in **'blue zones'** consume a healthy diet and live long.

8. **Exercise and lifestyle** – Regular exercise with exclusion of addictions like tobacco, alcohol and drugs is associated with healthy and prosperous old age.

9. **Social connections** – Social activity leads to longevity. Married people live longer than single. Social connections play a vital role in developing harmonious personality and thereby augments brain function to creative vistas. Stimuli from various activities such as talking with family and friends, reading, following the news, discussing, watching movies etc. lead to an active mind. Maintaining an active mind is the impetus towards reaching the summit of healthy longevity.

Thus, interaction between genetic and environmental factors i.e. **exposome** (the sum of person's experiences due to exposures from birth to death) may strikingly and sufficiently contribute to longevity.

Diseases of Old Age – Both chronic and acute diseases can especially affect the elderly. In the setting of chronic disease, a superadded acute illness can prove fatal. Many diseases which are especially prevalent in the elderly are:

1. **Cardiovascular disease** – coronary artery disease and hypertension

2. **Cerebrovascular disease** like stroke causing hemiparesis (reduced muscle power in half the body) or hemiplegia (total paralysis of half the body)

3. **Diabetes -** Maturity onset diabetes starts in middle age or beyond. Diabetes is extremely common in India. In fact, our country is known as 'diabetes capital of the world'.

4. **Chronic obstructive pulmonary disease (COPD)** and other respiratory diseases like chronic bronchitis and emphysema, asthma etc. cause suffering in day - to - day life of old people.

Besides the above diseases other infectious diseases like influenza, pneumonia and tuberculosis can affect old people and may be the cause of death. Influenza and pneumonia vaccines are prescribed in old age.

5. **Cancer -** Most cancers are more prevalent in elderly people. Common cancers are those of lung, prostate, oral cavity, stomach and rectum in males, and breast, cervix and ovary cancer in females.

6. **Septicemia** – Old persons suffering from diabetes or chronic kidney diseases, become prone to septicemia – an acute generalized infection of the blood stream which can be fatal if not treated urgently and intensively.

7. **Kidney disease** – Chronic renal failure often ensues secondary to long standing diabetes and uncontrolled high blood pressure.

8. **Diseases of joints and bones** – arthritis, osteoporosis, etc. occur in old age. Osteoarthritis of the knee is extremely common and presents as pain, stiffness and/or swelling of one or both knees. Fractures occur more easily in old age due to brittleness and rarefaction (osteoporosis) of bones. A fall in the elderly leading to **fracture of the thigh bone** (femur) and **prolonged confinement to bed** is a common sequence of events often culminating in death. In fact, being bedridden itself is a risk factor for further osteoporosis (rarefaction of bones), pneumonia and venous thrombosis.

9. **Sarcopenia** – This refers to gradual loss of muscle mass performance and strength with aging. After the age of 30 years, people typically lose about 3% - 5% of their muscle mass each decade. The loss is greater in inactive people, and it becomes more noticeable and speeds up at around age 60. Sarcopenia can be retarded by consuming a healthy diet including high - quality proteins - about 20 to 35 grams of protein in each meal. Another measure is exercise - maintaining a physically active lifestyle that includes exercises such as resistance training and walking.

10. **Mental disorders – depression** and **dementia** are two mentals' disorders very common in old age. Dementia means a decline in mental abilities occurring at a faster rate than normal. Old people due to melancholy get disenchanted with life and often loose the will to live.

Financial independence is very important in old age. An ageing person should plan for enough money in the post - retirement period so that as far as possible they are not financially dependent on others.

11. **Alzheimer's disease** is a type of dementia associated with deposits of certain proteins in the brain. Most patients (> 70%) are 75 years old and older. The brain progressively shrinks, and brain cells die. There is a gradual decline in cognition, memory, behavior and social skills. The early signs of the disease include forgetting recent events. Over time, there are serious memory problems and inability to perform everyday tasks. Although medicines can slow the progression of symptoms, there is no cure for Alzheimer's so far. In advanced stages, malnutrition, dehydration and infection are the usual cause of death.

How to promote healthy aging (Secrets of Long Life) – Achieving longevity has been vividly illustrated by Dan Buettner in an article "The Secrets of Long Life" published in National Geographic Magazine of 2005. In many societies people naturally live beyond a hundred years. He refers to **5 blue zones -** Okinawa, Japan; Sardinia, Italy; Loma Linda, California; The Nicoya Peninsula, Costa Rica; Ikaria, Greece, where many people living greater than 100 years remain dynamic and active. On the other hand, Non - Latino Americans and African Americans usually do not live more than 70 years and the original inhabitants of America and Britain live up to 80 - 85 years. The distinctive features of balanced and moderate lifestyle followed by Blue Zone people are analyzed as follows –

Nutrition and Weight – Some old people are fond of taking refined sugar and flour and foods with high **glycemic index** and saturated fats. Instead, if they take diet rich in vitamin C, vitamin E, Beta - carotene and **antioxidants**, they will easily neutralize free radicals (unstable molecules of oxygen) in their body. A high fiber plant - based diet containing plenty of fruits, nuts, vegetables, legumes and whole grains, are believed to support beneficial microbes in the gut. Such microbes help break down fibers into short chain fatty acids, shown to stimulate immune cell activity. Elderly people should be aware of ideal weight for their height, not get obese and try to achieve and maintain this through a balance between calorie intake and exercise.

80% Rule – The Confucius custom or *mantra* prevalent in people of **Okinawa** (Japanese island where people live long) is '**Hara hachi bu**' (i.e. stop eating when you are 80% full), serving only small quantity of food, eating less after dusk, chomping and masticating the food slowly and thoroughly and thus not letting fat build up in the body. The traditional Okinawa diet is high in carbohydrates but low in calories viz; quinoa, oats, buckwheat, legumes – beans like lentils, chickpeas, black beans, starchy vegetables like beet, potato, sweet potato, corn, pea, fruits like banana, grape, apple, pineapple, mango, orange, blueberry, dried fruit, thus almost excluding fat. Vegetables and soy products are preferred along with small amounts of noodles, rice, pork and fish. Though certain blue zone people consume alcohol in meagre quantity, they abstain from drug abuse (tobacco, cannabis, opium, cocaine) and accomplish longevity because they eat balanced diet of beans, lentils and meagre amount of meat, pork etc. Avoiding excess eating "अति सर्वत्र वर्जयेत्", maintains the body sturdy and agile and opens the gateway to longevity. In the Indian tradition longevity can be accomplished by following 3 principles as – "eating the food according to weather and climate" *Rit Bhukh* (**ऋतभुख**); "eating the food easily absorbable in the body" *Hit Bhukh* (**हितभुख**); "eating less than actual hunger" *Mit Bhukh* (**मितभुख**). Sanskrit Mantra in *Kathopanishad* (**कठोपनिषद**) recites as following "**ॐ सहनाववतु, सहनौभुनक्तु। सह वीर्य करवावहै, तेजस्विनावधीतमस्तु, मा विद्विषावहै, ॐ शान्तिः शान्तिः शान्तिः** Explanation – meals taken in the congregation of family and members of society help abate physical, psychosomatic and worldly sorrows and agony

Supplements – It may be beneficial to take supplements of all such minerals and vitamins which may not be present in required amounts in our diet. For example, vitamin D deficiency is extremely common even in a sunny country like ours and this essential nutrient is probably best supplemented.

Exercise – Regular physical activity is one of the most important things an elderly person can do for maintaining good health. Health benefits increase with more physical activity. Exercise can prevent or delay many health problems that come with aging and helps strengthen muscles. Running marathon is not needed, just keeping on moving, gardening etc. are good ways to maintaining good health. Continuing with day - to - day activities also makes the elderly less dependent on others.

According to the Centre for Disease Control USA, in general, adults aged 65 years or beyond need at least **150 minutes a week** of **moderate - intensity activity** such as brisk walking or aerobic exercises or alternatively 75 minutes a week of **vigorous - intensity activity** (such as hiking, jogging, or running). In addition, at least **2 days a week** of activities that **strengthens muscles like** working all major muscle groups including legs, hips, back, abdomen, chest, shoulders and arms. Activities to **improve balance** (such as standing on one leg) are also beneficial. If the elderly person has chronic conditions which make these recommendations difficult to follow, they should still be as physically active as their abilities allow.

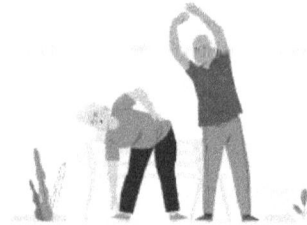

Yog – This is an ancient Indian practice which includes certain postures (आसन्, *Asana*), breathing (प्रणायाम्, *Pranayam*), concentration on single object (धारण, *Dharan*) contemplation (ध्यान, *Dhyan*) and meditation (समाधि, *Samadhi*). Scientific studies show that yoga improves strength, balance and flexibility; helps relieve back pain and arthritis symptoms, benefits heart health, relaxes the individual, improves mood and helps manage stress.

Though people not acquainted with the Indian science of *Yog* interpret it only a type of exercise, this is to reiterate that *Yog* is a science, a way of life which if practiced according to prescribed rules may capacity build the elderly person towards wellness. *Ayurveda* and *Yog* if followed with devotion add longevity to stipulated life years (refer to Chapter 11).

Rest & sleep – Adequate sleep is a critical predictor of better mental well - being, improved ability to perform day to day activities, reduced risk of falls, better self - reported health status, and reduced risk of hospitalization. During sleep the **melatonin** hormone is secreted in the body which repairs the worn - out cells and activates the body and mind for the coming day. Thus, sleep provides solace to the body and mind and increases muscular strength. Sleep is anti - inflammatory and it heals the wounds of our body.

As all adults, the elderly also need about 7 to 9 hours of sleep each night. However, older people tend to fall asleep earlier but also wake earlier than they did when young. **Insomnia** is a common problem in the elderly.

Ways to counter insomnia are:

(i)   Sticking to a consistent sleep routine i.e. going to bed and waking up at the same time each day

(ii)   Cutting down on caffeine, which is a stimulant and diuretic i.e. increases the need to urinate during the night

(iii) Remaining physically active - Regular exercise like walking, running or swimming not only helps one to fall asleep faster, but also helps attain a higher proportion of restorative deep sleep and awaken less often during the night

(iv)   Limiting daytime naps - Prolonged daytime sleep can disrupt the natural sleep cycle

(v)   Quitting tobacco as its nicotine affects sleep.

Enhancing Mental activity: Our memory and cognitive abilities can decline with age, as do concentration, attention span and ability to adapt to new situations. Keeping our minds active and engaged is a way to combat this decline. Ways to keep the mind invigorated are to read more – as by joining a book club; play mind stretching games like puzzles, chess, bridge or computer games, opt for mental maths rather than using a calculator or learn a new skill such as knitting, embroidery or even gardening.

So, cultivation of an absorbing **hobby** is a way towards promoting healthy old age. In old age cognitive mechanics gets reduced, but cognitive pragmatics is increased, similarly abstract reasoning is diminished but crystallized intelligence is augmented. Momentum of advancing old age can be diminished by aerobic exercises, dancing - skipping - hopping etc.

Dimensions of prospective memory can be increased by cultivating creative pursuits. Memory of ageing people can be augmented if they teach language, geography, mathematics etc. to children. Ageing people may live in the atmosphere of social harmony by practicing creative genius.

For example, Helen Small was applauded in the Campus of UT – Dallas, USA for completing a research project in psychology in the age of 92 years. Similarly, Pablo Casals, Birju Maharaj, Bismillah Khan practiced their art forms till advanced old age and respectively bestowed mesmerizing and world - acclaimed performance on cello, *kathak* and *shehnai*.

Super Agers are adults reaching over age 80 years, who have the mental capacity of individuals who are at least 3 decades younger. The super agers have greater memory ability and develop very strong social relationship bonds. They have certain brain regions packed with spindly neurons called **Economo neurons** which play the role of social processing and awareness. Super Agers' brains age at a much slower rate than average.

The following article will rekindle a pragmatic view in super agers to achieve optimism.

https://www.org/health/brain - health/info - 2023/minds - of - super - agers.html

So, youngsters must learn to imbibe those attributes which may bless them with 'super ageing' after 80 years.

Social inclusion & Activity – Indian ethos: Having close family ties is important to promote healthy ageing. Recent research is providing sufficient evidence that **social linkages** are important determinants in augmenting healthy longevity. Preparation for old age includes cultivating friendships and relations by activities like potluck parties, local choir or gardening club, book club, going out with friends to the theatre, cinema or shops, continue working or doing voluntary work. In India, many elderly people perform daily prayers in groups or go and live in *ashrams* where they meet others doing spiritual activity. Taking retreat in reclusive living, severing of family relations and social ties have been denounced by the seers and philosophers in India from ages. Indian philosophers hold the view that escape from the stress of real - world is neither laudable and nor does it pay dividends.

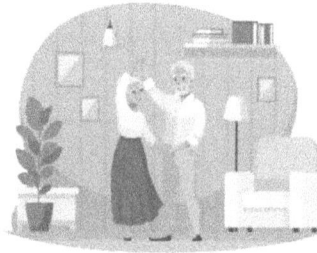

They plead for 4 ashramas viz; **Brahmacharya** (celibate age 5 - 25), **Grahastha** (family life age 26 - 50), **Vanaprastha** (austere life at home age 51 - 75) and **Sanyas** (solitary life age 76 onwards) but hold that the person is entitled to take recourse to *vanaprastha* or *sanyas ashram* only after fulfilling all the obligations of life and society.

Ikigai: This is a Japanese concept which means "a motivating force; something or someone that gives a person a sense of purpose or a reason for living". More generally it may refer to something that brings pleasure or fulfilment. The concept encourages people to **discover what truly matters** to them and to live a life filled with purpose and joy. Finding your ikigai involves a journey of **self - exploration -** reflecting on what you love, what you're good at, what the world needs, and what you can be paid for. Finding one's purpose in life even at an advanced age is to follow one's passion and find ultimate bliss.

Hector Garcia and Francesc Miralles have written a book entitled **Ikigai** wherein the authors elucidate the **secret "How to live a long life"** by the following equation:

Love your work → Passion for work → Develop skill → Profession → Remuneration → Vocation → Vocational Occupation becomes the need

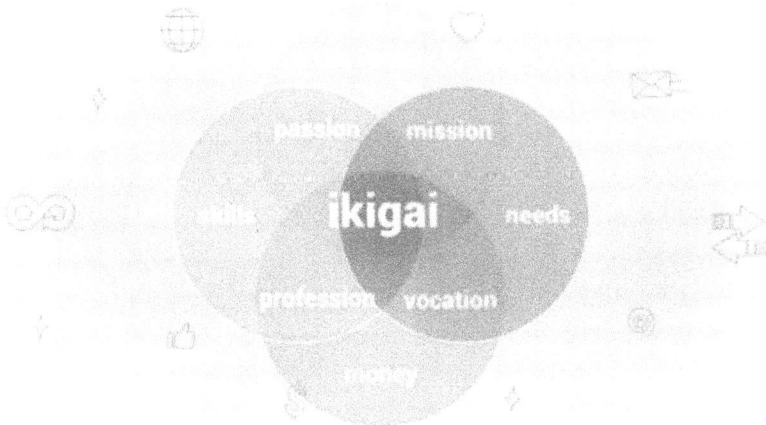

People in Okinawa believe that if everybody learns how to share love and good behavior within the tribe or society, he/she will not only flow in the wave of pleasure and happiness but also will earn esteem for himself as well as for the society, this is what the *Ikigai* of the society is. When one's vocation becomes the demand of society, he achieves the mission of his life which is reflected through his happiness, this is what the *Ikigai* of a man is! *Ikigai* in Japanese people reverberate through them till they realize the **final goal**.

Incessantly searching for Ikigai keeps Okinawans enthralled and happy. They do not believe in accumulation, discard materialism, maintain mental equilibrium and embrace spiritualism. Blue zone people are never tormented with the occurrence of disasters and calamities, they are not overpowered with chaos, confusion, misery or agony. Their social life is never blemished with perennial sadness, they believe that depression reduces life expectancy.

Social service and being a good Samaritan: In the final advanced years of life, it gives a lot of inner satisfaction and joy to help others not as fortunate as oneself. This could be in the form of financial help or spending time and energy to make their lives easier.

There is no other gain – maybe not even the gratitude of the beneficiary. It is the instant inner feeling of pure joy at being able to make a difference to anyone or a group or community and making good use of your time and efforts.

Achieving longevity is the goal of every human in this world. Living long proceeds from living a life enriched with quality – The Science of Ethics and Aesthetics hold that the longevity of human life is upheld by the righteous thinking and righteous conduct, unrighteous or sinful conduct leads to unhealthy life and abridgement of life years. Here comes the role of **Quality of Life** which is analyzed below.

Quality of life - every person must devote themselves to pursue only those maxims and tenets which add years to their life. According to UNDP - Report "the evaluation of national economic development is estimated on certain indicators viz; per capita income, gross national income (GNI), **purchasing power parity** (PPP)". As per these indicators now the nations of the world are categorized in following 4 tiers viz: upper most tier, upper tier, middle tier and lowest tier.

Nations placed at the lowest tier are indicated in the index lacking in literacy and education which make them fall short of good health and wellness in social life, thus life expectancy is relatively low in these societies.

The World Health Organization (WHO) defines health as "**a state of complete physical, mental and social wellbeing and not merely the absence of disease and infirmity**". **Wellness** is the ability of people to be aware and make choices leading to a successful life. The assessment of wellness of an individual is the assessment of his **Quality of Life – QOL** which is how he lives or spends his life in daily routine. The concept of QOL originated in the USA in the 1970s, by Flanagan. WHO thus defines Quality of life as "an individual's perception of their own position in life as a whole in the context of the culture and value systems in which they live in relation to their goals, expectations, standards and concerns".

Although the definition of QOL is still evolving, it is considered as "a broad range of human experiences related to one's overall well - being".

The WHO, over several years, developed a QOL scale (questionnaire) – the WHOQOL. This was developed in over 15 different cultural settings of the world, so as to be applicable cross– culturally.

The QOLS has been tested for its psychometric properties like reliability and validity.It is a 100 - question assessment that currently exists in 29 languages. It generates a multi - dimensional profile of scores across various domains and sub - domain (facets). A shorter version WHOQOL - BREF (BREF stands for brief version), with 26 items has also been developed.

Quality of life (QOL) measures have become an important part of health outcomes assessment. For populations with chronic disease, measurement of QOL provides a meaningful way to determine and compare the impact of diseases or health care interventions when cure is not possible. Over the past two decades, hundreds of instruments have been developed by researchers that aim to measure QOL in different chronic illnesses. **Health - related quality life - HRQOL** of individuals may be understood by taking into account various forms of diseases, disabilities or disorders by which they have been assaulted.

In conclusion, focusing solely on material wealth and physical well - being risks leading society toward moral and spiritual decay.

Humanity's true progress lies in fostering an atmosphere of peace, unity, and harmony, where spiritual values guide us. The wisdom passed down by elders reflects this truth: "Do not search for happiness in external pursuits." Those who understand this inner wisdom often create a fulfilling, joyful life in their later years, finding contentment within their families and communities. Such individuals live long, loved and respected, knowing the secret of a life well - lived.

Chapter 49

Death – The Inevitable Truth

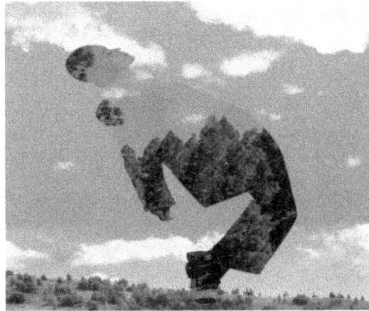

Learning Objectives:

- Cause of death, information of death, death certificate
- Brain death - The window for cadaveric organ donation
- Persistent vegetative state
- Euthanasia – active and passive
- The difference between prolonged grief and disenfranchised grief on the death of loved ones
- Realizing and harmonizing with the feelings of a dying person

The fear of death is universal. In our daily lives, we treat life as an undeniable truth, often ignoring the reality of death as we chase after our desires, ambitions, and worldly achievements. However, when confronted with the impending death of a loved one or our own mortality, we are often struck with deep distress and melancholy, questioning the purpose and meaning of our existence.

In those moments, the realization of life's fleeting nature can make everything feel futile.

Confirmation of death – Death should be confirmed clinically by:

i) absence of any pulse – peripheral (radial) and central (carotid) for 2 minutes

ii) absence of any respiratory movements on '**Look, listen and feel**' for at least 2 minutes

iii) fixed dilated pupil with absence of any response to light, and,

iv) absence of corneal reflex – lack of blinking on touching the cornea with a thread.

Death Certificate: This is a legal document that must be signed by a Medical Officer. It usually has the following information –

i) Name, Age and Sex of the individual

ii) Date and time of death

iii) Location of death

iv) Manner of death – natural, accident, homicide, suicide or undetermined

v) Method of body disposition – burial, cremation etc.

vi) Cause of death – Underlying, intermediate and immediate cause/s with duration of each.

Cause of Death – The World Health Organization (WHO) publishes the **International Classification of Diseases** (ICD) **and causes of death** – the global standard for diagnostic health information. The latest version of ICD – the ICD 11 was released in 2024. All hospitals and health facilities should attempt to classify the diagnosis of patients according to ICD. This allows for collation and comparison of data from different parts of the world.

Cause of death data are an important source of information on human health. Knowing the reasons why people die are important for targeting where, when, and how resources should be expended.

The cause of death can be the **proximate cause** (starting point for unbroken chain of events which lead to death), **immediate cause** or **contributory cause**.

The World Health Organization has standardized the cause of death section in the death certificate.

There are 2 parts - Part 1 is used for diseases or conditions that form part of the sequence of events leading directly to death. The **immediate** (direct) cause of death is entered on the first line. There must always be an entry on line 1 (a) and it may be the only condition reported in Part 1 of the certificate. Where there are two or more conditions that form part of the sequence of events leading to death, each event in the sequence should be recorded on a separate line **(intermediate causes)**. There is also a column for duration i.e. the time interval between the onset of each condition that is entered on the certificate and death.

Part 2 is used for conditions that do not belong in Part 1 but whose presence contributed to death. As an example, leukemia may be the initial illness (underlying cause) which led to low blood counts (intermediate cause) and this led to pneumonia (immediate cause) which finally caused death. **Contributory cause** can be malnutrition. Cardio - respiratory arrest should not be listed as a cause of death as it is the final common pathway leading to death.

A death certificate is usually written by the doctor or hospital attending at the time of death. This death certificate besides having patients' name, age, sex, unique Id, address and other demographic data also mentions the underlying cause of death like cancer, stroke, septicemia, injury or heart attack.

For epidemiological purposes in communities where no death certificates are entered, the cause of death information may be deciphered through **Verbal Autopsy -** a procedure of gathering information about cause of death of an individual by interviewing the family members about symptoms and circumstances leading to death.

Registration of death is mandatory in most countries. It is essential to register death to establish the fact of death, to document the date and time of death, to relieve the person from legal and official obligations, to allow settlement of inheritance, and authorize the family to collect insurance benefits etc.

For this, provisions have been made to issue certificates lawfully. According to the **Registration of Births & Deaths Act, 1969, India** every death must be registered with the concerned State/UT Government within 21 days of its occurrence. The person registering the death could be the head of the family if it occurred at home; by the doctor in - charge if it occurred in a hospital; by jail in - charge if the death occurred in a jail; and by the headman of the village or the in - charge of the local police station in case the body is found deserted in that area of jurisdiction.

Brain death – The brain is the organ responsible for all actions, thoughts, learning and internal functions of the body. **Once brain death occurs, the patient cannot be revived** and for all purposes is dead. The heart and lung may continue to function with or without external support (like ventilator). Brain death may occur ahead of cardiac and respiratory failure. The heart may continue to beat and blood supply to various organs continues. This is a **unique state** when fully functional organs like kidney of the patient can be harvested and donated to another patient for prolonging life.

This offers a 'window' of opportunity' for **human cadaveric organ donation.** Recently, a Parliamentary Act upheld that declaration of brain death is legal for fulfilling the provisions and formalities of organ donation. If there is clinically no response from the patient, pupils are fixed and dilated, and all other brain stem reflexes are lost the person is declared "**brain dead**". Different countries have their own criteria for declaration of brain death. Some require a flat electro - encephalogram (EEG).

Organ Donation – sometimes dying person and their close relatives express their desire for organ donation when the death is imminent. A few motivated and dedicated persons in every society having the ambition to serve humanity commit and fill the necessary documents of kidney, eye and other organ donation after death. At other times many hospitals have good Samaritan organ donation advocacy personnel who at an opportune time open up a dialogue for organ donation with the patients and their near and dear as and when appropriate.

Notably, big hospitals with transplantation programs have patients in - waiting to receive organs like cornea and kidney etc.

Post death (cadaveric) donation is the only form of organ donation practiced in advanced countries and is also becoming popular in India. Organ donation for transplantation and body donation for anatomical studies are noble causes indeed.

Persistent Vegetative State: This refers to a condition of chronic brain dysfunction in which a person in coma has awake and sleep cycles, may open eyes, move or make sounds but shows no signs of awareness of surroundings. The patient is unable to speak, to eat, has no control over movements and cannot follow basic commands. Vegetative patients retain their reflexes and might grind their teeth or grimace; their eyes may rove about the room but won't fix on anything. Cause may be head trauma or other illness or stroke with irreversible damage to the brain. Treatment is usually supportive care. If a person has been in this state for 3 months, improvement is extremely rare. The patient can survive in this state for years, however, – in long term care facilities or hospitals till families decide to end life support.

Euthanasia or **Mercy killing - *Daya Mrityu*** or *Karuna Mrityu* is administered to those terminally ill patients who are in hospital suffering from irreversible and incurable disease and have lost all hopes of meaningful life. Administering death of a person by medical procedures is called **euthanasia** (दयामृत्यु मृत्यु/करूणा मृत्यु). Though euthanasia has been bestowed legal recognition in many countries, yet it is not legal in many societies or countries. The societies or the countries not acceding to this practice of euthanasia, advocate that liberty to life is the natural right of man and thus life breath of ailing man should not be brought to an end.

In all such cases the doctors and specialists conduct a thorough clinical examination and confer with each other about the **prognosis** of the patient. Then the family is informed and next of kin discuss with each other and may take the collective decision about '**do not resuscitate' (DNR)** consent. This means that hospital staff is issued instructions that resuscitation in the event of a cardiac or respiratory arrest should not be started. It does not involve withdrawing life support system where a patient is already on ventilator or drugs to maintain blood pressure.

Euthanasia is categorized into two types:

Passive Euthanasia: This is a medical procedure in which medical support system giving sustenance to the patient is removed. Thus, removal of life - sustaining interventions like ventilators, feeding tubes, oxygen, heart support systems and other medical support systems, allows the dying patient to pass away naturally and peacefully as per the advice of the doctors and collective deliberation of family members. Withdrawal of life support is ethical and permissible in brain dead. Palliative treatment should proceed towards providing efficacious relief from pain.

Relief from breathlessness is also provided. Drugs like narcotics and opioids are administered and they are accorded a dignified farewell.

Active Euthanasia: This is a medical procedure in which certain drugs or medical procedures are administered to the ailing person so that they may leave this world in painless state of mind. Active euthanasia is a procedure in which death is administered out of sympathy and compassion. Active euthanasia is a process of collective decision - making in which a group of persons participate and deliberate with each other viz; family members, doctors, the legal experts like advocates, magistrates, social workers participate in inducing comfortable death to the suffering patient. Before administering active euthanasia to the acutely suffering patient the physician or the specialist is obliged to carry out complete examination of patient's body and mind function.

Legal validity of Passive Euthanasia in India – Aruna Shanbaug was a nurse – a victim of sexual assault (rape) in 1973 at King Edward Memorial (K.E.M.) Hospital in Mumbai. On November 27, 1973, while changing clothes in the hospital's basement after her duty, she was sexually assaulted then strangled with a chain. After thorough medical examination she was declared to be in **vegetative state**. During vegetative state her cardiac and respiratory system and other significant systems of the body continued functioning. She was provided all the necessary diet and medicines through food pipe. Aruna Shanbaug lived through coma for a long period of 42 years.

In the end she passed away due to pneumonia on May 18, 2015. A petition filed by a non - governmental organization in the year 2005 in Hon'ble

Supreme Court of India, made the prayer to allow passive euthanasia (voluntary stopping of life support) to the patient suffering due to vegetative state. This petition started the debate on passive euthanasia in India and ultimately the court upheld that **passive euthanasia** is not infringement of the **fundamental right.** With this decision passive euthanasia became legal in India –thus, in India, passive euthanasia is legally permissible, but active euthanasia is not.

Reactions to death of a loved one – When someone in the family, a dear friend, a relative, or one's own child, spouse, etc., passes away, feeling of melancholy often seeps deep down into the heart and mind of the family and society. The death of someone close can sometimes deeply affect us for a long period, leading to sadness, depression, and various physical and mental illnesses. Death is an eternal truth but we hardly recognize this reality occurring in every generation. However, when the goals of life go unfulfilled or the pursuits not realized, incompleteness persists with sorrow and melancholy which result in crying and agony. We get alienated from society. Sometimes, the events of death seem submerging in endless sorrows like the vast ocean spread all around us. Gradually, choices melt down, ways leading to achieve the pursuits seem slipping away and as a result we stand baffled. What to do! What not to do! prevail deep down into our mind and thought, torments us every now and then. Elisabeth Kubler - Ross analyses the phenomenon of death occurring on continuously – the acknowledgement or repudiation of this phenomenal eternity by the human being may be **in 5 different stages**, such as:

- **Denial and Isolation -** Not acknowledging the evidence of the death of a family member or dear friend.

- **Anger -** After recognizing death, manifesting anger towards the well - wishers viz; doctors, healthcare workers, and other family members while worrying about unfulfilled obligations due to existential incapacities and inadequacies.

- **Bargaining/Negotiation** – After giving conscious assent to the phenomena of imminent death, cry for saving the life of the patient or beloved family member inviting expert advice from doctors, astrologers.

- **Depression** – After the extinction of all the possible alternatives of bailing out life, the overwhelming sorrow pervades the mind and body through and through.

- **Acceptance** – thus, acknowledging the eternity of death whether the phenomenon relates to yourself, or any family member is giving approval to testimony of death. Scientists of succeeding generations not acceding to the arguments of *Kubler - Ross* repudiate the validity of the five stages against which humans usually struggle.

Spiritual leaders and mystics hold that death is not a terrifying or dreadful happening, but a magnificent and endless play in Nature. Death is neither demonic design, nor a diabolic maneuvering, nor an inferno created by some ghost or phantom, lamenting death of a person dear to you is not crying for a lost thing or object, death is an unfading separation or an ineffaceable bereavement from your loved ones. Death is a gradual dissolution of solid into subtle, matter into ether, physical into spiritual, perishable into imperishable, permanent into non - existent. **Consciousness** is an expression of Cosmic energy – revealed in many ways that we are unable to catch.

The moment we try to catch Consciousness or Cosmic Energy, it slips from our catch. Consciousness of Cosmic Energy is manifested in infinite possibilities where from life begins and wherein it ends, energy gets restored into its natural form. Death is the restoration of that energy which we enjoyed as a life. But the cycle of life and death being infinite, after death life takes a new beginning. Life and death are two sides of the same coin, two digits of the same play.

Life is the direct march of Ultimate Reality on the earth, death is the retreat of that very Ultimate Reality in its own unfathomed bosom. Life and death are the two phases of the same phenomena manifested through the Ultimate Reality. Life and death are the two aspects appearing in and through the Ultimate Reality from where Creation and Cataclysm keep on manifesting in innumerable colors and shades like a mysterious enigma. Creation is a Whole taken out of the Whole (Ultimate Reality) and Dissolution or Death of a being is the Whole returned into the Whole.

Mystics call and attribute the Ultimate Reality the Supreme Consciousness which never depletes either in the process of creation or in the process of dissolution or death or complete inundation taken over the universe.

The famous Indian poet *Gopal Das Neeraj* has beautifully shed ample light on the phenomena of life and death in the following poem:

भाई! जरा देख के चलो, आगे ही नहीं पीछे भी

दायें ही नहीं बायें भी, ऊपर ही नहीं नीचे भी, ए भाई!

तू जहां, आया है वो तेरा – घर नहीं, गाँव नहीं

गली नहीं, कूचा नहीं, रस्ता नहीं, बस्ती नहीं

दुनिया है और प्यारे, दुनिया एक सर्कस है

और इस सर्कस में – बड़े को भी, छोटे को भी

खरे को भी, खोटे को भी, मोटे को भी, पतले को भी नीचे
से ऊपर को, ऊपर से नीचे को आना–जाना पड़ता

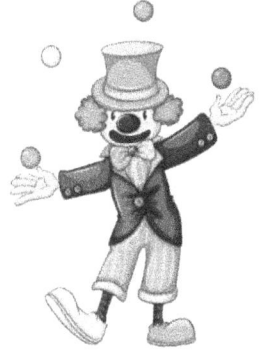

In this grand circus of life there is no permanent home, village, street or city.

The world itself is the stage and everyone whether rich or poor, good or bad, fat or thin is participating in the ever - marching process of Life & Death!

Death is the only eternal phenomenon where the entire universe converges, where all beings are absorbed into the One Eternal Cosmic Energy. The loss of life, especially in childhood or young adulthood, represents an irreplaceable blow to both society and the nation. Yet, death is a smooth and peaceful transition from the fleeting and transient to the eternal - a return to Pure Consciousness, the Absolute Reality. Human life, with its average lifespan of around 60 years, is marked by a natural desire to live actively and to face life's challenges with strength and purpose. No one wishes to depart in weakness or illness, burdened by sorrow and pain. We all hope for a dignified exit from this world, a departure that reflects peace and acceptance rather than fear.

Death, as the poet reflects, is not something to resist or dread but a process parallel to life itself - a release from the physical to the transcendental.

The poem encourages a serene acceptance of death, reminding us that while life is impermanent, death is a gentle resolution of all struggles. In its final stanza, the poet urges us not to fear or view death as terrifying but to embrace it as an ever - present, natural occurrence. In taking our last breath, we are liberated from life's agonies and find peace.

Proceeding towards death breath by breath – depicting empathetically the suffering of a patient lying on the ICU bed, Professor Trilok Chandra Goel illustrates… "Let me not feed through my central vein, nay, do not resuscitate me from embracing death the eternal truth, nor do I wish to have my mouth and nose hooked to a ventilator and nay! not my heart be supported on a balloon pump…. let me! let me!! my Lord have the peaceful bliss of death near my bed - नहीं चाहिए मुझे कृत्रिम श्वसन, कृत्रिम स्पंदन, नसों में कृत्रिम भोजन, मुझे चाहिए मृत्यु शय्या का परमानन्द…. may it not be painful, may it be the time of departure from life. Everyone wishes such a time to be minimal.

Fighting death with medical interventions is a sorrowful and painful state which nobody wants to embrace when he is taking his last breath. Death is a peaceful state of mind, it is a state of bliss, and it is emancipation from the fetters of lust and passions – death is a journey from infinity to infinity.

Chapter 50

Health Insurance & Mediclaim

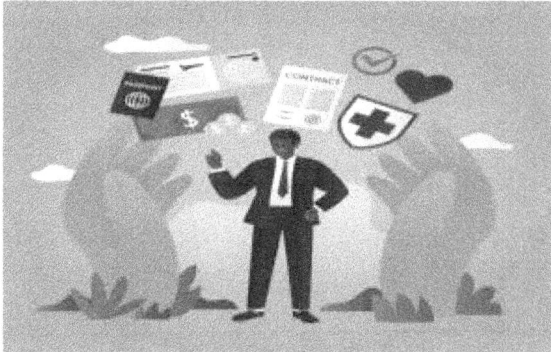

Learning Objectives:

- Why health insurance?
- Claim submission for the expenditure incurred on the treatment as per Mediclaim insurance list
- The role of the third-party administrator in scrutiny and disposal of Mediclaim expenditure
- The role of the Grievance Redressal Officer and impartiality of Insurance Ombudsman in the disposal of Mediclaim bills
- Reinforcement and rejuvenation of health insurance by IRDAI

Health is the fundamental right of citizens. Government run health care facilities may not fulfill the total demand . Indolence, infirmity and disease may affect almost anybody at some stage in life. Government and employer may provide health facility or treatment reimbursement.

Investing in a health insurance policy provides financial protection, access to quality health care and peace of mind. Medical emergencies are covered and such incidents should not deplete finances and essential daily expenses.

Lower middle - class people tend to fall below poverty line if an adverse health event strikes. Government encourages citizens to take private health insurance by giving tax deduction on the insurance premium. Some health insurance schemes provide preventive health check - ups, blood tests and cancer screening. Chronic diseases management like asthma, hypertension, diabetes, mental disorders may not be covered. We also recommend that one should purchase health insurance policy if not covered by government or employer, especially if one is not so wealthy.

Diseases are prevalent in every society, and the rising costs of medicines and healthcare materials make treatment more expensive. The Government of India has a network of public health facilities which provide health care at reduced costs, but for various reasons the vast majority of the population avail of private health care facilities, resulting in substantial 'out of pocket' expenses. On average, families spend about 10% of their income on medical issues. To provide relief from this financial burden, governments and various banking institutions have introduced health insurance systems.

The insurer pays regular **premiums** to the insurance company and the company pays for medical expenses incurred as and when needed. Health insurance in general means a wide and comprehensive coverage of treatment related expenditure.

- Health Insurance covers **hospital - related expenses** such as room rent, doctor's or surgeon's fees, medication, nursing charges, operation theatre charges, and cost of implants etc. Usually, the policy reimburses medicines taken 30 days before hospitalization and up to 60 days after discharge. Medical claims must be submitted within 15 - 30 days after discharge. Most health insurance policies do not cover dental treatment, eye check - up, eye glasses and out - patient treatment of short illnesses. Chronic illnesses like diabetes, hypertension, rheumatism, mental disorders etc. also may not be covered. Upon hospitalization, it is essential to notify the insurance company or the **third - party administrator (TPA)** in writing. The TPA is responsible for reviewing and processing the insurance claims. The patient - caretaker should take cognizance of the facilities being granted during admission in clinics or hospitals as follows:

- Must consist of at least 15 patient beds (10 beds in those cities where population is < 10 lacs),

- Skilled doctors and nursing staff being available round the clock (24 hours) well - equipped and disinfected operation theatre with qualified surgeons. **Registration** of the hospitals in the local authority is mandatory.

- Case file and records of day - to - day treatment must be maintained by hospital.

This system operates on the "**law of averaging**," where the pooled premiums of policyholders cover the medical expenses of individuals. Health insurance programs embody the principle of "*Health for All*," as outlined by the World Health Organization (WHO), ensuring equitable access to healthcare.

Previously, health insurance claims could only be made if the patient remained hospitalized for 24 hours or more, but advancements in medical technology have made such conditions less relevant. Procedures like appendectomy, eye surgery, radiotherapy, chemotherapy, coronary angiography, angioplasty, fracture treatment, lumbar puncture, fissure and piles surgeries, prostate procedures, hernia and hydrocele surgeries and even gall bladder surgery are now - a - days can be safely done as day care procedures which reduces the expenses of extra day hospitalization. Expensive tests like PET CT scans are often completed within a single day.

Health insurance claims are also extended to treatments provided in Ayurvedic, Unani, and Homeopathic hospitals. Additionally, ambulance and physiotherapy expenses are reimbursed under health insurance policies for in - patient treatment. Pre - existing conditions are covered and reimbursed if these are mentioned at the time of taking the policy or after 2 - 4 years of continuous policy coverage. However, certain expenses, such as for cotton, bandaging, syringes, and disposables, are not reimbursed. Similarly, treatments for general weakness, dental treatment, venereal diseases, self - inflicted injuries, pregnancy, conditions caused by tobacco or alcohol use, fat - reduction therapies, and cosmetic surgeries are not eligible for reimbursement under most health insurance policies.

One should declare and make sure that any pre - existing congenital or chronic disease and habits like tobacco, alcohol or drug abuse are mentioned in the policy document.

Buying Health Insurance and awareness – Mediclaim Policy Insurance Rules 2016 & 2017 have been promulgated by **Insurance Regulatory & Development Authority of India** (**IRDAI**), according to which proposal - application should be duly completed with utmost integrity while filling all the required columns along with former diseases, duration and claims thereof. Agents and middle men who sell health insurance policies may give allurements of lower premium and fill the form with incomplete data and usually cheat on not disclosing pre - existing chronic disease and other habits like tobacco and alcohol. At the time of claim these things become apparent and treatment reimbursement is denied. Similarly, porting health insurance from one company to another may be treated as as a breach of contract in the continuity of old insurance plan. The history of the insurance company's disposal and settlement of treatment expenditure, its conditions and its market credibility should be cross checked wisely. The photocopy of the records of claim application and its receipt should be maintained with the claimant as several enquires may be put up by the TPA before settling the claim. It may be the strategy of the health insurance companies to give a tough time in settling claims and in this process some people give up. Perseverance usually wins. Complaints concerning rejection of treatment cost or heavy deduction or delay in reimbursement should be sent to the Chief Executive Officer (CEO) or **Grievance Redressal Officer** of the company. Further complaints may be lodged in the office of the **Insurance Ombudsman** if the previous complaint sent to the CEO is not replied to within 30 days or if the reply is unsatisfactory. Pleading by advocate is not recognized in the disposal or settlement of the complaints. It is incumbent upon the claimant to solicit the unfeigned and righteous claim and prove it with the help of treating doctor or hospital.

Functioning of the office of Insurance Ombudsman – Health insurance policyholder may register his complaints free of charge in writing to the Office of the Insurance Ombudsman, in simple language along with the photocopy of the policy, mobile number, email id, full address, the settlement of which is generally done within 90 days in a single hearing.

The health insurance company is bound to comply with the orders or the decrees of the Hon'ble Insurance Ombudsman within 30 days. Address, phone and email of the state Insurance Ombudsman can be obtained online.

Recent changes and upgradation in health insurance policies - Health insurance sector in India is dedicated to empowering poor people. Inclusive and accessible healthcare ecosystems will ensure protection against unforeseen medical expenses. Insurance companies have been incentivized to diversify healthcare product.

Salient features of recent changes that are generally not known to people developed by **Insurance Regulatory and Development Authority of India (IRDAI)** are as follows

1. Cap on buying health insurance policies has been eliminated, new procedures have been introduced empowering the poor to obtain comprehensive coverage.

2. Maximum age restriction for purchasing health insurance is scrapped – elderly can purchase health insurance from April 01, 2024.

3. As per IRDAI Gazette notification F No IRDAI/Reg/8/202/2024 dt. 22.03.2024 health insurance providers shall introduce tailored policies for specific demographics, and ensure due diligence in settling claims and grievances thereof, specifically in case of senior citizens and other groups like students, children, maternity etc.

4. Health policies for pre - existing medical conditions like cancer, heart disease, chronic renal failure, AIDS etc. shall be offered.

5. Life insurance companies may launch extended health policies lasting up to 5 years, whereas general insurers/stand alone health insurers are limited to offer policies for up to 3 years in a single go.

6. Health insurance waiting period has been decreased from 48 months to 36 months – all pre - existing medical conditions should be covered after 36 months, whether the policy holder discloses them initially or subsequently.

7. After completing 60 consecutive months of health coverage, including portability and migration, insurers cannot challenge policies or claims due to non - disclosure or misrepresentation, except in cases of established fraud.

8. Life insurers are barred from introducing indemnity - based health policies, which compensate for hospital expenses. Instead, they are only permitted to provide benefit - based policies.

9. Life insurers have the liberty to bundle health plans with ULIPs (Unit Linked Insurance Plans).

10. Premium adjustments during the policy term are prohibited, however, the same is not prohibited on factors like age and risk. Insurance companies are allowed to offer premium payment in instalments.

11. Travel policies can only be offered by general and health insurance companies. There is no limit on *AYUSH* treatment coverage. Treatments under *AYUSH* will receive coverage up to the sum insured without any cap. Policyholders with benefit - based policies can file multiple claims with various companies, enhancing flexibility and options like a top - up policy.

Ayushman Bharat under PMJAY – is dedicated initiative of government of India focusing on 2 objectives viz:

(i) Promoting universal health coverage (**UHC**) especially among the poor population throughout India. Thus, under this scheme Health and Wellness Centers (**HWCs**) are being established out of which 1.5 lacs Ayushman Bharat Health and Wellness centers are already functioning.

(ii) National public health insurance scheme entitled Pradhan Mantri Jan Arogya Yojana (**PM - JAY**) has been launched for low - an income earner which eventually covers 50% of the country's population, where family may obtain up to **Rs five lacs** per year for indoor treatment in private hospital and nursing homes. The reimbursement to the hospitals is done as per the rate list of the Ayushman Bharat.

This scheme covers wide scope in the sphere of medical care spanning prevention, promotion and ambulatory care – across primary, secondary and tertiary levels, catering to the vast population of the country. The scheme has been recently extended to all Indian citizens who have attained the age of 70 years irrespective of income.

In conclusion, the recent initiatives by IRDAI represent a major advancement in India's health insurance sector. By eliminating age restrictions for policy purchases, reducing waiting periods for pre - existing conditions, and mandating coverage for a broader range of medical treatments, the regulatory body has made healthcare more inclusive and accessible. These reforms empower individuals to obtain comprehensive coverage suited to their specific needs while encouraging insurance companies to innovate and diversify their products.

As a result, the health insurance sector in India is not only providing financial protection but also promoting the overall well - being of the common masses. Tax rebate on health insurance premium and low rates of health insurance in India are additional benefit.

ABOUT THE AUTHORS

Dr Sandeep Kumar is an Ex Professor of Surgery, King George's Medical University, Lucknow and Founder Director, All India Institute of Medical Sciences, Bhopal. He is a renowned surgeon, a breast specialist and a surgical oncologist. He is the Editor - in - Chief of Indian Journal of Surgery and South Asian Journal of Geriatric Medicine, Surgery, Palliative Care and Hospice. Published over 150 research papers with high impact and Research Gate scores that are widely quoted. Has contributed chapters in text books. A recipient of **National Medical Sciences Academy of India Award**. He is a prolific speaker and has been invited to speak in several Universities and Colleges in India and abroad. He helped establish a Hospice and a free School for poor children. His other books are *Raag Georgian, Achhe Ilaj ke 51 Nuskhe* or *51 Secretes of Getting Medical Treatment*. His you - tube channel - *Swasthya ki Pathshala* presents his simple style and explanations of medical topics for educating masses.

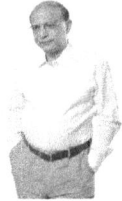

Ajay Kumar Agrawal retired Joint Director, Department of Culture, Government of Uttar Pradesh. Studied Sanskrit, English literature, Philosophy and Political Science eruditely. Post - graduate in Philosophy and Political Science from the University of Allahabad. *Lok Rang – UP* is a literary work piece and documentation by him – the widely exhibited book illustrates various aspects of folk music and festivals of Uttar Pradesh. Another book *Ramayana Traditions and National Cultures in Asia* by him from the Culture Department is an eternal heritage of the world created on life episode of Lord Ram. His academic achievements include creation of e - calendar, artist and music e - directory, e - booking of departmental auditoria and music & theatre workshops of the State, Hindi version of websites for KGMU, Lucknow and AIIMS, Bhopal and several newspaper articles. He has won accolades in copywriting and producing brochures of literary and cultural events.

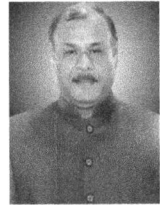

ABOUT THE BOOK

This book serves as a beacon, guiding readers towards leading a healthier life! It is a comprehensive resource that everyone should have in their personal library. As you delve into its contents, you will gradually master the art of maintaining a healthy lifestyle, and understanding how to access optimal treatment options. The topics covered within are commonly featured in various magazines, but seldom does one find a single book encompassing such a wide range of subjects.

The book introduces various types of health services, teaching readers how to safeguard their own health and that of their families. It capacity builds and instils a sense of responsibility and determination to fight infirmity, indolence and disease. It provides an insider's perspective on how doctors work and health policies. Moreover, it offers essential information about an array of concerns – from common place female diseases to various infectious diseases, accidents, injuries, cancer, blood pressure, diabetes, prevention and immunity. It encourages the pursuit of a healthy old age and elucidates the concept of a peaceful demise. After turning the final pages one will smiling, realizing that you have become, in a sense, your own **'Half Doctor'**. This book is a must read for anyone striving to take control of their health journey.